Malaria: New Insights

Malaria: New Insights

Edited by Kyler Hall

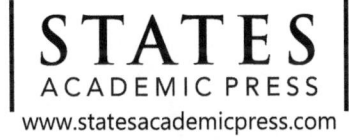

STATES
ACADEMIC PRESS

www.statesacademicpress.com

States Academic Press,
109 South 5th Street,
Brooklyn, NY 11249, USA

Visit us on the World Wide Web at:
www.statesacademicpress.com

ISBN: 978-1-63989-338-6

Trademark Notice: Registered trademark of products or corporate names are used only for explanation and identification without intent to infringe.

Cataloging-in-Publication Data

Malaria : new insights / edited by Kyler Hall.
    p. cm.
Includes bibliographical references and index.
ISBN 978-1-63989-338-6
1. Malaria. 2. Malaria--Prevention. 3. Fever. 4. Protozoan diseases. I. Hall, Kyler.
RC156 .M35 2022
616.936 2--dc23

Table of Contents

Preface

This book was inspired by the evolution of our times; to answer the curiosity of inquisitive minds. Many developments have occurred across the globe in the recent past which has transformed the progress in the field.

Malaria is an infectious disease that is spread by mosquitoes and affects humans and other animals. Common symptoms of malaria are tiredness, headaches, vomiting and fever. Severe symptoms can involve seizures, yellow skin, coma or death. Normally, the symptoms start to occur ten to fifteen days after the infected mosquito bites. If the malaria infection is not treated properly, it can reoccur but the reinfection causes milder symptoms. Malaria is caused by the micro-organisms of Plasmodium group and is most commonly spread by an infected female Anopheles mosquito. When an infected female Anopheles mosquito bites, it introduces the parasites into the person's blood from its saliva. There are five species of Plasmodium that can infect and be spread by humans. This book is a compilation of chapters that discuss the clinical approaches of malaria. It brings forth some of the unexplored aspects of this disease. This book includes contributions of experts and scientists which will provide innovative insights into this field.

This book was developed from a mere concept to drafts to chapters and finally compiled together as a complete text to benefit the readers across all nations. To ensure the quality of the content we instilled two significant steps in our procedure. The first was to appoint an editorial team that would verify the data and statistics provided in the book and also select the most appropriate and valuable contributions from the plentiful contributions we received from authors worldwide. The next step was to appoint an expert of the topic as the Editor-in-Chief, who would head the project and finally make the necessary amendments and modifications to make the text reader-friendly. I was then commissioned to examine all the material to present the topics in the most comprehensible and productive format.

I would like to take this opportunity to thank all the contributing authors who were supportive enough to contribute their time and knowledge to this project. I also wish to convey my regards to my family who have been extremely supportive during the entire project.

Editor

1

Pre-Erythrocytic Vaccine Candidates in Malaria

Ken Tucker, Amy R. Noe, Vinayaka Kotraiah,

Timothy W. Phares, Moriya Tsuji,

Elizabeth H. Nardin and Gabriel M. Gutierrez

Abstract

A vaccine providing sterile immunity against malaria has been shown to be possible with antigens from the pre-erythrocytic stages of malaria. Therefore, it is reasonable to focus vaccine development efforts on the pre-erythrocytic stages, consisting of both sporozoites and liver stage parasites, where it is expected that sterile immunity against the parasite can be elicited to block the development of blood stage infection, clinical disease, and resulting parasite transmission. Accordingly, we will review the preclinical and clinical studies of malaria pre-erythrocytic efforts as well as highlight the advances, trends, and roadblocks encountered in these efforts.

Keywords: *Plasmodium falciparum*, malaria, vaccine, clinical trial, CSP, TRAP, CelTOS, LSA, EP1300, STARP, EXP-1, immune response, humoral, cellular, CD4+, CD8+

1. Introduction

Immunity to malaria correlates with age and develops only after years of repeated exposure to bites from infected mosquitoes [1, 2]. Most adolescents in malaria-endemic regions have developed a level of protective immunity that provides resistance to clinical disease but does not fully eliminate infection [1]. This lack of sterile immunity does not prevent further spread of the disease, as some level of parasitemia persists in these individuals. A complete understanding of how the malaria parasite avoids clearance remains unknown. However, mechanisms such as extreme allelic variation, strain diversity, as well as the unique complexity of the malaria parasite life cycle are undoubtedly involved. In this regard, identification of the conserved, critical epitopes of the parasite that are directly associated with eliciting protection may provide the best viable target node for vaccine development. In addition, recent data from mouse models of malaria suggest that T cell exhaustion significantly impairs development of effective immune responses and contributes to chronic malaria infection [3–5]. Notwithstanding the fleeting immunity that individuals receive from frequent infection with the parasite, it suggests that there are targets for the immune system to attack.

Importantly, exposure to attenuated sporozoites that can infect hepatocytes but do not develop into the blood-phase of malaria can induce immunity that eliminates parasitic infection (i.e., sterile immunity). This has been demonstrated by conducting immunizations with irradiated sporozoites both in mouse models of malaria [6] as well as in humans with different strains of *Plasmodium falciparum* [7–10]. Similarly, induction of sterile immunity can occur in individuals undergoing chloroquine or mefloquine chemoprophylaxis. The resulting "chemically attenuated" *Plasmodium falciparum* sporozoites (CPS-CQ or CPS-MQ), which undergo full liver stage development but do not develop to clinical blood-stage infection [11, 12], can induce sterile immunity [12–15]. Of note is that sterile protection may not fully develop when sporozoites do not progress at least partially through liver stage development, potentially providing stage transcendent protection [16, 17]. These discoveries demonstrate that a vaccine providing sterile immunity against malaria is possible with antigens from the pre-erythrocytic stages of malaria. Therefore, it is reasonable to focus vaccine development efforts on the pre-erythrocytic stages, consisting of both sporozoites and liver stage parasites, where it is expected that sterile immunity against the parasite can be elicited to block the development of blood stage infection, clinical disease, and resulting parasite transmission.

1.1. Correlates of immunity

The correlates of immunity for sterile protection to malaria are not well defined [18, 19]. In both mice and humans immunized with irradiated sporozoites, sterile protective immunity is believed to be directed to both sporozoites and liver stages of malaria [1, 18]. Antibodies to sporozoites can opsonize sporozoites or neutralize invasion into hepatocytes, and potentially act synergistically with T cells to confer sterile immunity [20]. Additionally, several monoclonal antibodies against the major sporozoite surface antigen, the circumsporozoite protein (CSP), are capable of mediating protection upon passive transfer into animals [21].

Regarding cellular response, studies in mice involving depletion of CD4+ and CD8+ T cells indicate a T cell response is essential for protective immunity [22–24]. In mice immunized with irradiated sporozoites, IFN-γ produced by CD4+ and CD8+ T cells is believed to be the main antiparasitic effector produced by the immune response [18, 23, 25, 26]. IFN-γ may activate effector cells, such as natural killer cells and macrophages that can target and kill parasite-infected liver cells. CD8+ CTLs that recognize *Plasmodium* antigens presented by major histocompatibility complex (MHC) class I molecules on parasite-infected liver cells also may target those cells for destruction [25, 27–29]. This has led to identifying epitopes and vaccination approaches against malaria that elicit CD8+ T cell-mediated IFN-γ secretion and development of CTLs [25, 28, 30]. However, it is important to note that in studies of mice with incapacitated CD8+ T cell function, CD4+ T cell-dependent sterile immunity can be elicited upon immunization with irradiated sporozoites [31]. Additionally, studies evaluating peptide vaccines in mice indicate that CD8+ T cells may not be necessary for sterile immunity but rather CD4+ T cells provide a critical role in immunity [18, 32–35]. Thus, in mice there is not a definitive marker for sterile immunity, and it is plausible that different immune responses may jointly contribute to protection.

In humans, immunization with irradiated sporozoites induces protective immunity consisting of both humoral and cell-mediated responses. Cell-mediated immunity comprises of a mixed population of CD4+ and CD8+ T cells producing IFN-γ and cytotoxic activity, both of which have been shown to possess antiliver stage activity [19, 25]. However, upregulation of CD8+ T cells does not always correlate with protective immunity in humans [10, 19, 25]. For example, immunity elicited in humans under chloroquine chemoprophylaxis with *Plasmodium falciparum* sporozoites is associated with CD4+ T cell production of IFN- γ, TNF, and IL-2 [12, 14], but not with upregulation of CD8+ T cells. Although the role of CD8+ T cells in mediating sterile protection in humans is still unclear, it appears that multiple factors including antibody, CD4+ and CD8+ T cells collectively contribute to overall protective immunity in humans.

1.1.1. Immunological challenges

Two genetic restrictions impact development of vaccines to malaria. The first genetic restriction is related to the extreme heterogeneity of the *Plasmodium* genome and resulting proteome, and existence of a large variety of different circulating strains (particularly for *P. falciparum*) that produce antigens that vary in sequence. As a result of this extreme heterogeneity, in many cases, efforts to identify antigens that can elicit protection against a broad range of malaria strains have been limited to the antigens that are the least variable. In this case, proteins selected for vaccine development are restricted to those relatively conserved across strains, which limits the available vaccine targets. The second restriction involves the population of HLA alleles on each person's cells that recognize these vaccine candidates and are involved in the induction of an immune response. Because of HLA polymorphism, individuals in a population will not generally recognize the same epitopes in an antigen. That is, a single individual in a given population will have HLAs that are capable of binding only a subset of the epitopes present in a vaccine. This means that a single epitope may only stimulate an effective immune response in a small percentage of any population, depending on the representation of the relevant HLA allele(s) in that population [28, 36–38]. The combined effect of these two restrictions is that an effective vaccine must provide many antigenic epitopes to ensure an effective immune response to the spectrum of circulating *Plasmodium* strains is elicited in a significant percentage of a population.

The need for a multiantigen vaccine has resulted in a number of studies identifying conserved epitopes in *Plasmodium* proteins that can stimulate CD4+ or CD8+ T cells from individuals either exposed to malaria or immunized with sporozoites [36–38]. The approach has been refined to identify promiscuous peptides capable of binding more than one type of HLA, resulting in antigens that can affect immune response in a larger percentage of the population. Incorporation of these epitopes into chimeric recombinant proteins for processing by immune cells to produce the peptides and stimulate T cells has been done [39, 40]. Examples of this approach are the multiepitope strings in ME-TRAP [41] and EP1300 (Section 4). Unfortunately, in these constructs, the epitope strings produced low immune responses, even when other whole proteins in these vaccine compositions elicited a robust immune response [42–45].

Another confounding element to vaccine development, in general, is the elicitation of regulatory T cells (Tregs). It is understood that Tregs represent a "self-check" for providing immune tolerance to self and preventing the damaging effects of immune overreaction. For example, Tregs are involved in shutting down immune responses after they have successfully eliminated invading infectious agents, as well as their endogenous role of preventing autoimmunity [46]. However, some pathogens have been found to exploit development of Treg responses in order to evade elimination and persist in the human host. Tregs can also be induced by vaccination and some vaccine development efforts, such as those against tumors and chronic infection (e.g., tuberculosis), have included steps to overcome the constraints of such vaccination-induced Treg responses that result in suppression of immunity [47]. One somewhat successful approach pursued by biotechnology and pharmaceutical companies is development of adjuvant formulations, small molecules, and monoclonal antibodies to overcome the induction of and/ or inhibit Treg function [48]. This area of study is also important regarding the development of malaria vaccines, as there is a growing set of data to support the conclusion that induction of Tregs during acute malaria infection limits the generation of immune memory and increases susceptibility to infection [49]. Of particular concern for malaria vaccine development efforts is that in the infant target population, functional Tregs are present in high numbers [49]. Therefore, tools to identify and remove Treg epitopes from malaria vaccines could be critical to the development of candidates that induce strong T cell responses.

1.1.2. Antigen discovery efforts

The understanding that infection with attenuated sporozoites can confer sterile immunity led to a new focus on discovery of liver-stage antigens [1]. Serological approaches to antigen discovery have been used in malaria research; however, sera from chronically infected individuals predominantly recognize the blood-phase of infection [50]. Therefore, discovery of liver-stages antigens has required methodologies that exploit recent discoveries of immunity targeting the liver-phase of infection. For example, immunological approaches using sera from individuals on antimalarial therapy (CPS-CQ or CPS-MQ) while in malaria-endemic regions were applied to screen libraries expressing *Plasmodium* peptides [51, 52]. Later, similar approaches were applied using blood from individuals immunized with irradiated sporozoites to evaluate expression libraries for reactivity with antibodies [53, 54], or T cell responses with peripheral blood mononuclear cells (PBMCs) [55]. These types of approaches continue to be a source of new antigens [56].

The availability of numerous genomic sequences from *Plasmodium* species has greatly facilitated such studies and made possible further large-scale genomic screening approaches that apply transcriptional analysis using isolated sporozoites with targeted comparisons to different phases in the *Plasmodium* lifecycle [57–61]. When applied to vaccine discovery, the genomic screens typically include a selection of proteins shown to react with antibodies or responsive T cells from individuals immune to *Plasmodium*. On a smaller scale, specific stages of the parasite's lifecycle have been evaluated using proteomic analysis [54, 62, 63]. These efforts have been augmented by extensive cross-comparison of results to prioritize those antigens identified by more than one approach. Many of these antigens, which show a relatively conserved primary protein structure, are being evaluated and developed as components of subunit vaccines against malaria (Section 5).

1.1.3. Surrogate models of protection

One of the challenges in vaccine development is the need for an animal model that clearly correlates to immunity and efficacy in humans. Mice are frequently used to evaluate antigens for both the resulting immune response and efficacy to preventing infection. Both inbred and outbred strains have been evaluated. While inbred strains (e.g., BALB/c and C57BL/6) provide more consistent results, outbred strains (e.g., CD1 and ICR) are believed to better represent the diversity of the immune response that is encountered in humans due to the polymorphism of the MHC (HLA in human). As *Plasmodium* strains that infect humans do not infect rodents, mouse models of malaria either require (1) use of rodent malaria species (e.g., *P. berghei*, and *P. yoelii*) and immunization with the rodent malaria ortholog of the target antigen, which is generally divergent from the corresponding vaccine target from a *Plasmodium* species that infects humans (e.g., *P. falciparum* and *P. vivax*); or (2) development of chimeric parasites where the rodent malaria ortholog of the target antigen has been replaced by the corresponding protein from a human malaria species. In some cases, orthologs of the vaccine targets do not exist in the rodent malaria species, making evaluation in animal models difficult (e.g., LSA-1 and SIAP2 [61], and SIAP2 [61, 64]). While chimeric rodent malaria strains that express the *P. falciparum* antigen have still been used in this type of scenario [33], the impact upon the physiology of the parasite, the host-pathogen interaction, and resulting response to vaccination is not clear. In rare cases, orthologs are sufficiently similar between the rodent and human malaria species to permit immunization using the human malaria antigen and challenge using a wild-type rodent malaria species [65]. While mouse models of malaria can be useful, immune response and level of protection to a target antigen can vary when different rodent malaria strains/species or chimeric models are used, making analysis difficult as it is not clear which of these datasets may be most applicable to or predictive of *P. falciparum* in humans [19, 28].

The use of nonhuman primate (NHP) models provides a more phylogenetically related model of human disease for both the host and parasite. However, cost and the regulations concerning research with NHPs have limited the use of these models. Even when used to evaluate immunity and safety of vaccines, NHPs are typically not challenged with sporozoites, so vaccine efficacy cannot be determined [66–68]. Further, interpretation of results using a NHP model must be balanced with the realization that old-world monkeys do not have the ortholog to the human HLA-C locus, which is one of the three classical human MHC class I loci [69]. In humans, HLA-A and HLA-B (the other two classical human MHC class I loci) exhibit extreme diversity through extensive allelic polymorphism in each class I gene [70]. Whereas in *Rhesus macaque* (the best characterized old-world monkey), there are very limited morphotypes for class I genes, but relative to humans there are more types of class I genes and extensive diversity of the combination of the genes resulting in a potential 10-fold greater diversity of proteins in NHPs [70, 71]. Therefore, the limited overlap of NHP and human MHC, with each species containing unique MHC genes, and the much larger repertoire of MHCs in NHP makes it difficult to extrapolate results in NHP immune response to predict the response in humans. Thus, the immune response of NHPs to peptides developed for a human vaccine must be cautiously interpreted, and extrapolation of the results to define an appropriate dosage for use in humans may be problematic. Because of these limitations, many antigens have rapidly progressed to testing in humans with very limited efficacy testing in animals.

Lastly, it is noteworthy that several research groups have recently developed humanized mouse models that mimic human immune system for the purpose of testing human malaria vaccines. These humanized mice can mount both human T cell and antibody-mediated immunity in the context of HLA-restriction [72–74]. Other efforts have been made toward creating a mouse model having human liver [75–79]. These humanized liver mice can sustain development of human malaria parasites from sporozoites to blood stages.

2. Pre-erythrocytic vaccines based on CSP

2.1. Structure and antigenicity

One of the most studied of malaria proteins is the sporozoite surface antigen CSP, which forms a dense coat surrounding the parasite. This protein is involved in sporozoite motility and invasion where contact of the N-terminal region of CSP with hepatocytes triggers cleavage of the N-terminal region from the remainder of the protein [80–82]. This cleavage event is required for sporozoite infection of hepatocytes [80, 81, 83]. Apart from the central repeat region, CSP contains two regions of high conservation: Region 1 in the N-terminal third of the protein that includes the proteolytic cleavage site, and Region II in the C-terminal third of the protein; the latter has some hepatocyte binding activity [82, 84] and is located in a section of CSP enriched in T cell epitopes (**Figure 1**).

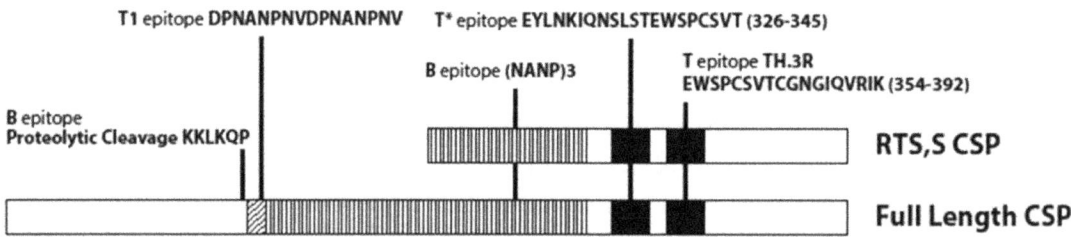

Figure 1. Schematic of full-length CSP identifying important epitopes.

Over 30 years ago, NANP repeats in the central repeat region of the protein were identified as the target of protective antibodies [85–88]. The T1 epitope, which is located in the *P. falciparum* CS minor repeat region, comprised of alternating NANPNVDP repeats, was originally identified by human CD4+ Th1-type T cells from a volunteer immunized with irradiated *P. falciparum* sporozoites [87]. Multiple CD4+ and CD8+ T cell epitopes have been identified in the C-terminal region of CSP, and these are recognized by murine and human cells. Several CD4+ T cell epitopes in this region, labeled as T*, UTC, or TH2 in various publications, include one or more epitopes termed "universal" as they are recognized by a broad spectrum of HLA class II molecules. The T* epitope is present in the C-terminus of CSP amino acids 326–345 and promotes both cytotoxic and helper CD4+ T cell responses. The T* epitope was identified using CD4+ T cell clones derived from volunteers immunized by multiple exposures to the bites of irradiated *P. falciparum* (NF54 strain) infected mosquitos [89]. The T* epitope spans part of a polymorphic region as well as a portion of the conserved Region II. Different CD4+ T cell clones selected from these irradiated sporozoites volunteers recognized truncated peptides (8–18 amino acids long), all of which contained the RII sequence [89]. Importantly, the T* epitope, unlike the T1 epitope, is presented *in vitro* by multiple DR alleles reflecting a broad MHC class II binding pattern, thus suggesting a "universal CD4+ T cell epitope" for malaria [89, 90].

It has been speculated that CSP-specific T cells are required to provide protection through help for antibody production and CTL function, as well as direct cytokine-mediated antiparasite activity [22, 91]. However, the regions of CSP containing immunodominant T cell epitopes are also highly polymorphic among circulating *P. falciparum* strains [92], which is problematic regarding their use in vaccines.

2.1.1. RTS,S (Mosquirix)

The most advanced malaria vaccine (RTS,S) is a virus-like particle (VLP) consisting of a fragment (central repeat and C-terminal regions, amino acids 207–395) of the CSP fused to a hepatitis B virus surface antigen (**Figure 1**). Phase 3 clinical trials of RTS,S/AS01 (commercially known as Mosquirix), a liposomal adjuvant formulation AS01 which contains monophosphoryl lipid A (MPLA) and QS-21, have provided evidence for high levels of antiCSP antibody correlating with reduced clinical malaria episodes [93]. Interestingly, individuals immunized with irradiated sporozoites or RTS,S generate antibodies to the repeat region, which represents the immunodominant region of the protein under these circumstances; however, adults in endemic regions naturally infected with the parasite, and thus partially immune from disease, have high levels of antibodies against the C-terminus and other nonrepeat regions [94]. In malaria nonexposed individuals immunized the with RTS,S vaccine, protection correlated with CD4+ and CD8+ T cells responses to the C-terminal region of CSP [95], while in other studies, sterile immunity was correlated with antirepeat antibodies [96]. In endemic areas, protection against clinical disease in RTS,S immunized infants also correlated with antiCSP antibodies [97]. Altogether, the protective efficacy of the CSP-based RTS,S/AS01 vaccine is a clear demonstration that a recombinant subunit vaccine containing a portion of the protein delivered on a heterologous VLP carrier can provide partial protection in humans. As 30–50% protection against clinical disease was obtained in RTS,S immunized infants and children in endemic areas, it is clear that there is room for improvement upon the RTS,S vaccine.

2.2. Vaccines containing CSP repeats

Whereas there are several multiantigen pre-erythrocytic vaccines that include CSP repeat units along with other CSP epitopes, the vaccines described in this section contain only CSP repeat units or CSP repeat units combined with epitopes from other malaria antigens. One of the earliest vaccine trials with epitopes from CSP was a Phase I trial with controlled human malaria infection (CHMI) where 35 volunteers were immunized with a three-unit NANP repeat peptide $(NANP)_3$ conjugated to tetanus toxoid (TT) and adjuvanted with alum [98]. As the CSP repeats are a known B cell epitope, the three volunteers with the highest ELISA and immunofluorescence assay (IFA) titers were challenged with *P. falciparum* sporozoites (strain NF54); one of these volunteers was sterilely protected. A second trial with CHMI was conducted with this same vaccine where 202 volunteers were immunized and four volunteers with the highest titers were challenged; however, no sterile protection was seen in the challenged volunteers [99]. The results from these trials spurred development of vaccines containing minimal epitopes from CSP that contain CSP repeat units as well as the combination of CSP repeat units with epitopes from other malaria antigen vaccine targets.

One effort to explore combination of CSP repeat units with another malaria vaccine target includes development of a series of influenza virosome-based vaccines. However, virosome-based antigen developed contains a slight variation of the CSP repeat units, NPNA rather than NANP [100]. The resulting vaccine incorporating a constrained $(NPNA)_3$ repeat was termed PEV302. In a Phase I study, 16 volunteers received PEV302 and eight volunteers received a combination vaccine containing PEV302 as well as an influenza virosome containing a portion of domain III from AMA-1, termed PEV301 [101]. Sera collected from volunteers were used to assess ELISA and IFA titer to the constrained repeat peptide and *P. falciparum* (NF54) sporozoites, respectively. Of the 21 volunteers immunized with PEV302, 19 demonstrated titers $\geq 10^2$ after three immunizations [102]; however, a challenge was not conducted as part of this study. A second trial that included CHMI was conducted with these vaccines where the PEV301 and PEV302 epitopes were combined (known as PEV3A) and administered together to 12 volunteers [103]. In this same trial, 13 volunteers were co-immunized with PEV3A and ME-TRAP. Both groups were challenged; however, all volunteers developed parasitemia. The ELISA titers to UK-39 constrained repeat peptide and IFA titers *P. falciparum* (NF54) sporozoites elicited in both studies were similar with all individuals in the second study demonstrating titers $\geq 10^2$.

2.3. Vaccines containing minimal CSP epitopes

It has been suggested that malaria, along with other infectious diseases (e.g., HIV), has resisted classical vaccine strategies by utilizing a method of stimulating either strain-specific or incomplete, nonprotective immunity, which appears to have arisen from having co-evolved with humans for millions of years [104]. Further, studies with CSP in particular have suggested mechanisms other than allelic variation for parasite escape, even suggesting that the immune-dominant repeat region presents as an immunogenic "decoy" that elicits nonneutralizing antibody responses [105]. In general, the majority of vaccine developed strategies have targeted pathogens that display little antigenic variation, are highly conserved among isolates, and are readily inhibited by immune responses stimulated by native antigens, which is not the case for malaria. Furthermore, that only partially protective immune responses result after years of malaria exposure suggests that the parasites may be utilizing a "cloaking" strategy to hide in plain sight of the host immune system such as incorporation of human-like protein sequences to induce Treg expansion [106]. Indeed, for vaccine targets, it has been shown that the degree of cross-conservation of predicted epitopes with the human genome inversely correlates with their immunogenicity [107], and in the case of malaria, Tregs (via PD1 upregulation) are responsible for a low frequency of precursor T cells [5]. Therefore, utilizing a minimal, well-designed epitope set for one or more targeted antigens may provide the most effective means to circumvent the parasites' avoidance mechanisms.

Efforts to combine the CSP repeat unit with other CSP epitopes include development of a series of synthesized peptide constructs containing $(NANP)_3$ (also known as B), the T1 epitope $(NANPNVDP)_2$, and in later studies, the T* epitope (**Figure 1**). A Phase I trial of a synthetic multiple antigenic peptide (MAP) immunogen, which includes four linked T1B peptides adjuvanted in alum with or without QS21, found that better ELISA and IFA titers were achieved with QS21 formulations [108]. This study also demonstrated that recognition of the T1 epitope by T cells is highly MHC-restricted with T cell responses limited to high responder MHC class II genotypes (present in only 25–35% of the population). None of the volunteers in this study were challenged. To address limitations of the T1 epitope, the T* epitope (which is recognized in the context of many human MHC class II molecules) was included in a branched synthetic peptide immunogen containing four linked T1BT* peptides as well as a linked Pam3Cys as endogenous adjuvant [109]. In a small Phase I trial of the tetra-branched T1BT* peptide in 10 volunteers of diverse HLA types, the majority of the volunteers (8/10) seroconverted following the first dose and reached peak antirepeat antibody titers of 10^3–10^4 following three immunizations [110]. The immunized volunteers developed T*-specific Th1- type CD4+ T cell responses. CD4+ T cell clones derived from PBMC up to 10 months after peptide immunization recognized the T* epitope in the context of multiple HLA DR and DQ molecules and secreted high levels of IFN-γ and variable levels of TNF-α [111]. The immunized volunteers in this study were not challenged. Note that up to 1 mg of immunogen was safely administered per dose in these clinical studies.

Additional clinical trials have investigated novel delivery platforms and adjuvants to enhance immunogenicity of CSP minimal T and B cell epitopes. A VLP based on the hepatitis B virus core antigen, ICC 1132, was engineered to express the T1, B $(NANP)_3$, and T* epitopes [112]. A total of four clinical studies were conducted with this antigen. Phase I trials using alum as adjuvant elicited suboptimal antibody and cellular responses [113, 114]. Use of a more potent water-in-oil emulsion-based adjuvant, Montanide ISA 720, enhanced not only immunogenicity, but also reactogenicity in a NHP model [115]. Two clinical studies were conducted with ICC 1132 formulated in Montanide ISA 720; however, due to the potential for increased reactogenicity, only a single administration was given. In the first study with ICC 1132 in ISA 720, escalating doses of antigen (from 20 to 50 µg) were administered [116]. Both ELISA and IFA titers with a single dose of ICC 1132 in ISA 720 were improved as compared to those achieved with three doses of ICC 1132 in alum. A second clinical study was conducted where a single 50µg dose of ICC 132 in ISA 720 was administered to 11 volunteers that were subsequently challenged; however, none of the volunteers were protected [117]. A summary of Phase I clinical studies, with CSP vaccine candidates, is provided in **Table 1**.

Category	RTS,S (AS02)	RTS,S (AS03)	RTS,S (AS04)	RTS,S (Alum)	Pf CS 282–383	NANP-TT	(T1B)4	(T1BT*)4	ICC-1132	ICC-1132	ICC-1132	ICC-1132
Epitopes	NANP, aa 302–395 (207–395)				NANP, aa 302–383 (282–383)	(NANP)3	NANP, NVDP (T1)	NANP, NVDP (T1), (T*) aa 326–345	NANP, NVDP (T1), (T*) aa 326–345			
Carrier/platform	HBsAg				None	TT fusion	MAP	Polyoxime	HBcAg (truncated)			
Formulation/adjuvants	AS02	AS03	AS04	Alum	ISA 720	Alum	Alum +/- QS21	Pam3Cys	Alum, saline Alum		ISA 720	ISA 720
Route	IM	IM	IM	IM	IM	IM	SC	SC	IM	IM	IM	IM
# Administrations	3 1–3	3	3 3	3	3	3	3	3	2–3	3	1	1
Dose	50μg 10μg, 25μg, 50μg	50μg	50μg	50μg	≥100μg	20μg, 50μg, 100μg, 160μg	500μg, 1000μg	1000μg	20μg, 50μg	20μg, 50μg	5μg, 20μg, 50μg	50μg
IFA: % titer >10² [group GMT]	100% [6400] 100% [3200–10500]	100% [4755]	75% [654] 100% [ND]	50% [ND]	100% [2364–2810]	23% [ND]	25–67% [5511]	25–67% (+QS21) 70% [216]	25–63% [57–226]	33–71% [ND]	38–100% [ND]	ND
ELISA: % Seroconv. (titer >10²), coat Ag	100%, NANP 100%, NANP	100%, NANP	100%, NANP 100%, NANP		100%, CS 282–383	33–57%, NANP	25–86% (+QS21), NANP (T1B)4	100%, (T1BT*)4	50–75%, (T1B)4	40–75%, (T1B)4	63–100%, (T1B)4	100%, NANP
Cellular proliferation	ND 50–86%		0% 10%		63% (ISA)	0%	86% (+QS21) spz	60%	47–75%	50%	ND	ND
Protection (# protected/# challenged)	86% (6/7) 50μg × 3 30% (3/10) 50μg × 1 50% (7/14) 50μg × 2 50% (3/6) 50μg ×3 57% (4/7) 25μg × 3 25% (1/4) 10 μg × 3	29% (2/7)	13% (1/8) 25% (2/8)	0% (0/6)	ND	33% (1/3)	ND	ND	ND	ND	ND	0% (0/11)
References	[121] [124]	[121]	[121] [122]	[122]	[119]	[98]	[123] [90]	[110] [90]	[113] [112]	[114]	[116]	[117]

Percentages indicate percent responders for IFA, ELISA, and cellular proliferation; ND, not determined; GMT, geometric mean titer.

Table 1. Summary of clinical trials of CSP vaccine candidates (including RTS,S CHMI studies).

2.4. Long synthetic CSP peptide vaccines

In addition to vaccine studies using minimal T and B cell epitopes, clinical studies have investigated immunogenicity of long synthetic peptides containing the entire N- or C-terminus of *P. falciparum* CSP [118]. Of interest is the Pf CSP 282-383 study where a long synthetic peptide including C-terminus amino acids 282–383 from CSP (PfCS102) was synthesized and administered to volunteers as a formulation in either alum or Montanide ISA 720 [119]. Elevated ELISA and IFA titers were seen with ISA 720 formulation as compared to alum. In a second clinical trial, PfCS102 formulated in ISA 720 or AS02A elicited IFN-γ secreting CD8+ T cells specific to malaria in some individuals [120]. Tenfold higher antibody and cellular responses were obtained with the AS02 adjuvant formulation. However, no volunteers were challenged in these studies. Note that synthesized peptide doses of ≥100μg were administered in this study.

2.5. Preclinical pipeline of novel CSP-based vaccines

Additional preclinical studies of VLP have utilized a woodchuck hepatitis core antigen engineered to express CSP repeats in the loop region and multiple universal T cell epitopes at the C-terminus, termed Mal-78-3T VLP [125]. Mice immunized intraperitoneally (i.p.) with Mal-78-3T VLP, formulated in alum/QS21 or ISA 720 adjuvant, developed high levels of antirepeat antibodies. Sterile immunity was obtained in Mal-78-3T immunized mice of three different strains following challenge by transgenic sporozoites expressing *P. falciparum* CSP repeats.

The minimal T and B cell epitopes have also been tested as a recombinant protein using a TLR5 agonist, flagellin, as adjuvant in murine studies [126, 127]. Chimeric flagellin protein containing multiple T1BT* modules, or nearly full-length *P. falciparum* CSP, elicited high levels of antirepeat antibody. The chimeric protein was immunogenic without addition of exogenous adjuvant when delivered subcutaneously or as a needle-free intranasal vaccine.

In addition to the TLR 5 agonist, a TLR-7 agonist, imiquimod, was also found to be a potent adjuvant for vaccines containing minimal T and B cell epitopes. Immunization of mice with the linear T1BT* peptide subcutaneously followed by application of topical TLR-7 agonist imiquimod induced protective antibody-mediated immunity as well as splenic CD4+ T cell responses [128]. Recent Phase I/II studies have demonstrated that topical imiquimod can also enhance immunogenicity and protective efficacy of a seasonal flu vaccine [129, 130], supporting the use of the murine model for identification of promising TLR agonist adjuvants for human trials.

Of interest are murine studies demonstrating that micro- and nanoparticle vaccines containing minimal T and B cell epitopes were immunogenic without the addition of exogenous adjuvants. Layer by Layer (LbL) microcapsules were constructed by sequential layering of positively charged poly-l-lysine and negatively charged poly-L-glutamic acid with derivatized peptides containing T1BT* epitopes added to the final layer [131]. Mice immunized with LbL microparticles in PBS elicited sporozoite neutralizing antibodies that blocked *in vitro* invasion of transgenic *P. berghei* sporozoites expressing *P. falciparum* CSP repeats into human hepatoma cells and reduced parasite liver burden following challenge by exposure to the bites of mosquitoes infected with the transgenic rodent parasites. Protection was comparable to levels obtained following immunization with T1BT* peptide in Freund's adjuvant.

Self-assembling proteins that form nanoparticles (SAPNs) have also been examined in murine studies [132, 133]. The SAPN is comprised of 60 monomers of a recombinant linear protein containing trimeric and pentameric coiled-coil domains separated by a flexible linker with T and B cell epitopes expressed at N- or C-terminus. Following expression in *Escherichia coli*, monomers self-assemble to form spherical SAPN of ~40 nm in diameter. A *P. falciparum* SAPN was constructed comprised of monomer containing four copies of the NANP repeats at the C-terminus and three previously identified *P. falciparum* CSP CD8+ T cell epitopes (KPKDELDY, MPNDPNRNV, and YLNKIQNSL) at the N-terminus, along with a designed pan-DR binding T cell epitope termed PADRE. All strains of mice immunized with two or three doses of SAPN developed high ELISA titers that persisted over 52 weeks and CD8+ T central memory cells secreting IL-2 and IFN-γ. Mice challenged by i.v. injection of transgenic rodent parasites expressing full length *P. falciparum* CSP protein showed 90–100% protection, with 50% of SAPN immunized mice still protected against sporozoite challenge at week 52. Protective immunity was mediated by both sporozoite neutralizing antirepeat antibodies and CD8+ T cells.

One notable target absent in most CSP-based constructs is the N-terminus of CSP, which contains both T and B cell epitopes as well as the highly conserved Region I (**Figure 2**). Further, within Region I, resides the proteolytic cleavage site and a ligand-binding domain which have been shown to be key requirements for sporozoite infection of hepatocytes [80, 81, 83]. Antibodies raised to this region have been shown to confer 90% protection in animal passive transfer studies [134]. Therefore, efforts are now being pursued to identify and incorporate this epitope into some of the strategies described in this section.

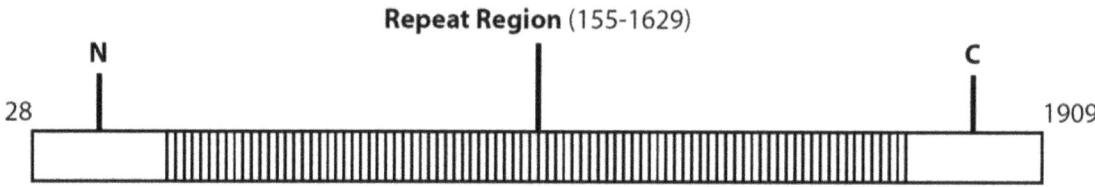

Figure 2. Diagram of LSA-1 (adapted from [164]).

3. Vaccines containing liver stage antigens

3.1. Cell-traversal protein for ookinetes and sporozoites (CelTOS)

3.1.1. Structure and antigenicity

As its name suggests, CelTOS is expressed in both the ookinetes and sporozoite stages of malaria, and functions in cell transversal [135]. This protein is highly conserved across multiple species of *Plasmodium* including those that cause malaria in rodents (*P. berghei*) and primates (*P. falciparum* and *P. vivax*) [135]. Identification of CelTOS (182 AA—GenBank: AAN36249.1) as a potential protective antigen built upon a previous proteomic analysis identifying expressed proteins in specific phases of the *P. falciparum* lifecycle [62]. Using prototypical HLA supertypes, algorithms were developed to identify potential peptides that could bind to HLA supertypes, and peptides from 27 proteins were screened for stimulating PBMCs from volunteers vaccinated with irradiated sporozoites and subsequently challenged with infection by *P. falciparum* [55]. From these, CelTOS was identified as stimulating the highest number of effector T cells producing IFN-γ overall [55]. Subsequently, Kaiser et al. identified CelTOS using a suppression-subtractive hybridization approach in *P. yoelii* sporozoites versus merozoites [58].

In malaria-naive volunteers infected with irradiated sporozoites, peptides from CelTOS stimulate IFN-γ production from effector T cells in eight out of 12 volunteers [55]. Six out of 35 Ghanaian adults demonstrated effector T cells to CelTOS [136]. In mice immunized with irradiated sporozoites, low levels of IFN-γ producing CelTOS-specific CD8+ T cells are induced [137].

3.1.2. Preclinical and clinical trials of CelTOS vaccine

Vaccines comprised of CelTOS recombinant protein or expression vectors (i.e., DNA and viral vectors) have demonstrated protective efficacy against malaria in mouse models. CelTOS administered as a recombinant protein with the adjuvants Montanide ISA 720 or glucopyranosyl lipid A stable emulsion (GLA-SE) elicited CelTOS-specific antibodies, CD4+ and CD8+ T cells, and protection (10–76% protection, depending on dose and mouse strain) from infective challenge with *P. berghei* in BALB/c and CD1 mice [65, 138, 139]. This protection was demonstrated using homologous and heterologous challenge, demonstrating the unique level of conservation of CelTOS even across species of the parasite [65, 138]. Note that a challenge was not conducted with GLA-SE formulations. In mice vaccinated with recombinant CelTOS, protective immunity did not correlate with the level of antibody production, and passive immunization did not provide significant protection from infection [138]. In one study, self-adjuvanting bacterial vectors expressing CelTOS were used to vaccinate BALB/c mice and sterile immunity (40–60% protection, depending on dose) was demonstrated even though an antibody response to CelTOS was not detected [140]. In these studies, clearance of parasites infecting the liver plays a major role in protective immunity, which is likely potentiated by CD4+ and CD8+ T cells [138, 141]. Protective immunity in BALB/c mice was dependent on the mixed response of both the CD4+ and CD8+ T cells to CelTOS [138, 140, 141]. Studies using viral vectors encoding CelTOS did not demonstrate protective immunity in either BALB/c or CD1 mice, even though an antibody response and moderate levels of CelTOS-specific CD4+ and CD8+ T cells were induced, and control cohorts immunized with CSP in the same prime/boost protocol did demonstrate sterile immunity [33, 137].

Two Phase I trials with CHMI have been performed with a recombinant CelTOS protein produced in *E. coli* (FMP012) formulated with either GLA-SE or AS01B and tested for safety and efficacy (ClinicalTrials.gov: NCT01540474; ClinicalTrials.gov: NCT02174978). Malaria-naïve adults (18–50 years of age) were vaccinated three times with FMP012 GLA-SE or four times with FMP012 AS01B, and adverse events were monitored. Antibody titers to FMP012 were monitored. Vaccinated volunteers along with nonvaccinated controls were challenged with *P. falciparum* to determine the efficacy of the immune response as determined by time to parasitemia evaluated by blood smear. Results for neither trial have been published.

3.2. Exported protein-1 (EXP-1)

3.2.1. Structure and antigenicity

Exported protein 1 (EXP-1) (162 AA—GenBank: AAN35808.1) was discovered by screening an *E. coli* expression library of blood stage antigens using a monoclonal antibody to *P. falciparum* and was designated antigen 5.1 (Ag5.1) [142]. It was subsequently rediscovered by other screening approaches and designated circumsporozoite-related antigen (CRA), EXP-1, QF116, and *P. yoelii* hepatocyte erythrocyte protein 17 (HEP17) [143–147]. Adults in malaria-endemic regions produced antibodies to the protein and EXP-1-dependent CD4+ and CD8+ T cells [37, 38, 143]. EXP-1 was incorporated in some of the earliest subunit vaccines for malaria tested in humans [148], and peptides from this protein continue to be incorporated into vaccines for malaria, such as ex23 used in ME-TRAP [44].

EXP-1 is conserved across strains of specific *Plasmodium* species [143, 147]. The demonstration that this protein elicited an immune response that provided protection across a diverse spectrum of murine malaria strains in challenged mice [149] led to analysis identifying supertype-peptides that elicited response from a variety of HLA types [37]. In addition to being a vaccine target, the protein is a glutathione S-transferase that has been associated with artesunate metabolism, making it a potential drug target for malaria [150].

The immune responses of people in malaria endemic regions demonstrate that EXP-1 elicits antibody and IFN-γ responses from CD4+ and CD8+ T cells. Indonesian and African adults had detectable antibodies that react with EXP-1 [151–153]. In African children in malaria endemic regions, the presence of antibody responding to an EXP-1 peptide encompassing amino acids 101–162 were associated with decreased infection [154]. Low level IFN-γ and CD4+ T cells were seen in response to EXP-1 in West Africans, although CD8+ T cells were not detected [151]. A similar limited response of CD8+ T cells and low level CD4+ T cells by Kenyans was noted with only one peptide, EXP-10, stimulating CD8+ T cells [37, 38]. Adults from Gambia and Tanzania with natural immunity to malaria develop EXP-1-dependent CTL and the EXP-1 peptide EX23 has also been shown to elicit a CTL response [155]. In another study, African children naturally exposed to malaria only developed low levels of EXP-1-dependent IFN-γ expression [156]. However, the peptides used for this study (EXP2, EXP80, and EXP91) were previously demonstrated to give no CD8+ T cell response in African adults [37], and may not reflect the potential for EXP-1 as a vaccine component. This potential is demonstrated in Caucasian adults, that when immunized with irradiated sporozoites developed EXP-1-dependent CD8+ T cells as well as CD4+ T cells [37, 55].

3.2.2. Preclinical and clinical trials of EXP-1

EXP-1 provided protection from malaria in a mouse model where protection was dependent on the development of CD8+ T cells and expression of IFN-γ or nitric oxide [149]. This study resulted in an early emphasis on CD8+-dependent IFN-γ production in the development of subunit vaccines against malaria.

5.1-(NANP)19 is a recombinant protein expressed in *E. coli* that contains EXP-1 fused with 19 repeats of the tetramer NANP from CSP [157]. Thirteen adults were vaccinated subcutaneously with 5.1-(NANP)19 using two or three immunizations containing 50 or 400 μg of protein without adjuvant [148]. The vaccine was safe and only caused reactions at the site of injection. All volunteers developed antibody to the NANP peptide, and six developed 5.1-(NANP)19-spectific effector T cells. Seven volunteers were subsequently challenged with *P. falciparum* by bites from infected mosquitoes. While all seven volunteers developed parasitemia, one did not develop symptoms of malaria.

In a study with 194 semiimmune children (6–12 years old) immunized with 5.1-(NANP)19, all but eight children had considerable levels of antibody to EXP-1 [158]. None of the nonvacci-nated children developed malaria in this study over the 12 weeks of observation, and the protective efficacy of the vaccine could not be determined.

EXP-1 has been tested in a number of clinical trials as a component of multiantigen vaccines: EP1300, L3SEPTL, ME-TRAP, and MuStDP5. See the discussion in Section 5, **Table 3**.

3.3. Liver-stage antigen-1 (LSA-1)

3.3.1. Structure and antigenicity

Liver stage antigen 1 (LSA-1) is expressed after parasites have invaded hepatocytes and antigen accumulates in the parasitophorous vacuole [52, 159]. The function of this antigen is not known. LSA-1 was discovered using antisera from volunteers who remained on chloroquine while in a malaria endemic region to obtain antibodies to the liver stage of malaria. The antisera were used to screen recombinant DNA expression libraries [52]. Subsequently, a peptide ls94 from LSA-1 was found to bind to HLA-B53, which is MHC class I associated with resistance to severe malaria in West Africa. This indicated that class-I restricted CD8+ T cells are important for protective immunity against malaria in Africans [160, 161].

LSA-1 (UniProtKB/Swiss-Prot: Q25893) is a 1909 amino acid protein from the *P. falciparum* strain NF54 [162]. Even though strain 3D7 is derived from NF54 [163], the 3D7 strain produces a protein that is 1162 amino acids in length. The amino terminal and carboxyl terminal ends of the protein are nonrepetitive, whereas the middle of the protein contains multiple repeats (**Figure 2**). This repeat region results in significant variation of the protein between strains of *P. falciparum* [162].

LSA-1 antigen stimulates IFN-γ producing T cells, composed of CD4+ and CD8+ T cells, and CTL was demonstrated from volunteers in regions with endemic malaria [36, 37, 151, 164–166]. The immune response to LSA-1 typically increased with age and exposure to the parasite

[165–168]. In Gabonese children, LSA-1-dependent IFN-γ producing T cells were correlated with reduced disease severity [169]. Further, naturally infected individuals often express antibodies to LSA-1, targeting primarily the central repetitive region of the protein [170], and antibody to LSA-1 is associated with a reduction in disease severity [171–173].

Immunization of malaria-naive volunteers with irradiated sporozoites produced an immune response to LSA-1 that included CD4+ and CD8+ T cells, and a weak antibody response [37, 38, 55, 174]. However, when volunteers were challenged with infection, the volunteers who responded to LSA-1 were not protected from malaria [55]. Further, in malaria-naive volunteers immunized by exposure to bites from infected mosquitoes while receiving chloroquine, 74% of the volunteers produced antibodies to LSA-1; however, the humoral response did not provide sterile protection from malaria [175].

3.3.2. Preclinical and clinical trials of LSA-1 vaccine

Rodent strains of *Plasmodium* do not contain orthologs of LSA-1 [64, 176], and animal models evaluating LSA-1 are limited to NHPs. Analysis of immunity to peptides from LSA-1 in combination with LSA-3, SALSA, and STARP in NHPs has been the focus of several studies wherein immunity to the peptides is altered by lipidating the peptides or incorporating the peptides in Montanide ISA-51 [66, 177, 178]. High levels of B cells and CD4+ T cells producing IFN-γ in response to LSA-1 were demonstrated. One of the peptides for LSA-1 (LSA1-J) elicited CD8+ CTLs. The NHPs were not challenged with infection by *Plasmodium*, so the impact of this immune response is not known.

Analysis of LSA-1 vaccination using prime/boost approaches using DNA viral vehicles is limited. A prime boost of LSA-1 in chimpanzee adenovirus 63 (ChAd63) and modified vaccine Ankara (MVA) in BALB/c and CD-1 mice demonstrated sterile protection using a chimeric strain of *P. berghei* expressing the *P. falciparum* LSA-1 protein [33]. Seven out of eight mice, for both the BALB/c and CD-1 mice, demonstrated a significant delay in time to onset of parasitemia. LSA-1-dependent IFN-γ production by CD4+ and CD8+ T cells, and antibodies were detected; however, the mediators for protection were not clear. In BALB/c mice where CD4+ or CD8+ T cells were depleted, protection was not dependent on CD8+ T cells; however, results suggested that CD4+ T cells play a significant role. Analysis of the immune response developed in rhesus monkeys using DNA priming and pox virus boosting (using the nonreplicating canary pox virus ALVAC-Pf7) was carried out using an antigen cocktail containing LSA-1, CSP, TRAP, AMA1, and MSP1 [179]. This resulted in a predominant CD4+ T cell response with secretion of IL-2. Low-level IFN-γ production was attributed to CD4+ T cells and CD8+ T cells were low and only present in animals with high CD4+ T cell responses. No antibodies to LSA-1 were detected. The animals were not challenged with infection by *Plasmodium*, so the impact of this immune response is not known.

Recombinant protein LSA-NRC was developed to assess efficacy of an LSA-1 vaccine in the clinic. LSA-NRC incorporates *P. falciparum* NF54 LSA-1 nonrepetitive N-terminal and C-terminal regions, and includes two 17-amino-acid repeats from the repetitive central region of the protein (**Figure 3**). This antigen was administered with AS01B (a liposomal formulation with MPLA and QS-21) in rhesus monkeys and elicited high titers of antibodies and CD4+ T cells producing IL-2 alone or IL-2 with IFN-γ, but CD8+ T cells were not detected [180]. The NHPs were not challenged with infection by *Plasmodium*, so the impact of this immune response is not known.

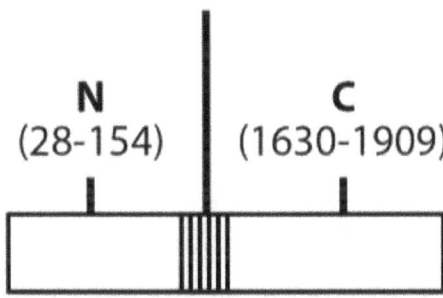

17AA Repeat x 2
(EQQSDLEQERLAKEKLQERLAKEKLQEQQRDLEQ)

Figure 3. Diagram of LSA-NRC (adapted from [181]).

Phase I trials with CHMI were carried out in malaria naïve volunteers using a recombinant LSA 1 protein (FMP011). LSA-NRC adjuvanted with either AS01B or AS02A was well tolerated, safe, and immunogenic at both low and high doses of the antigen [64]. All volunteers developed antibodies after the first dose of the vaccine. Vaccinated volunteers developed LSA-1 specific CD4+ T cells following the second dose. The low dose of LSA-NRC, with either AS01B or AS02A, resulted in LSA-1-dependent CD4+ T cells that produced both IL-2 and IFN-γ. However, the LSA-1 high-dose groups had fewer CD4+ T cells and little to no IFN-γ response relative to the low-dose cohort. None of the groups produced LSA-1-dependent CD8+ T cells. These results were similar to the immune response seen in the preclinical studies in mice (BALB/c and A/J mice) and rhesus monkeys [180, 182]. Only the high-dose groups were challenged along with nonvaccinated volunteers using the homologous 3D7 strain of P. *falciparum*. All 22 volunteers that were challenged became parasitemic without delayed onset of the erythrocytic infection.

Several clinical trials of multiantigen pre-erythrocytic vaccines that included LSA-1 as an antigen (EP1300, L3SEPTL, ME-TRAP, MuStDP5, and NYVAC-Pf7) have been conducted and are discussed in Section 4, **Table 3**.

3.4. Liver-stage antigen-3 (LSA-3)

3.4.1. Structure and antigenicity of LSA-3

While LSA-3 is included with the liver-stage antigens, some report it is actually a blood stage antigen [183]. Using malaria-naive volunteers immunized with irradiated P. *falciparum*, LSA-3 was identified by comparing antibody response of protected and nonprotected volunteers to a recombinant DNA expression library [53].

LSA-3 is composed of three nonrepeating regions (NR-A, NR-B, and NR-C) flanking two short repeat regions (R1 and R3) and one long repeat region (R2) (see **Figure 4**) [53]. The nonrepeat regions are well conserved across geographically diverse strains of *P. falciparum* [184]. The most significant variation is in the repeating regions, but this is due to the organization and the number of repeating subunits rather than composition of the repeating regions [184]. Vaccine development draws upon the protein from *P. falciparum* strains T9/96 and 3D7 (1586 AA GenBank: ACT22567.1).

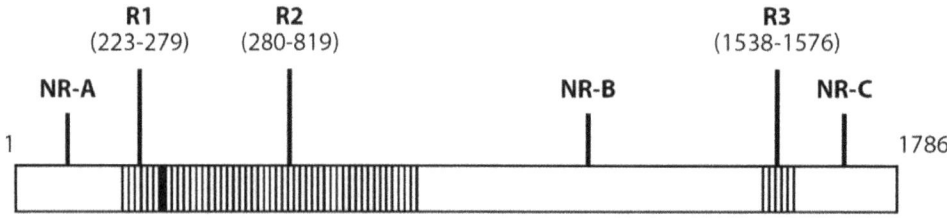

Figure 4. Diagram of the domains of LSA-3 (adapted from [185]).

In individuals exposed to *P. falciparum*, LSA-3 elicits antibodies, and CD4+ and CD8+ T cells. West African adults demonstrated CD4+, and class I–LSA-3-dependent CTLs [151, 155]. Antibodies to LSA-3 were demonstrated in children from West Africa, and increased with age [171, 185], and malaria-naive Europeans develop antibodies to LSA-3 when immunized with irradiated sporozoites [53].

3.4.2. Preclinical and clinical trials of LSA-3

Rodent strains of *Plasmodium* do not contain orthologs of LSA-3 [176], and animal models evaluating LSA-3 are limited to NHPs. A murine model with the infectious challenge using a strain of *P. berghei* that was genetically modified to contain the *P. falciparum* LSA-3 gene has been reported [33]. BALB/c and CD1 mice were primed with ChAd63 and boosted with MVA encoding LSA-3, but sterile immunity was demonstrated in only 13% of the BALB/c mice. The BALB/c mice developed antibodies and moderate levels of PBMCs producing LSA-3-specific IFN-γ were developed. Both CD4+ and CD8+ T cells were produced against the antigen, and CD8+ T cells predominated.

Vaccination with LSA-3 has been shown to elicit sterile immunity in chimpanzees [53]. This study demonstrated sterile immunity using various forms of LSA-3, albeit only one chimpanzee was used for each specific antigen. LSA-3 was expressed as GST-fused recombinant peptides in three segments: DG (encompassing AA 1–60), NN (encompassing AA 369–447), and PC (encompassing AA 869–1786). The mixture of these three peptides (designated as LSA-3 GST) elicited sterile immunity when administered with the adjuvant SBAS2 (SBAS2 is an adjuvant containing MPLA and QS21) or with Montanide ISA 51. The synthetic lapidated peptides CT1, NR1, NR2, and RE were also evaluated. Vaccination with NR2 alone elicited sterile immunity. Further, NR2 administered with NR1 and Montanide ISA 5, or with NR1 and CT1 with Montanide ISA 51 also elicited sterile immunity. Studies in chimpanzees using the same LSA-3 peptides in combination with peptides derived from LSA-1, STARP, and SALSA demonstrated that the LSA-3 peptides elicited IFN-γ production with a mixed response of CD4+ and CD8+ T cells [66].

Later studies in chimpanzees immunized with plasmid expressing the nearly full length LSA-3 also demonstrated LSA-3 provided protection, with three of the four immunized chimpanzees demonstrating sterile immunity [186]. In this study, only low levels of IFN-γ were detected from a mixed class I and class II response, and no antibodies were detected. Studies in *Aotus* monkeys immunized with recombinant LSA-3 without adjuvant also developed low but sustained levels of antibodies to LSA-3, and LSA-3 dependent IFN-γ production; however, neither correlated with protection [187]. Subsequent challenge with *P. falciparum* demonstrated that three of the five immunized monkeys were sterilely protected. Interestingly, immuno-fluorescence assay titers to *P. falciparum* sporozoites were highest in monkeys that were protected. These results were repeated when *Aotus* monkeys were immunized using two peptides of LSA-3, amino acids 100–222 in the amino-terminal nonrepeat region, and amino acids 501–596 in the repeat-2 region of the protein from *P. falciparum* strain T9/96 [187]. In this later study, monkeys were immunized with the recombinant peptides adjuvanted with AS02, eliciting antibody and high IFN-γ responses with sterile immunity in four out of four immunized animals.

A Phase I clinical trial with challenge evaluating the safety and efficacy of recombinant LSA-3 protein adjuvanted with aluminum hydroxide or Montanide ISA 720 was carried out, but the results of the study have not been published [188].

Clinical trials for multistage pre-erythrocytic vaccines that contain LSA-3 include L3SEPTL, ME-TRAP, and MuStDP5 and are discussed in Section 4, **Table 3**.

3.5. Sporozoite threonine-asparagine-rich protein (STARP)

3.5.1. Structure and antigenicity

STARP (GenBank: CAA81224.1) was identified by screening a lambda library with antibodies developed in malaria exposed missionaries under chloroquine treatment [51]. It is a 604-amino acid protein with a central hydrophilic region (amino acids 85–489) that contains a complex repetitive structure that can vary in size between different strains of *P. falciparum*. Two peptides from this repetitive region (Rp10 and Rp45) have been evaluated in vaccines [51]. Even with variation in the repetitive structure, the protein is highly conserved across a variety of geographically separated strains [51, 189].

People in malaria endemic regions produce antibody to STARP [190–192], with the percentage of the population related to the rate of exposure to malaria [193]. The main STARP antibody response in Africans naturally exposed to malaria or volunteers immunized with irradiated sporozoites was to the Rp10 peptide, and purified antibody prevented 90% of the sporozoites from infecting human liver cells *in vitro* [193]. In West African children, the presence of antibody to STARP was associated with protection from malaria [171]. A conserved HLA class I epitope eliciting a CTL response in adults naturally infected with *P. falciparum* has been identified and was incorporated in the multiple epitope used as part of the vaccine ME-TRAP [36, 41] (Section 4, **Table 3**).

3.5.2. Preclinical and clinical trials of STARP

A limited number of T cell epitopes have been identified in STARP. The conserved epitope st8 was demonstrated to elicit a CD8+ T cell CTL response in an African adult exposed to *P. falciparum* [36]. The Rp10 epitope is both a B cell and class I T cell epitope [189]. However, in a NHP model, the Rp10 epitope elicits low levels IFN-γ response but no detectable CTL; note that the NHPs were not challenged with infection in these studies [66, 178].

Homologues of STARP have been identified in *P. yoelii* (PY00217 and PY05105) and *P. reichenowi* (PRCDC_0700500) [176, 189]. However, no studies of animals vaccinated with STARP and challenged with infection are published.

Clinical trials for multiantigen vaccines that include STARP, L3SEPTL, and ME-TRAP, are discussed in Section 4, **Table 3**.

3.6. Thrombospondin-related anonymous protein (TRAP)

3.6.1. Structure and antigenicity of TRAP

The TRAP protein was initially identified based on peptide motifs in common with thrombo-spondin and properdin [194]. Subsequently, it was demonstrated that TRAP contributed to the binding of sporozoites to hepatic cells [195], and antibodies to the protein block binding of sporozoites to hepatic cells [196]. In addition to TRAP referring to "thrombospondin-related anonymous protein," the literature refers to TRAP as "thrombospondin-related adhesion protein" [42] and as sporozoite surface protein-2 (SSP2) [196]. TRAP antigen from *P. falciparum* T9/96 (559 AA-PRF: 226137) differs by 6% from the amino acid sequence of TRAP in the 3D7 strain (574 AA-CAD52497.1). The major difference between the strains is the protein from the 3D7 strain contains hepta-repeat of the PPN sequence while T9/96 only contains a single PPN.

Early development of TRAP as a component in a malaria vaccine focused on identifying peptides that were recognized by MHC 1 and elicited a CTL response from individuals exposed to the parasite [36–38, 41, 197, 198]. Evaluation of the immune response to TRAP in naturally infected African donors demonstrated CD4+ and CD8+ T cells. Gambian and Kenyan adults demonstrated CD8+ T cell-dependent CTL activity against TRAP [36–38, 151, 197]. In a study in Kenya, TRAP-dependent IFN-γ producing T cells correlated with reduced disease severity in children [199]. Additionally, it has been demonstrated that a CD4+ T cell response dominated over a CD8+ T cell response to TRAP in Kenyan children and adults, and the CD4+ T cells reactive with TRAP were correlated with reduced risk of clinical malaria [200].

Analysis of the immune response to TRAP in malaria-naive volunteers immunized with irradiated sporozoites (using the 3D7 clone of *P. falciparum* strain NF54) demonstrated CD8+ T cell-dependent CTL activity against TRAP [37, 198], and TRAP-specific CD4+ T cells [38]. In a separate study using 12 malaria-naive Caucasian male volunteers immunized with irradiated sporozoites, TRAP was recognized by five of the volunteers and resulted in the development of TRAP responsive CD4+ T cells, CD8+ T cells, and antibodies [55].

While antibodies are recognized as important in protection from the erythrocytic phase of malaria and reducing the severity of disease, their role in providing sterile protection in the liver-stage is controversial. *In vitro*, antibodies to TRAP can block binding of sporozoites to human hepatocytes, and it has been postulated that antibodies could help to prevent infection of the liver [201]. In a study using malaria-naive volunteers infected with *P. falciparum* while receiving chloroquine to provide sterile immunity, volunteers did not produce antibodies to TRAP or detectable memory B cells [175]. A recent study, using malaria-naive volunteers vaccinated with irradiated sporozoites and subsequently challenged with the homologous strain of *P. falciparum* (3D7 clone of NF54) correlated the magnitude of the antibody response to TRAP with sterile protective immunity [54]. In this study, both sterilely protected individuals (six volunteers) and individuals who developed blood-stage parasitemia (five volunteers) developed antibodies to TRAP and other *P. falciparum* antigens, but the magnitude of the immune response was significantly higher in the protected volunteers. In a similar but separate study using 12 volunteers immunized with irradiated sporozoites, while a subset of the volunteers responded to TRAP, the immune response to TRAP was associated with volunteers who did not develop sterile immunity [55].

3.6.2. Preclinical and clinical trials of TRAP vaccine

Recent studies have tested TRAP alone and in combination with RTS,S in malaria naive adults [202]. The expressed protein was a truncated form of TRAP consisting of amino acids 26–511 with an additional hepta-histidine at the carboxyl-terminus. Volunteers immunized with TRAP in AS02 developed antibodies and modest CD4+ and CD8+ T cell responses (46 SFU/10^6 PBMCs). In an effort to determine if there was a synergistic effect of immune responses to TRAP and CSP, a clinical study with CHMI was conducted where volunteers were immunized with two 25 µg doses of TRAP or two doses of both TRAP and RTS,S (25 and 50 µg, respectively) in AS02. Following challenge, 1/11 volunteers (9%) developed sterile immunity in the cohort vaccinated with TRAP and RTS,S with no significant delayed patency in remaining volunteers. The level of protective efficacy was lower than was previously reported for immunization with RTS,S alone, suggesting potential antigenic competition.

Clinical trials of multiantigen vaccines containing TRAP, including EP1300, L3SEPTL, ME-TRAP, MuStDP5, and NYVAC-Pf7 are discussed in Section 4, **Table 3**.

4. Multiantigen pre-erythrocytic vaccines

Early studies with multiantigen vaccines were based on the rational that a combination of antigens would elicit a broad immune response more comparable to that elicited by whole sporozoite vaccine. A number of multiantigen vaccines comprised of DNA, polyprotein, and recombinant viral vectors containing combinations of epitopes or entire pre-erythrocytic antigens have been tested in clinical trials (listed in alphabetical order).

4.1. EP1300

EP1300 is a multivalent DNA vaccine composed of a total of 38 CTL and 16 HTL epitopes derived from TRAP, CSP, EXP-1, and LSA-1 expressed as a single protein, and the NANP repeating epitope from CSP for antibody development (**Figure 5**). The epitopes are linked using spacers that facilitate proteolytic processing of the protein into individual epitopes in the body; while this worked in animals, processing may not have occurred correctly in humans.

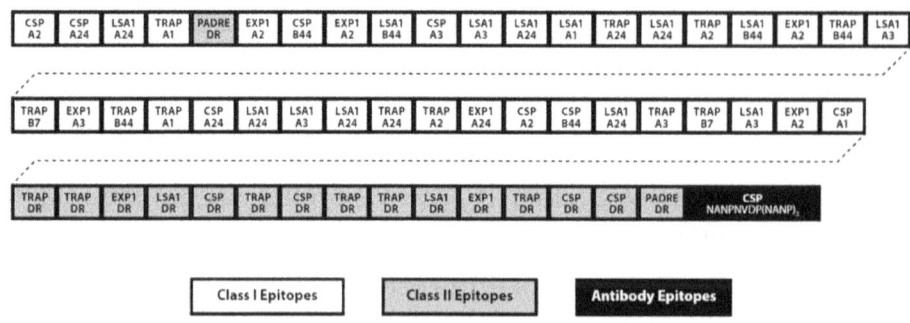

Figure 5. Arrangement of epitopes from CSP, EXP-1, LSA-1, and TRAP in EP1300.

A Phase Ia dose-escalating study in healthy malaria-naive adults (18–40 years of age) was initiated in 2010 to evaluate the safety and immunogenicity of EP1300. EP1300 was delivered using electroporation. This trial was completed in 2015 [203]. The trial demonstrated the vaccine was safe and well tolerated but did not elicit a significant immune response in the volunteers (Unpublished Results, ClinicalTrials.gov: NCT01169077).

4.2. L3SEPTL polyprotein vaccine

L3SEPTL polyprotein is comprised of six pre-erythrocytic-stage antigens, LSA-3, STARP, EXP-1, Pfs16, TRAP, and LSA1-N/C, linked together to produce a 3240-aa-long polyprotein (**Figure 6**) [204]. In this construct, LSA-1 is modified so that only one repeat is included flanked by the conserved amino-end (amino acids 1–148) and the carboxyl-end (amino acids 1523–1909). The nucleic acid sequence expressing the recombinant fused protein is delivered as plasmid DNA using the human cytomegalovirus promoter, or in the viral vehicles MVA and Fowlpox (FP9), to provide the vaccines PP, MVA-PP, and FP9-PP, respectively.

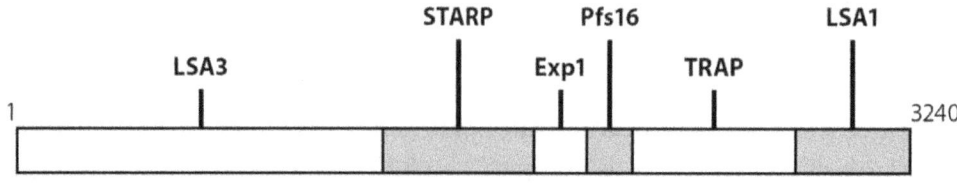

Figure 6. Diagram of the L3SEPTL fusion protein (adapted from [204]).

The MVA-PP and FP9-PP vaccines were evaluated in a Phase I with challenge dose-escalation human clinical trial using malaria-naive volunteers [205]. Generally, the vaccine was well tolerated, but the immunity was lower than expected. Priming with MVA resulted in a stronger immune response than did FP9, and when FP9 was used for priming (FP9/FP9/MVA), the immune response was not significantly elicited until the MVA vehicle was used to deliver the antigens [205]. This was in contrast with the results seen in the preclinical study using FP9-PP for the priming. When delivered using MVA priming, all six proteins elicited IFN-γ-producing T cells, with stronger and more frequent responses seen for LSA-3, LSA-1, TRAP, and STARP. However, the number of IFN-γ-producing T cells was lower than had been reported in other studies [205]. Following challenge, none of the 15 vaccinated volunteers demonstrated protection or delayed onset of disease relative to the six nonvaccinated volunteers.

4.3. ME-TRAP

The most extensively tested multiantigen vaccine, ME (multiepitope)-TRAP vaccine, was designed to elicit T cell responses to target the hepatic stages of the malaria parasite. Nucleic acid encoding an ME string was designed to include CD8+ and CD4+ T cell epitopes from TRAP, CSP, EXP-1, LSA-1, LSA-3, and STARP (**Table 2**) [36, 41, 197, 198]. The ME were fused in-frame to the nucleic acid sequence encoding the entire TRAP antigen from *P. falciparum* strain T9/96, encoding a polypeptide of 789 amino acids referred to as multi-epitope thrombospondin-related adhesion protein (ME-TRAP) [44].

Antigen	Designation	Amino acid sequence	Epitope
CSP	cp6	MNPNDPNRNV	HLA class I antigens
CSP	cp26	KPKDELDY	
CSP	cp39	YLNKIQNSL	
EXP-1	ex23	ATSVLAGL	
LSA1	ls6	KPIVQYDNF	
LSA1	ls8	KPNDKSLY	
LSA1	ls50	ISKYEDEI	
LSA1	ls53	KSLYDEHI	
LSA3	la72	MEKLKELEK	
STARP	st8	MINAYLDKL	
TRAP	tr26	HLGNVKYLV	
TRAP	tr29	LLMDCSGSI	
TRAP	tr39	GIAGGLALL	
TRAP	tr42/43	ASKNKEKALII	
CSP (*P. berghei*)	pb9	SYIPSAEKI	Mouse MHC class I antigen
CSP	NANP	NANPNANPNANPNANP	B cell epitopes
TRAP	TRAP-AM	DEWSPCSVTCGKGTRSRKRE	Heparin binding motif
CSP	CSP	DPNANPNVDPNANPNV	Class II antigens (BCG and Tetanus toxin are not malarial antigens)
BCG		QVHFQPLPPAVVKL	
Tetanus toxin	QFIKANSKFIGITE		

Table 2. Peptides used in the multi-epitope domain of ME-TRAP [41].

Vaccine	Antigens (adjuvants)	Delivery regimen	Efficacy (# protected/# participants)	Immune response	Population	References
L3SEPTL (peptide)	LSA, STARP, Exp1, Pfs16, TRAP, and LSA1	FFM	0% protection (0/8)	85 SFU/10^6 PBMCs	Malaria naïve adults	[205]
		MMF	0% protection (0/7)	96 SFU/10^6 PBMCs		
ME TRAP	TRAP and peptides from CSP, LSA-1, LSA-3, EXP-1, STARP expressed as a single protein.	DDDMM	0% protection (8/8 delayed patency)	158-316 SFU/10^6 PBMCs	Malaria Naïve adults	[44]
		DDMM	0% protection, (6/6 delayed patency)	234 SFU/10^6 PBMCs		
		DDD	0% protection (0/5)	33 SFU/10^6 PBMCs		
		MMM	0% protection (0/4)	44 SFU/10^6 PBMCs		
		DDM	12.5% protection (1/8 sterile immunity, 7/8 delayed patency)	423 SFU/10^6 PBMCs; low titer antibodies	Malaria naïve adults	[42]
		DDM	10% protective efficacy relative to control group	250 SFU/10^6 PBMCs	Gambian adults	[219]
		FFM	12.5% protection (2/16 sterile immunity, 14/16 delayed patency)	430 SFU/10^6 PBMCs, mixture of CD4+ and CD8+ T cells	Malaria naïve adults	[45, 207]
		MMM	0% protection (0/4)	0 SFU/10^6 PBMCs		
		FM	0% protection (0/5)	380 SFU/10^6 PBMCs, mixture of CD4+ and CD8+ T cells		
		MF	0% protection (0/5)	100 SFU/10^6 PBMCs, mixture of CD4+ and CD8+ T cells		
		DDMF	0% protection (4/4 delayed patency)	200 SFU/10^6 PBMCs, CD4+ T cells		
		DDFM	0% protection (0/3)	300 SFU/10^6 PBMCs, CD4+ T cells		
		FFM	0% protection (73% infection in vaccines, 80% infection in controls; no statistically significant decrease)	107 SFU/10^6 PBMCs	Kenyan children	[210]
		CM	21% protection (3/14 sterile immunity, 5/14 delayed patency)	1300 SFU/10^6 PBMCs, CD4+ and CD8+ T cells producing IFN-γ, IL2, TNF-α (protection associated with CD8+ IFN-γ producing T cells)	Malaria naïve adults	[212]
		CM	13% protection (2/15 sterile immunity, 5/15 delayed patency)	2000 SFU/10^6 PBMCs, and antibodies detected	Malaria naïve adults	[213]

Vaccine	Antigens (adjuvants)	Delivery regimen	Efficacy (# protected/# participants)	Immune response	Population	References
		CM	67% protection (18% infection in vaccines, 47% infection in controls)	1450 SFU/10^6 PBMCs, CD4+ and CD8+ T cells producing IFN-γ, IL2, TNF-α	African adults	[105, 214]
MuStDO5	TRAP, CSP, EXP1, LSA1, and LSA3	DDD	0% protection (0/8)	For both regimens: class I— 41 SFU/10^6 PBMCs; class II— 59 SFU/10^6 PBMCs, no antibodies detected	Malaria naïve adults	[215, 216]
		DDD & plasmid with hGM-CSF	0% protection (0/23)			
NYVAC-Pf7	CSP, TRAP, LSA-1, MSP1, SERA, AMA1 and Pfs25	NNN	3% protection (1/35 sterile immunity, 34/35 delayed patency)	9/38 volunteers developed CTL to TRAP; 2/38 volunteers developed CTL to LSA1; 50% of volunteers developed antibody to TRAP and LSA1	Malaria naïve adults	[218]

*Regimens are the sequence of immunization using the vehicles D (plasmid DNA), F (attenuated fowlpox virus FP9), M (modified vaccinia virus Ankara), C (chimpanzee adenovirus 63), and N (attenuated vaccinia virus NYVAC) to provide gene sequences encoding the described antigens.
**T cells isolated by FAC, antigen-dependent T cell count not provided. SFU refers to antigen-specific IFN-γ producing T cells.

Table 3. Summary of the efficacy of multi-antigen pre-erythrocytic vaccines tested in clinical trials.

Expressing the ME-TRAP antigen *in situ* using DNA vaccines (plasmids) or viral vehicles has been employed to provide low-cost vaccination. While results in animal models using plasmids to deliver antigens were promising, the immunity elicited in humans was typically low. Heterologous prime/boost combinations, wherein the antigen remained constant but was delivered using different vehicles, reduced the development of immunity to the vehicle while provided a boost to the immune system with the target antigens [206]. In humans, the order of vehicle used for immunization was demonstrated to affect overall immune response [45, 207]. Thus, studies have focused on identifying the appropriate combination and order of vehicles that can be used to produce an elevated and expanded immune response. Plasmids encoding ME-TRAP only elicited a low-level immune response [44], and subsequent efforts have focused on viral vehicles for both priming and boosting (**Table 3**).

The MVA strain has proven to be a strong vehicle for boosting, and clinical trials using ME-TRAP subsequently focused on identifying an optimal priming vehicle and dosing regimen (see **Table 3**). Using an attenuated fowlpox virus vehicle (FP9) with MVA elicited strong immunity in malaria-naive volunteers and limited protection [207], but provided only low-level immunity in people in malaria-endemic regions without providing significant protection [208–210] (see **Table 3**). The recent addition of a chimpanzee adenovirus 63 (ChAd63) for priming has provided encouraging results (see **Table 3**). AdCh63 priming elicits both CD4+ and CD8+ T cells at much higher levels than DNA or FP9 priming [211], and also results in a much higher proportion of IFN-γ-secreting monofunctional CD8+ T cells that were correlated to sterile protection [212]. This combination has provided protection from infection in malaria-naive volunteers comparable to the immunity provided by CSP using the same delivery platform [212, 213]. Further, ME-TRAP using the ChAd63/MVA regimen elicited a strong immune response and provided significant protection in Africans who had prior exposure to malaria [43, 214]. Using a Cox regression analysis, vaccine efficacy was 67% during the 56 days of monitoring.

4.4. Multistage DNA vaccine operation five antigens (MuStDO5)

The MuStDO5 cocktail is composed of sequences encoding the antigens TRAP, CSP, EXP-1, LSA-1, and LSA-3 using sequences based on *P. falciparum* strain 3D7 [215, 216]. LSA-1 only encodes the nonrepetitive amino and carboxyl ends of the protein (462 amino acids), with the repetitive 727 amino acid middle domain removed. Each antigen is encoded on a separate plasmid using the same vector VCL-25 (Vical Inc., San Diego, CA, USA), with expression controlled by the promoter/enhancer of the human cytomegalovirus. The cocktail of plasmids is used for vaccination to provide each of the five antigens. In this study, the impact of including a plasmid expressing human granulocyte-macrophage colony-stimulating factor (hGM-CSF) as an immune enhancer was evaluated. This vaccine is safe and well tolerated. However, protective immunity was not demonstrated, and the addition of hGM-CSF decreased the response to class I epitopes.

4.5. NYVAC-Pf7 attenuated vaccinia virus

NYVAC-Pf7 is composed of an attenuated vaccinia virus NYVAC engineered to express seven antigens (Pf7) to target pre-erythrocytic, blood stages, and transmission stages of the parasite [217]. The seven antigens include three pre-erythrocytic antigens (CSP, TRAP, and LSA-1), three blood stage antigens (MSP1, SERA, and AMA1), and the Pfs25 antigen found on the sexual stage ookinete. CSP, TRAP, LSA-1, AMA1, and Pfs25 are derived from *P. falciparum* 3D7 strain. The *lsa-1* gene was modified to produce a protein linking amino acids 1–458 with 1630–1909, removing the sequence encoding the repeat region of the protein. Each gene is under a separate poxvirus promoter and expressed as a separate protein as follows: CSP under H6, TRAP under 42K, LSA-1 under C10LW, MSP1 under H6, SERA under 42K, AMA1 under I3L, and Pfs25 under I3L (**Figure 7**). Each gene was inserted into defined sites in the genome of the attenuated vaccinia strain NYVAC by *in vivo* recombination to produce NYVAC-Pf7.

A Phase I/II clinical trial was carried out with malaria-naive adults [218]. Volunteers were immunized with either high dose (1×10^8 pfu) or low dose (1×10^7 pfu) of NYVAC-Pf7 at 0, 4, and 26 weeks. Vaccination with NYVAC-Pf7 resulted in delayed onset of parasitemia following challenge in all volunteers who received the vaccine, as compared to nonvaccinated volunteers. The CTL response or antibody titer did not demonstrate a relationship to the time of delay to onset of parasitemia. One vaccinated volunteer from the low-dosage group demonstrated sterile immunity. About 50% of the volunteers in each of the dosage groups developed antibodies to TRAP and LSA-1, regardless of the dosage. Low levels of CTL were developed to TRAP, with no statistical significance due to the dosage. A CTL response to LSA-1 was only seen in the low-dosage group. However, the CTL response did not correlate with the time to onset of parasitemia, and the one volunteer exhibiting sterile immunity did not develop a detected CTL response.

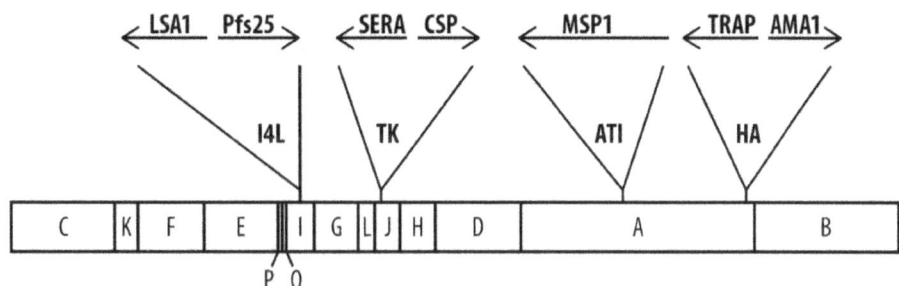

Figure 7. Genomic Organization of the NYVAC-Pf7 (adapted from [217]). The poxvirus promoters are represented with solid boxes.

5. New proteins for pre-erythrocytic malaria vaccines

New malarial proteins have been discovered through screens for pre-erythrocytic phase sporozoites, including identifying mRNA or proteins expressed in specific stages of the lifecycle of the parasite (e.g., sporozoites for the mosquito salivary glands), and typically included monitoring the immune response to the specific proteins using antibodies or T cells from volunteers vaccinated with sporozoites that were either irradiated or suppressed with chemotherapy, as discussed in the Introduction. Section 5 summarizes the preclinical studies carried out focusing on antigens analyzed beyond the initial identifying screen.

5.1. DNA vaccine encoding SAP1

Sporozoite asparagine-rich protein 1 (SAPI) was identified using suppressive-subtractive hybridization to identify *P. berghei* genes that are up-regulated in the sporozoite as it transitions from the mosquito midgut into the salivary gland [60]. In targeted deletion studies, *P. yoelii* SAP1 knockout sporozoites can invade hepatocytes but arrest in early liver stage development [220]. The *P. yoelii* genome sequence encoding the SAP1 protein domain corresponding to amino acids 3063–3227, and flanked by two CpG motifs to enhance the immune response, was cloned into pcDNA3.1(+) [221]. SAP1encoded in plasmid DNA was evaluated for protective immunity against challenge with a homologous strain of *P. yoelii*. BALB/c mice were immunized intramuscularly with 100 µg plasmid three times with 3 weeks between each vaccination. Controls included mice vaccinated with phosphate buffered saline. For the protection study, each group was composed of ten mice. BALB/c mice were challenged by bites from mosquitoes infected with *P. yoelii* 2 weeks after the final immunization. Onset of parasitemia was evaluated using blood smears. Mice without parasitemia 14 days after challenge were considered completely protected. The mice immunized with DNA encoding SAP1 produced SAP1-

specific antibodies and moderate levels of T cells secreting IFN-γ. All 10 of the control mice vaccinated with phosphate buffered saline developed parasitemia. Two of 10 (20%) of the mice vaccinated with pcDNA3.1(+)/SAP1 did not develop parasitemia.

5.2. Adenovirus vectored pre-erythrocytic antigens

This was an exploratory study to evaluate the protective immunity of newly identified pre-erythrocytic-stage antigens, selected from sporozoite and liver stage libraries based on the predicted signal sequences [137]. The *P. yoelii* orthologues of P36p (PY01340; Py52), Ag5 (PY00410; hypothetical protein), Sporozoite Invasion-Associated Protein-1 (PY00455; SIAP1), Kruepple-like protein (PY00839; KLP), and TRAP-like protein (PY01499; TLP), CelTOS or CSP were delivered in 10^{10} virus particles of adenovirus encoding each individual antigen [137]. Protection was evaluated as the parasite burden in the liver following infection. Immunization of female BALB/c (H2-K^d) mice with adenovirus vector (Ad) expressing P36p, CelTOS, or Ag5 elicited a high IFN-γ T cell response that was comparable to the response to CSP. Following challenge, only mice immunized with Ad-CSP reduced the parasite burden. None of the other antigens reduced the burden of parasites as compared to nonvaccinated mice.

5.3. Heterologous prime boost with DNA and vaccinia viral vector

The protective immunity of the individual antigens CSP, Falstatin, PY03661, and UIS3, as well as combinations of the antigens, were evaluated using the *P. yoelii* model [222]. CD1 mice (14 per group) were vaccinated intramuscularly with a priming dose of the DNA vaccine, and boosted with the vaccinia vector vaccine. Parasitemia was evaluated by blood smears following challenge with 300 *P. yoelii* sporozoites. The combination of Falstatin and UIS3 and PY03661 provided protective immunity (57%) against challenge. Heterologous prime boost with CSP protected 36% of the mice. The addition of plasmid expressing murine GM-CSF to immunization scheme did not enhance protective immunity.

5.4. Heterologous prime boost with viral vectors ChAd63 and MVA

Humoral responses in mice were evaluated using recombinant ChAd63 and MVA viral vectors expressing eight individual *P. falciparum* 3D7 antigens [33]. Responses elicited following immunization with five newly identified antigens, upregulated in sporozoite 3 (UIS3), Falstatin, liver-stage associated protein 1 (LSAP1), liver-stage associated protein 2 (LSAP2), and the early transcribed membrane protein 5 (ETRAMP5) were compared to three previously characterized antigens, LSA-1, LSA-3, and CelTOS.

Protective efficacy was evaluated in both BALB/c (inbred) and CD1 (outbred) mice, with each antigen evaluated in a separate cohort of mice using heterologous prime boosts with ChAd63/ MVA. Mice were challenged with *P. berghei* transgenic parasites that were modified to express the cognate *P. falciparum* antigen. The immunity and protective efficacy against infection was evaluated for each antigen using nonvaccinated controls for comparison.

The BALB/c mice developed antibodies to all the antigens except LSAP1. High levels of IFN-γ (>1000 SFU/10^6 PBMCs) developed in mice immunized with UIS3 and LSA1. Moderate levels of IFN-γ (>250 SFU/10⁶ PBMCs) were developed against ETRAMP5, CelTOS, LSAP2, Falstatin, and LSA-3. LSAP1 elicited very low levels of IFN-γ (<100 SFU/10⁶ PBMCs). CD8+ T cells predominated for UIS3, LSA-1, and LSA-3 cellular responses, while CD4+ T cells predominated for Falstatin. Highest levels of protection were found in BALB/c or CD1 mice immunized with LSAP2 (85 and 70%, respectively) or LSA-1 (87.5% for both murine strains). Mice immunized with CSP gave 37.5 and 33.3% sterile immunity in BALB/c and CD1 mice, respectively. Strain variation noted, with 30% of CD1, but none of the BALB/c, mice were protected following immunization with TRAP or LSAP1. Minimal or no protection was obtained in mice immunized with ETRAMPS, CelTOS, UIS3, Falstatin, or LSA-3.

6. Conclusions

Trends, advances, and roadblocks for malaria pre-erythrocytic vaccine development identified by the preclinical and clinical studies summarized in this chapter include:

- The hallmarks for protective immunity are not clear and the elements associated with sterile immunity vary in humans. Antibodies, IFN-γ, CD4+ T cells, CD8+ T cells, and cytolytic lymphocytes are believed to play essential roles in immunity, but are not always collectively demonstrated in immunity that protects from infection by *Plasmodium*.

- To achieve effective immunity that induces T cells across a wide population of people will require multiple and diverse T cell epitopes. Many of the studies that identified T cell epitopes in humans demonstrated that, within the limited number of volunteers in a Phase I clinical trial, only a limited subset of individuals respond to any single protein.

- Vaccines that string T cell epitopes from different proteins together in a composite recombinant protein (e.g., multiepitope strings) do not elicit significant T cell responses in humans. This is found even when other proteins in the vaccine do elicit strong immune response.

- For protective immunity in humans, the means and route of administration effect efficacy of the antigens. For example, irradiated sporozoites are more effective by intravenous verses intradermal administration, and TRAP delivered using heterologous vehicles of chimpanzee adenovirus followed by a modified vaccinia virus (heterologous prime boost regimen) provides more effective immunity than immunization using only one of these vehicles, or using other combinations of vehicles.

- Adjuvant formulations remain a critical factor for pre-erythrocytic vaccines, as highly purified subunit vaccine lack the pathogen-associated molecular patterns that trigger the innate immune responses required for initiation of adaptive immunity. Alum has been found to be a poor adjuvant for malaria subunit vaccines in Phase I/II trials. Oil-based adjuvants, e.g., ISA 50 or ISA 720, while enhancing immune responses, have been limited by increased reactogenicity. Precisely targeted adjuvants, such as TLR agonists, have been shown to enhance immunogenicity and protective efficacy of pre-erythrocytic vaccines, and hold promise as future adjuvant formulations.

- While cost competitiveness is a goal for malaria vaccines, it is unlikely that this has been a primary consideration in the early development plan for many candidates as much of the focus is on efficacy. Multiple platforms and approaches have been described in this chapter including DNA-based platforms, viral vehicles, recombinant proteins, and chimeric proteins composed of peptides. In consideration of vaccine design and development, production may be an initial focus to contain costs per dose. This includes consideration for adjuvants and processes to stabilize the vaccine for delivery to the clinic. However, it is not always obvious in early development which approaches may be the most cost effective for commercial vaccine production as efficiencies may be realized through optimizing processes and scaling of production so as to reduce costs significantly relative to the costs to produce research material. Further contributors to the direct cost for vaccination are transportation and storage requirements for the vaccine, the dosage, and number of boosters required to achieve protective immunity. This cost analysis may also need to consider compliance if complex or protracted boosting schedules are required. While development may strive to contain these direct costs, the vaccine still must be effective at preventing the morbidity and mortality caused by malaria.

Acknowledgements

This publication was made possible through support provided by the Office of Health, Infectious Diseases, and Nutrition, Bureau for Global Health, U.S. Agency for International Development, under the terms of the Malaria Vaccine Development Program (MVDP) Contract AID-OAA-C-15-00071, for which Leidos, Inc. is the prime contractor. The opinions expressed herein are those of the author(s) and do not necessarily reflect the views of the U.S. Agency for International Development.

Author details

Ken Tucker[1], Amy R. Noe[1], Vinayaka Kotraiah[1], Timothy W. Phares[1], Moriya Tsuji[2], Elizabeth H. Nardin[3] and Gabriel M. Gutierrez[1*]

*Address all correspondence to: gabriel.m.gutierrez@leidos.com

1 Leidos Life Sciences, Leidos Inc., Frederick, MD, USA

2 HIV and Malaria Vaccine Program, Aaron Diamond AIDS Research Center, Affiliate of the Rockefeller University, New York, NY, USA

3 Division of Parasitology, Department of Microbiology, New York University School of Medicine, New York, NY, USA

References

[1] Crompton PD, Moebius J, Portugal S, Waisberg M, Hart G, Garver LS, et al. Malaria immunity in man and mosquito: insights into unsolved mysteries of a deadly infectious disease. Annu Rev Immunol. 2014;32:157–87. DOI: 10.1146/annurev-immunol-032713-120220

[2] Gupta S, Snow RW, Donnelly CA, Marsh K, Newbold C. Immunity to non-cerebral severe malaria is acquired after one or two infections. Nat Med. 1999;5:340–3. DOI: 10.1038/6560

[3] Horne-Debets JM, Faleiro R, Karunarathne DS, Liu XQ, Lineburg KE, Poh CM, et al. PD-1 dependent exhaustion of CD8+ T cells drives chronic malaria. Cell Rep. 2013;5:1204–13. DOI: 10.1016/j.celrep.2013.11.002

[4] Ryg-Cornejo V, Ioannidis LJ, Ly A, Chiu CY, Tellier J, Hill DL, et al. Severe malaria infections impair germinal center responses by inhibiting T follicular helper cell differentiation. Cell Rep. 2016;14:68–81. DOI: 10.1016/j.celrep.2015.12.006

[5] Wykes MN, Horne-Debets JM, Leow CY, Karunarathne DS. Malaria drives T cells to exhaustion. Front Microbiol. 2014;5:249. DOI: 10.3389/fmicb.2014.00249

[6] Nussenzweig RS, Vanderberg J, Most H, Orton C. Protective immunity produced by the injection of x-irradiated sporozoites of plasmodium berghei. Nature. 1967;216: 160–2.

[7] Clyde DF, McCarthy VC, Miller RM, Hornick RB. Specificity of protection of man immunized against sporozoite-induced falciparum malaria. Am J Med Sci. 1973;266:398–3.

[8] Hoffman SL, Goh LM, Luke TC, Schneider I, Le TP, Doolan DL, et al. Protection of humans against malaria by immunization with radiation-attenuated Plasmodium falciparum sporozoites. J Infect Dis. 2002;185:1155–64. DOI: 10.1086/339409

[9] Rieckmann KH, Carson PE, Beaudoin RL, Cassells JS, Sell KW. Letter: sporozoite induced immunity in man against an Ethiopian strain of Plasmodium falciparum. Trans R Soc Trop Med Hyg. 1974;68:258–9.

[10] Seder RA, Chang LJ, Enama ME, Zephir KL, Sarwar UN, Gordon IJ, et al. Protection against malaria by intravenous immunization with a nonreplicating sporozoite vaccine. Science. 2013;341:1359–65. DOI: 10.1126/science.1241800

[11] Bijker EM, Bastiaens GJ, Teirlinck AC, van Gemert GJ, Graumans W, van de Vegte-Bolmer M, et al. Protection against malaria after immunization by chloroquine prophylaxis and sporozoites is mediated by preerythrocytic immunity. Proc Natl Acad Sci U S A. 2013;110:7862–7. DOI: 10.1073/pnas.1220360110

[12] Roestenberg M, McCall M, Hopman J, Wiersma J, Luty AJ, van Gemert GJ, et al. Protection against a malaria challenge by sporozoite inoculation. N Engl J Med. 2009;361:468–77. DOI: 10.1056/NEJMoa0805832

[13] Behet MC, Foquet L, van Gemert GJ, Bijker EM, Meuleman P, Leroux-Roels G, et al. Sporozoite immunization of human volunteers under chemoprophylaxis induces functional antibodies against pre-erythrocytic stages of Plasmodium falciparum. Malar J. 2014;13:136. DOI: 10.1186/1475-2875-13-136

[14] Bijker EM, Schats R, Obiero JM, Behet MC, van Gemert GJ, van de Vegte-Bolmer M, et al. Sporozoite immunization of human volunteers under mefloquine prophylaxis is safe, immunogenic and protective: a double-blind randomized controlled clinical trial. PLoS One. 2014;9:e112910. DOI: 10.1371/journal.pone.0112910

[15] Schats R, Bijker EM, van Gemert GJ, Graumans W, van de Vegte-Bolmer M, van Lieshout L, et al. Heterologous protection against malaria after immunization with *Plasmodium falciparum* sporozoites. PLoS One. 2015;10:e0124243. DOI: 10.1371/journal.pone. 0124243

[16] Silvie O, Semblat JP, Franetich JF, Hannoun L, Eling W, Mazier D. Effects of irradiation on *Plasmodium falciparum* sporozoite hepatic development: implications for the design of pre-erythrocytic malaria vaccines. Parasite Immunol. 2002;24:221–3.

[17] Suhrbier A, Winger LA, Castellano E, Sinden RE. Survival and antigenic profile of irradiated malarial sporozoites in infected liver cells. Infect Immun. 1990;58:2834-9.

[18] Doolan DL, Hoffman SL. The complexity of protective immunity against liver-stage malaria. J Immunol. 2000;165:1453–62.

[19] Perlaza BL, Sauzet JP, Brahimi K, BenMohamed L, Druilhe P. Interferon-gamma, a valuable surrogate marker of *Plasmodium falciparum* pre-erythrocytic stages protective immunity. Malar J. 2011;10:27. DOI: 10.1186/1475-2875-10-27

[20] Dups JN, Pepper M, Cockburn IA. Antibody and B cell responses to Plasmodium sporozoites. Front Microbiol. 2014;5:625. DOI: 10.3389/fmicb.2014.00625

[21] Fernandez-Arias C, Mashoof S, Huang J, Tsuji M. Circumsporozoite protein as a potential target for antimalarials. Expert Rev Anti Infect Ther. 2015;13:923–6. DOI: 10.1586/14787210.2015.1058709

[22] Rodrigues M, Nussenzweig RS, Zavala F. The relative contribution of antibodies, CD4+ and CD8+ T cells to sporozoite-induced protection against malaria. Immunology. 1993;80:1–5.

[23] Schofield L, Villaquiran J, Ferreira A, Schellekens H, Nussenzweig R, Nussenzweig V. Gamma interferon, CD8+ T cells and antibodies required for immunity to malaria sporozoites. Nature. 1987;330:664–6. DOI: 10.1038/330664a0

[24] Weiss WR, Sedegah M, Beaudoin RL, Miller LH, Good MF. CD8+ T cells (cytotoxic/ suppressors) are required for protection in mice immunized with malaria sporozoites. Proc Natl Acad Sci U S A. 1988;85:573–6.

[25] Todryk SM, Walther M. Building better T-cell-inducing malaria vaccines. Immunology. 2005;115:163–9. DOI: 10.1111/j.1365-2567.2005.02154.x

[26] Tsuji M, Miyahira Y, Nussenzweig RS, Aguet M, Reichel M, Zavala F. Development of antimalaria immunity in mice lacking IFN-gamma receptor. J Immunol. 1995;154:5338– 44.

[27] Huang J, Tsao T, Zhang M, Rai U, Tsuji M, Li X. A sufficient role of MHC class I molecules on hepatocytes in anti-plasmodial activity of CD8 (+) T cells in vivo. Front Microbiol. 2015;6:69. DOI: 10.3389/fmicb.2015.00069

[28] Lalvani A, Aidoo M, Allsopp CE, Plebanski M, Whittle HC, Hill AV. An HLA-based approach to the design of a CTL-inducing vaccine against *Plasmodium falciparum*. Res Immunol. 1994;145:461–8.

[29] Overstreet MG, Cockburn IA, Chen YC, Zavala F. Protective CD8 T cells against Plasmodium liver stages: immunobiology of an 'unnatural' immune response. Immunol Rev. 2008;225:272–83. DOI: 10.1111/j.1600-065X.2008.00671.x

[30] Tsuji M. A retrospective evaluation of the role of T cells in the development of malaria vaccine. Exp Parasitol. 2010;126:421–5. DOI: 10.1016/j.exppara.2009.11.009

[31] Oliveira GA, Kumar KA, Calvo-Calle JM, Othoro C, Altszuler D, Nussenzweig V, et al. Class II-restricted protective immunity induced by malaria sporozoites. Infect Immun. 2008;76:1200–6. DOI: 10.1128/iai.00566-07

[32] Charoenvit Y, Majam VF, Corradin G, Sacci JB Jr, Wang R, Doolan DL, et al. CD4(+) T-cell- and gamma interferon-dependent protection against murine malaria by immunization with linear synthetic peptides from a *Plasmodium yoelii* 17-kilodalton hepatocyte erythrocyte protein. Infect Immun. 1999;67:5604–14.

[33] Longley RJ, Salman AM, Cottingham MG, Ewer K, Janse CJ, Khan SM, et al. Comparative assessment of vaccine vectors encoding ten malaria antigens identifies two protective liver-stage candidates. Sci Rep. 2015;5:11820. DOI: 10.1038/srep11820

[34] Tsuji M, Romero P, Nussenzweig RS, Zavala F. CD4+ cytolytic T cell clone confers protection against murine malaria. J Exp Med. 1990;172:1353–7.

[35] Weiss WR, Sedegah M, Berzofsky JA, Hoffman SL. The role of CD4+ T cells in immunity to malaria sporozoites. J Immunol. 1993;151:2690–8.

[36] Aidoo M, Lalvani A, Allsopp CE, Plebanski M, Meisner SJ, Krausa P, et al. Identification of conserved antigenic components for a cytotoxic T lymphocyte-inducing vaccine against malaria. Lancet. 1995;345:1003–7.

[37] Doolan DL, Hoffman SL, Southwood S, Wentworth PA, Sidney J, Chesnut RW, et al. Degenerate cytotoxic T cell epitopes from *P. falciparum* restricted by multiple HLA-A and HLA-B supertype alleles. Immunity. 1997;7:97–112.

[38] Doolan DL, Southwood S, Chesnut R, Appella E, Gomez E, Richards A, et al. HLA-DR-promiscuous T cell epitopes from *Plasmodium falciparum* pre-erythrocytic-stage antigens restricted by multiple HLA class II alleles. J Immunol. 2000;165:1123–37.

[39] Thomson SA, Khanna R, Gardner J, Burrows SR, Coupar B, Moss DJ, et al. Minimal epitopes expressed in a recombinant polyepitope protein are processed and presented to CD8+ cytotoxic T cells: implications for vaccine design. Proc Natl Acad Sci U S A. 1995;92:5845–9.

[40] Whitton JL, Sheng N, Oldstone MB, McKee TA. A "string-of-beads" vaccine, comprising linked minigenes, confers protection from lethal-dose virus challenge. J Virol. 1993;67:348–52.

[41] Gilbert SC, Plebanski M, Harris SJ, Allsopp CE, Thomas R, Layton GT, et al. A protein particle vaccine containing multiple malaria epitopes. Nat Biotechnol. 1997;15:1280–4. DOI: 10.1038/nbt1197-1280

[42] Dunachie SJ, Walther M, Epstein JE, Keating S, Berthoud T, Andrews L, et al. A DNA prime-modified vaccinia virus ankara boost vaccine encoding thrombospondin-related adhesion protein but not circumsporozoite protein partially protects healthy malaria-naive adults against *Plasmodium falciparum* sporozoite challenge. Infect Immun. 2006;74:5933–42. DOI: 10.1128/iai.00590-06

[43] Kimani D, Jagne YJ, Cox M, Kimani E, Bliss CM, Gitau E, et al. Translating the immunogenicity of prime-boost immunization with ChAd63 and MVA ME-TRAP from malaria naive to malaria-endemic populations. Mol Ther. 2014;22:1992–03. DOI: 10.1038/mt.2014.109

[44] McConkey SJ, Reece WH, Moorthy VS, Webster D, Dunachie S, Butcher G, et al. Enhanced T-cell immunogenicity of plasmid DNA vaccines boosted by recombinant modified vaccinia virus Ankara in humans. Nat Med. 2003;9:729–35. DOI: 10.1038/nm881

[45] Vuola JM, Keating S, Webster DP, Berthoud T, Dunachie S, Gilbert SC, et al. Differential immunogenicity of various heterologous prime-boost vaccine regimens using DNA and viral vectors in healthy volunteers. J Immunol. 2005;174:449–55.

[46] Shevach EM. Regulatory T cells in autoimmmunity*. Annu Rev Immunol. 2000;18:423–49. DOI: 10.1146/annurev.immunol.18.1.423

[47] Coleman MM, Keane J, Mills KH. Editorial: Tregs and BCG-dangerous liaisons in TB. J Leukoc Biol. 2010;88:1067–9. DOI: 10.1189/jlb.0710419

[48] Mills KH. Designer adjuvants for enhancing the efficacy of infectious disease and cancer vaccines based on suppression of regulatory T cell induction. Immunol Lett. 2009;122:108–11. DOI: 10.1016/j.imlet.2008.11.007

[49] Ndure J, Flanagan KL. Targeting regulatory T cells to improve vaccine immunogenicity in early life. Front Microbiol. 2014;5:477. DOI: 10.3389/fmicb.2014.00477

[50] Chia WN, Goh YS, Renia L. Novel approaches to identify protective malaria vaccine candidates. Front Microbiol. 2014;5:586. DOI: 10.3389/fmicb.2014.00586

[51] Fidock DA, Bottius E, Brahimi K, Moelans II, Aikawa M, Konings RN, et al. Cloning and characterization of a novel *Plasmodium falciparum* sporozoite surface antigen, STARP. Mol Biochem Parasitol. 1994;64:219–32.

[52] Guerin-Marchand C, Druilhe P, Galey B, Londono A, Patarapotikul J, Beaudoin RL, et al. A liver-stage-specific antigen of *Plasmodium falciparum* characterized by gene cloning. Nature. 1987;329:164–7. DOI: 10.1038/329164a0

[53] Daubersies P, Thomas AW, Millet P, Brahimi K, Langermans JA, Ollomo B, et al. Protection against *Plasmodium falciparum* malaria in chimpanzees by immunization with the conserved pre-erythrocytic liver-stage antigen 3. Nat Med. 2000;6:1258–63. DOI: 10.1038/81366

[54] Trieu A, Kayala MA, Burk C, Molina DM, Freilich DA, Richie TL, et al. Sterile protective immunity to malaria is associated with a panel of novel *P. falciparum* antigens. Mol Cell Proteomics. 2011;10:M111.007948. DOI: 10.1074/mcp.M111.007948

[55] Doolan DL, Southwood S, Freilich DA, Sidney J, Graber NL, Shatney L, et al. Identification of *Plasmodium falciparum* antigens by antigenic analysis of genomic and proteomic data. Proc Natl Acad Sci U S A. 2003;100:9952–7. DOI: 10.1073/pnas.1633254100

[56] Aguiar JC, Bolton J, Wanga J, Sacci JB, Iriko H, Mazeika JK, et al. Discovery of novel *Plasmodium falciparum* pre-erythrocytic antigens for vaccine development. PLoS One. 2015;10:e0136109. DOI: 10.1371/journal.pone.0136109

[57] Ishino T, Yano K, Chinzei Y, Yuda M. Cell-passage activity is required for the malarial parasite to cross the liver sinusoidal cell layer. PLoS Biol. 2004;2:E4. DOI: 10.1371/journal.pbio.0020004

[58] Kaiser K, Matuschewski K, Camargo N, Ross J, Kappe SH. Differential transcriptome profiling identifies Plasmodium genes encoding pre-erythrocytic stage-specific proteins. Mol Microbiol. 2004;51:1221–32. DOI: 10.1046/j.1365-2958.2003.03909.x

[59] Lasonder E, Janse CJ, van Gemert GJ, Mair GR, Vermunt AM, Douradinha BG, et al. Proteomic profiling of Plasmodium sporozoite maturation identifies new proteins essential for parasite development and infectivity. PLoS Pathog. 2008;4:e1000195. DOI: 10.1371/journal.ppat.1000195

[60] Matuschewski K, Ross J, Brown SM, Kaiser K, Nussenzweig V, Kappe SH. Infectivity-associated changes in the transcriptional repertoire of the malaria parasite sporozoite stage. J Biol Chem. 2002;277:41948–53. DOI: 10.1074/jbc.M207315200

[61] Siau A, Silvie O, Franetich JF, Yalaoui S, Marinach C, Hannoun L, et al. Temperature shift and host cell contact up-regulate sporozoite expression of Plasmodium falciparum genes involved in hepatocyte infection. PLoS Pathog. 2008;4:e1000121. DOI: 10.1371/journal.ppat.1000121

[62] Florens L, Washburn MP, Raine JD, Anthony RM, Grainger M, Haynes JD, et al. A proteomic view of the *Plasmodium falciparum* life cycle. Nature. 2002;419:520–6. DOI: 10.1038/nature01107

[63] Tarun AS, Peng X, Dumpit RF, Ogata Y, Silva-Rivera H, Camargo N, et al. A combined transcriptome and proteome survey of malaria parasite liver stages. Proc Natl Acad Sci U S A. 2008;105:305–10. DOI: 10.1073/pnas.0710780104

[64] Cummings JF, Spring MD, Schwenk RJ, Ockenhouse CF, Kester KE, Polhemus ME, et al. Recombinant Liver Stage Antigen-1 (LSA-1) formulated with AS01 or AS02 is safe, elicits high titer antibody and induces IFN-gamma/IL-2 CD4+ T cells but does not protect against experimental Plasmodium falciparum infection. Vaccine. 2010;28:5135–44. DOI: 10.1016/j.vaccine.2009.08.046

[65] Bergmann-Leitner ES, Mease RM, De La Vega P, Savranskaya T, Polhemus M, Ockenhouse C, et al. Immunization with pre-erythrocytic antigen CelTOS from *Plasmodium falciparum* elicits cross-species protection against heterologous challenge with *Plasmodium berghei*. PLoS One. 2010;5:e12294. DOI: 10.1371/journal.pone.0012294

[66] BenMohamed L, Thomas A, Druilhe P. Long-term multiepitopic cytotoxic-T-lympho-cyte responses induced in chimpanzees by combinations of *Plasmodium falciparum* liver-stage peptides and lipopeptides. Infect Immun. 2004;72:4376–84. DOI: 10.1128/iai.72.8.4376-4384.2004

[67] Capone S, Reyes-Sandoval A, Naddeo M, Siani L, Ammendola V, Rollier CS, et al. Immune responses against a liver-stage malaria antigen induced by simian adenoviral vector AdCh63 and MVA prime-boost immunisation in non-human primates. Vaccine. 2010;29:256–65. DOI: 10.1016/j.vaccine.2010.10.041

[68] Ferraro B, Talbott KT, Balakrishnan A, Cisper N, Morrow MP, Hutnick NA, et al. Inducing humoral and cellular responses to multiple sporozoite and liver-stage malaria antigens using exogenous plasmid DNA. Infect Immun. 2013;81:3709–20. DOI: 10.1128/iai.00180-13

[69] Adams EJ, Parham P. Species-specific evolution of MHC class I genes in the higher primates. Immunol Rev. 2001;183:41–64.

[70] Otting N, Heijmans CM, Noort RC, de Groot NG, Doxiadis GG, van Rood JJ, et al. Unparalleled complexity of the MHC class I region in rhesus macaques. Proc Natl Acad Sci U S A. 2005;102:1626–31. DOI: 10.1073/pnas.0409084102

[71] Shen S, Pyo CW, Vu Q, Wang R, Geraghty DE. The essential detail: the genetics and genomics of the primate immune response. Ilar j. 2013;54:181–95. DOI: 10.1093/ilar/ilt043

[72] Danner R, Chaudhari SN, Rosenberger J, Surls J, Richie TL, Brumeanu TD, et al. Expression of HLA class II molecules in humanized NOD.Rag1KO.IL2RgcKO mice is critical for development and function of human T and B cells. PLoS One. 2011;6:e19826. DOI: 10.1371/journal.pone.0019826

[73] Huang J, Li X, Coelho-dos-Reis JG, Wilson JM, Tsuji M. An AAV vector-mediated gene delivery approach facilitates reconstitution of functional human CD8+ T cells in mice. PLoS One. 2014;9:e88205. DOI: 10.1371/journal.pone.0088205

[74] Huang J, Li X, Coelho-dos-Reis JG, Zhang M, Mitchell R, Nogueira RT, et al. Human immune system mice immunized with *Plasmodium falciparum* circumsporozoite protein induce protective human humoral immunity against malaria. J Immunol Methods. 2015;427:42–50. DOI: 10.1016/j.jim.2015.09.005

[75] Coelho-dos-Reis JGA, Li X, Silveira ELV, Mandraju R, Velmurugan S, Chakravarty S, et al. *Plasmodium falciparum* infection in "humanised liver" mice. MalariaWorld J. 2013;4:1–4.

[76] Foquet L, Meuleman P, Hermsen CC, Sauerwein R, Leroux-Roels G. Assessment of parasite liver-stage nurden in human-liver chimeric mice. Methods Mol Biol. 2015;1325:59–68. DOI: 10.1007/978-1-4939-2815-6_5

[77] Morosan S, Hez-Deroubaix S, Lunel F, Renia L, Giannini C, Van Rooijen N, et al. Liver-stage development of *Plasmodium falciparum*, in a humanized mouse model. J Infect Dis. 2006;193:996–04. DOI: 10.1086/500840

[78] Sack BK, Miller JL, Vaughan AM, Douglass A, Kaushansky A, Mikolajczak S, et al. Model for in vivo assessment of humoral protection against malaria sporozoite challenge by passive transfer of monoclonal antibodies and immune serum. Infect Immun. 2014;82:808–17. DOI: 10.1128/iai.01249-13

[79] Vaughan AM, Kappe SH, Ploss A, Mikolajczak SA. Development of humanized mouse models to study human malaria parasite infection. Future Microbiol. 2012;7:657–65. DOI: 10.2217/fmb.12.27

[80] Coppi A, Natarajan R, Pradel G, Bennett BL, James ER, Roggero MA, et al. The malaria circumsporozoite protein has two functional domains, each with distinct roles as sporozoites journey from mosquito to mammalian host. J Exp Med. 2011;208:341–56. DOI: 10.1084/jem.20101488

[81] Rathore D, Sacci JB, de la Vega P, McCutchan TF. Binding and invasion of liver cells by *Plasmodium falciparum* sporozoites. Essential involvement of the amino terminus of circumsporozoite protein. J Biol Chem. 2002;277:7092–8. DOI: 10.1074/jbc.M106862200

[82] Suarez JE, Urquiza M, Puentes A, Garcia JE, Curtidor H, Ocampo M, et al. *Plasmodium falciparum* circumsporozoite (CS) protein peptides specifically bind to HepG2 cells. Vaccine. 2001;19:4487–95.

[83] Coppi A, Pinzon-Ortiz C, Hutter C, Sinnis P. The Plasmodium circumsporozoite protein is proteolytically processed during cell invasion. J Exp Med. 2005;201:27–33. DOI: 10.1084/jem.20040989

[84] Sinnis P, Clavijo P, Fenyo D, Chait BT, Cerami C, Nussenzweig V. Structural and functional properties of region II-plus of the malaria circumsporozoite protein. J Exp Med. 1994;180:297–06.

[85] Dame JB, Williams JL, McCutchan TF, Weber JL, Wirtz RA, Hockmeyer WT, et al. Structure of the gene encoding the immunodominant surface antigen on the sporozoite of the human malaria parasite *Plasmodium falciparum*. Science. 1984;225:593–9.

[86] Enea V, Ellis J, Zavala F, Arnot DE, Asavanich A, Masuda A, et al. DNA cloning of Plasmodium falciparum circumsporozoite gene: amino acid sequence of repetitive epitope. Science. 1984;225:628–30.

[87] Nardin EH, Nussenzweig V, Nussenzweig RS, Collins WE, Harinasuta KT, Tapchaisri P, et al. Circumsporozoite proteins of human malaria parasites *Plasmodium falciparum* and *Plasmodium vivax*. J Exp Med. 1982;156:20–30.

[88] Zavala F, Tam JP, Hollingdale MR, Cochrane AH, Quakyi I, Nussenzweig RS, et al. Rationale for development of a synthetic vaccine against Plasmodium falciparum malaria. Science. 1985;228:1436–40.

[89] Moreno A, Clavijo P, Edelman R, Davis J, Sztein M, Sinigaglia F, et al. CD4+ T cell clones obtained from *Plasmodium falciparum* sporozoite-immunized volunteers recognize polymorphic sequences of the circumsporozoite protein. J Immunol. 1993;151:489–99.

[90] Calvo-Calle JM, Hammer J, Sinigaglia F, Clavijo P, Moya-Castro ZR, Nardin EH. Binding of malaria T cell epitopes to DR and DQ molecules in vitro correlates with immunogenicity in vivo: identification of a universal T cell epitope in the *Plasmodium falciparum* circumsporozoite protein. J Immunol. 1997;159:1362–73.

[91] Huang J, Tsao T, Zhang M, Tsuji M. Circumsporozoite protein-specific K(d)-restricted CD8+ T cells mediate protective antimalaria immunity in sporozoite-immunized MHC-I-K(d) transgenic mice. Mediators Inflamm. 2014;2014:728939. DOI: 10.1155/2014/728939

[92] Bailey JA, Mvalo T, Aragam N, Weiser M, Congdon S, Kamwendo D, et al. Use of massively parallel pyrosequencing to evaluate the diversity of and selection on

Plasmodium falciparum csp T-cell epitopes in Lilongwe, Malawi. J Infect Dis. 2012;206:580–7. DOI: 10.1093/infdis/jis329

[93] Kester KE, Cummings JF, Ofori-Anyinam O, Ockenhouse CF, Krzych U, Moris P, et al. Randomized, double-blind, phase 2a trial of falciparum malaria vaccines RTS,S/AS01B and RTS,S/AS02A in malaria-naive adults: safety, efficacy, and immunologic associates of protection. J Infect Dis. 2009;200:337–46. DOI: 10.1086/600120

[94] Calle JM, Nardin EH, Clavijo P, Boudin C, Stuber D, Takacs B, et al. Recognition of different domains of the *Plasmodium falciparum* CS protein by the sera of naturally infected individuals compared with those of sporozoite-immunized volunteers. J Immunol. 1992;149:2695–701.

[95] Sun P, Schwenk R, White K, Stoute JA, Cohen J, Ballou WR, et al. Protective immunity induced with malaria vaccine, RTS,S, is linked to *Plasmodium falciparum* circumsporozoite protein-specific CD4+ and CD8+ T cells producing IFN-gamma. J Immunol. 2003;171:6961–7.

[96] Stoute JA, Kester KE, Krzych U, Wellde BT, Hall T, White K, et al. Long-term efficacy and immune responses following immunization with the RTS,S malaria vaccine. J Infect Dis. 1998;178:1139–44.

[97] Olotu A, Lusingu J, Leach A, Lievens M, Vekemans J, Msham S, et al. Efficacy of RTS,S/AS01E malaria vaccine and exploratory analysis on anti-circumsporozoite antibody titres and protection in children aged 5–17 months in Kenya and Tanzania: a randomised controlled trial. Lancet Infect Dis. 2011;11:102–9. DOI: 10.1016/s1473-3099(10)70262-0

[98] Herrington DA, Clyde DF, Losonsky G, Cortesia M, Murphy JR, Davis J, et al. Safety and immunogenicity in man of a synthetic peptide malaria vaccine against *Plasmodium falciparum* sporozoites. Nature. 1987;328:257–9. DOI: 10.1038/328257a0

[99] Herrington DA, Clyde DF, Davis JR, Baqar S, Murphy JR, Cortese JF, et al. Human studies with synthetic peptide sporozoite vaccine (NANP)3-TT and immunization with irradiated sporozoites. Bull World Health Organ. 1990;68 Suppl:33–7.

[100] Moreno R, Jiang L, Moehle K, Zurbriggen R, Gluck R, Robinson JA, et al. Exploiting conformationally constrained peptidomimetics and an efficient human-compatible delivery system in synthetic vaccine design. Chembiochem. 2001;2:838–43.

[101] Genton B, Pluschke G, Degen L, Kammer AR, Westerfeld N, Okitsu SL, et al. A randomized placebo-controlled phase Ia malaria vaccine trial of two virosome-formulated synthetic peptides in healthy adult volunteers. PLoS One. 2007;2:e1018. DOI: 10.1371/journal.pone.0001018

[102] Okitsu SL, Silvie O, Westerfeld N, Curcic M, Kammer AR, Mueller MS, et al. A virosomal malaria peptide vaccine elicits a long-lasting sporozoite-inhibitory antibody

response in a phase 1a clinical trial. PLoS One. 2007;2:e1278. DOI: 10.1371/journal.pone.0001278

[103] Thompson FM, Porter DW, Okitsu SL, Westerfeld N, Vogel D, Todryk S, et al. Evidence of blood stage efficacy with a virosomal malaria vaccine in a phase IIa clinical trial. PLoS One. 2008;3:e1493. DOI: 10.1371/journal.pone.0001493

[104] Liu W, Li Y, Learn GH, Rudicell RS, Robertson JD, Keele BF, et al. Origin of the human malaria parasite *Plasmodium falciparum* in gorillas. Nature. 2010;467:420–5. DOI: 10.1038/nature09442

[105] Schofield L. The circumsporozoite protein of Plasmodium: a mechanism of immune evasion by the malaria parasite? Bull World Health Organ. 1990;68 Suppl:66–73.

[106] Nelson RW, Beisang D, Tubo NJ, Dileepan T, Wiesner DL, Nielsen K, et al. T cell receptor cross-reactivity between similar foreign and self peptides influences naive cell population size and autoimmunity. Immunity. 2015;42:95–07. DOI: 10.1016/j.immuni.2014.12.022

[107] Liu R, Moise L, Tassone R, Gutierrez AH, Terry FE, Sangare K, et al. H7N9 T-cell epitopes that mimic human sequences are less immunogenic and may induce Treg-mediated tolerance. Hum Vaccin Immunother. 2015;11:2241–52. DOI: 10.1080/21645515.2015.1052197

[108] Nardin E. The past decade in malaria synthetic peptide vaccine clinical trials. Hum Vaccin. 2010;6:27–38.

[109] Nardin EH, Calvo-Calle JM, Oliveira GA, Clavijo P, Nussenzweig R, Simon R, et al. *Plasmodium falciparum* polyoximes: highly immunogenic synthetic vaccines constructed by chemoselective ligation of repeat B-cell epitopes and a universal T-cell epitope of CS protein. Vaccine. 1998;16:590–600.

[110] Nardin EH, Calvo-Calle JM, Oliveira GA, Nussenzweig RS, Schneider M, Tiercy JM, et al. A totally synthetic polyoxime malaria vaccine containing *Plasmodium falciparum* B cell and universal T cell epitopes elicits immune responses in volunteers of diverse HLA types. J Immunol. 2001;166:481–9.

[111] Calvo-Calle JM, Oliveira GA, Nardin EH. Human CD4+ T cells induced by synthetic peptide malaria vaccine are comparable to cells elicited by attenuated *Plasmodium falciparum* sporozoites. J Immunol. 2005;175:7575–85.

[112] Birkett A, Lyons K, Schmidt A, Boyd D, Oliveira GA, Siddique A, et al. A modified hepatitis B virus core particle containing multiple epitopes of the *Plasmodium falciparum* circumsporozoite protein provides a highly immunogenic malaria vaccine in preclinical analyses in rodent and primate hosts. Infect Immun. 2002;70:6860–70.

[113] Gregson AL, Oliveira G, Othoro C, Calvo-Calle JM, Thorton GB, Nardin E, et al. Phase I trial of an alhydrogel adjuvanted hepatitis B core virus-like particle containing

epitopes of *Plasmodium falciparum* circumsporozoite protein. PLoS One. 2008;3:e1556. DOI: 10.1371/journal.pone.0001556

[114] Nardin EH, Oliveira GA, Calvo-Calle JM, Wetzel K, Maier C, Birkett AJ, et al. Phase I testing of a malaria vaccine composed of hepatitis B virus core particles expressing Plasmodium falciparum circumsporozoite epitopes. Infect Immun. 2004;72:6519–27. DOI: 10.1128/IAI.72.11.6519-6527.2004

[115] Langermans JA, Schmidt A, Vervenne RA, Birkett AJ, Calvo-Calle JM, Hensmann M, et al. Effect of adjuvant on reactogenicity and long-term immunogenicity of the malaria Vaccine ICC-1132 in macaques. Vaccine. 2005;23:4935–43. DOI: 10.1016/j.vaccine.2005.05.036

[116] Oliveira GA, Wetzel K, Calvo-Calle JM, Nussenzweig R, Schmidt A, Birkett A, et al. Safety and enhanced immunogenicity of a hepatitis B core particle *Plasmodium falciparum* malaria vaccine formulated in adjuvant Montanide ISA 720 in a phase I trial. Infect Immun. 2005;73:3587–97. DOI: 10.1128/IAI.73.6.3587-3597.2005

[117] Walther M, Dunachie S, Keating S, Vuola JM, Berthoud T, Schmidt A, et al. Safety, immunogenicity and efficacy of a pre-erythrocytic malaria candidate vaccine, ICC-1132 formulated in Seppic ISA 720. Vaccine. 2005;23:857–64. DOI: 10.1016/j.vaccine.2004.08.020

[118] Corradin G, Kajava AV, Verdini A. Long synthetic peptides for the production of vaccines and drugs: a technological platform coming of age. Sci Transl Med. 2010;2:50rv3. DOI: 10.1126/scitranslmed.3001387

[119] Lopez JA, Weilenman C, Audran R, Roggero MA, Bonelo A, Tiercy JM, et al. A synthetic malaria vaccine elicits a potent CD8(+) and CD4(+) T lymphocyte immune response in humans. Implications for vaccination strategies. Eur J Immunol. 2001;31:1989–98. DOI: 10.1002/1521-4141(200107)31:7<1989::aid-immu1989>3.0.co;2-m

[120] Audran R, Lurati-Ruiz F, Genton B, Blythman HE, Ofori-Anyinam O, Reymond C, et al. The synthetic *Plasmodium falciparum* circumsporozoite peptide PfCS102 as a malaria vaccine candidate: a randomized controlled phase I trial. PLoS One. 2009;4:e7304. DOI: 10.1371/journal.pone.0007304

[121] Stoute JA, Slaoui M, Heppner DG, Momin P, Kester KE, Desmons P, et al. A preliminary evaluation of a recombinant circumsporozoite protein vaccine against *Plasmodium falciparum* malaria. RTS,S Malaria Vaccine Evaluation Group. N Engl J Med. 1997;336:86–91. DOI: 10.1056/NEJM199701093360202

[122] Gordon DM, McGovern TW, Krzych U, Cohen JC, Schneider I, LaChance R, et al. Safety, immunogenicity, and efficacy of a recombinantly produced *Plasmodium falciparum* circumsporozoite protein-hepatitis B surface antigen subunit vaccine. J Infect Dis. 1995;171:1576–85.

[123] Nardin EH, Oliveira GA, Calvo-Calle JM, Castro ZR, Nussenzweig RS, Schmeckpeper B, et al. Synthetic malaria peptide vaccine elicits high levels of antibodies in vaccinees of defined HLA genotypes. J Infect Dis. 2000;182:1486–96. DOI: 10.1086/315871

[124] Kester KE, McKinney DA, Tornieporth N, Ockenhouse CF, Heppner DG, Hall T, et al. Efficacy of recombinant circumsporozoite protein vaccine regimens against experimental *Plasmodium falciparum* malaria. J Infect Dis. 2001;183:640–7. DOI: 10.1086/318534

[125] Whitacre DC, Espinosa DA, Peters CJ, Jones JE, Tucker AE, Peterson DL, et al. *P. falciparum* and *P. vivax* epitope-focused VLPs elicit sterile immunity to bnlood stage infections. PLoS One. 2015;10:e0124856. DOI: 10.1371/journal.pone.0124856

[126] Carapau D, Mitchell R, Nacer A, Shaw A, Othoro C, Frevert U, et al. Protective humoral immunity elicited by a needle-free malaria vaccine comprised of a chimeric *Plasmodium falciparum* circumsporozoite protein and a Toll-like receptor 5 agonist, flagellin. Infect Immun. 2013;81:4350–62. DOI: 10.1128/iai.00263-13

[127] Nacer A, Carapau D, Mitchell R, Meltzer A, Shaw A, Frevert U, et al. Imaging murine NALT following intranasal immunization with flagellin-modified circumsporozoite protein malaria vaccines. Mucosal Immunol. 2014;7:304–14. DOI: 10.1038/mi.2013.48

[128] Othoro C, Johnston D, Lee R, Soverow J, Bystryn JC, Nardin E. Enhanced immunogenicity of *Plasmodium falciparum* peptide vaccines using a topical adjuvant containing a potent synthetic Toll-like receptor 7 agonist, imiquimod. Infect Immun. 2009;77:739–48. DOI: 10.1128/iai.00974-08

[129] Hung IF, Zhang AJ, To KK, Chan JF, Li C, Zhu HS, et al. Immunogenicity of intradermal trivalent influenza vaccine with topical imiquimod: a double blind randomized controlled trial. Clin Infect Dis. 2014;59:1246–55. DOI: 10.1093/cid/ciu582

[130] Hung IF, Zhang AJ, To KK, Chan JF, Li P, Wong TL, et al. Topical imiquimod before intradermal trivalent influenza vaccine for protection against heterologous non-vaccine and antigenically drifted viruses: a single-centre, double-blind, randomised, controlled phase 2b/3 trial. Lancet Infect Dis. 2016;16:209–18. DOI: 10.1016/s1473-3099(15)00354-0

[131] Powell TJ, Tang J, Derome ME, Mitchell RA, Jacobs A, Deng Y, et al. *Plasmodium falciparum* synthetic LbL microparticle vaccine elicits protective neutralizing antibody and parasite-specific cellular immune responses. Vaccine. 2013;31:1898–904. DOI: 10.1016/j.vaccine.2013.02.027

[132] Guo Q, Dasgupta D, Doll TA, Burkhard P, Lanar DE. Expression, purification and refolding of a self-assembling protein nanoparticle (SAPN) malaria vaccine. Methods. 2013;60:242–7. DOI: 10.1016/j.ymeth.2013.03.025

[133] Kaba SA, McCoy ME, Doll TA, Brando C, Guo Q, Dasgupta D, et al. Protective antibody and CD8+ T-cell responses to the *Plasmodium falciparum* circumsporozoite protein induced by a nanoparticle vaccine. PLoS One. 2012;7:e48304. DOI: 10.1371/journal.pone.0048304

[134] Espinosa DA, Gutierrez GM, Rojas-Lopez M, Noe AR, Shi L, Tse SW, et al. Proteolytic cleavage of the *Plasmodium falciparum* circumsporozoite protein is a target of protective antibodies. J Infect Dis. 2015;212:1111–9. DOI: 10.1093/infdis/jiv154

[135] Kariu T, Ishino T, Yano K, Chinzei Y, Yuda M. CelTOS, a novel malarial protein that mediates transmission to mosquito and vertebrate hosts. Mol Microbiol. 2006;59:1369–79. DOI: 10.1111/j.1365-2958.2005.05024.x

[136] Anum D, Kusi KA, Ganeshan H, Hollingdale MR, Ofori MF, Koram KA, et al. Measuring naturally acquired ex vivo IFN-gamma responses to *Plasmodium falciparum* cell-traversal protein for ookinetes and sporozoites (CelTOS) in Ghanaian adults. Malar J. 2015;14:20. DOI: 10.1186/s12936-014-0539-5

[137] Mishra S, Rai U, Shiratsuchi T, Li X, Vanloubbeeck Y, Cohen J, et al. Identification of non-CSP antigens bearing CD8 epitopes in mice immunized with irradiated sporozoites. Vaccine. 2011;29:7335–42. DOI: 10.1016/j.vaccine.2011.07.081

[138] Bergmann-Leitner ES, Legler PM, Savranskaya T, Ockenhouse CF, Angov E. Cellular and humoral immune effector mechanisms required for sterile protection against sporozoite challenge induced with the novel malaria vaccine candidate CelTOS. Vaccine. 2011;29:5940–9. DOI: 10.1016/j.vaccine.2011.06.053

[139] Fox CB, Baldwin SL, Vedvick TS, Angov E, Reed SG. Effects on immunogenicity by formulations of emulsion-based adjuvants for malaria vaccines. Clin Vaccine Immunol. 2012;19:1633–40. DOI: 10.1128/cvi.00235-12

[140] Bergmann-Leitner ES, Hosie H, Trichilo J, Deriso E, Ranallo RT, Alefantis T, et al. Self-adjuvanting bacterial vectors expressing pre-erythrocytic antigens induce sterile protection against malaria. Front Immunol. 2013;4:176. DOI: 10.3389/fimmu.2013.00176

[141] Bergmann-Leitner ES, Li Q, Caridha D, O'Neil MT, Ockenhouse CF, Hickman M, et al. Protective immune mechanisms against pre-erythrocytic forms of *Plasmodium berghei* depend on the target antigen. Trials Vaccinol. 2014;3:6-10. DOI: 10.1016/j.trivac.2013.11.002

[142] Hope IA, Mackay M, Hyde JE, Goman M, Scaife J. The gene for an exported antigen of the malaria parasite *Plasmodium falciparum* cloned and expressed in Escherichia coli. Nucleic Acids Res. 1985;13:369–79.

[143] Coppel RL, Favaloro JM, Crewther PE, Burkot TR, Bianco AE, Stahl HD, et al. A blood stage antigen of *Plasmodium falciparum* shares determinants with the sporozoite coat protein. Proc Natl Acad Sci U S A. 1985;82:5121–5.

[144] Doolan DL, Hedstrom RC, Rogers WO, Charoenvit Y, Rogers M, de la Vega P, et al. Identification and characterization of the protective hepatocyte erythrocyte protein 17 kDa gene of *Plasmodium yoelii*, homolog of *Plasmodium falciparum* exported protein 1. J Biol Chem. 1996;271:17861–8.

[145]   Kara U, Murray B, Pam C, Lahnstein J, Gould H, Kidson C, et al. Chemical characteri-zation of the parasitophorous vacuole membrane antigen QF 116 from *Plasmodium falciparum*. Mol Biochem Parasitol. 1990;38:19–23.

[146]   Kara UA, Stenzel DJ, Ingram LT, Bushell GR, Lopez JA, Kidson C. Inhibitory mono-clonal antibody against a (myristylated) small-molecular-weight antigen from *Plasmo-dium falciparum* associated with the parasitophorous vacuole membrane. Infect Immun. 1988;56:903–9.

[147]   Simmons D, Woollett G, Bergin-Cartwright M, Kay D, Scaife J. A malaria protein exported into a new compartment within the host erythrocyte. Embo j. 1987;6:485–91.

[148]   Sturchler D, Just M, Berger R, Reber-Liske R, Matile H, Etlinger H, et al. Evaluation of 5.1-[NANP]19, a recombinant *Plasmodium falciparum* vaccine candidate, in adults. Trop Geogr Med. 1992;44:9–14.

[149]   Doolan DL, Sedegah M, Hedstrom RC, Hobart P, Charoenvit Y, Hoffman SL. Circum-venting genetic restriction of protection against malaria with multigene DNA immu-nization: CD8+ cell-, interferon gamma-, and nitric oxide-dependent immunity. J Exp Med. 1996;183:1739–46.

[150]   Lisewski AM, Quiros JP, Ng CL, Adikesavan AK, Miura K, Putluri N, et al. Superge-nomic network compression and the discovery of EXP1 as a glutathione transferase inhibited by artesunate. Cell. 2014;158:916–28. DOI: 10.1016/j.cell.2014.07.011

[151]   Dodoo D, Hollingdale MR, Anum D, Koram KA, Gyan B, Akanmori BD, et al. Meas-uring naturally acquired immune responses to candidate malaria vaccine antigens in Ghanaian adults. Malar J. 2011;10:168. DOI: 10.1186/1475-2875-10-168

[152]   Meraldi V, Nebie I, Moret R, Cuzin-Ouattara N, Thiocone A, Doumbo O, et al. Recog-nition of synthetic polypeptides corresponding to the N- and C-terminal fragments of *Plasmodium falciparum* Exp-1 by T-cells and plasma from human donors from African endemic areas. Parasite Immunol. 2002;24:141–50.

[153]   Porter KR, Aguiar J, Richards A, Sandjaya B, Ignatias H, Hadiputranto H, et al. Immune response against the exp-1 protein of *Plasmodium falciparum* results in antibodies that cross-react with human T-cell lymphotropic virus type 1 proteins. Clin Diagn Lab Immunol. 1998;5:721–4.

[154]   Meraldi V, Nebie I, Tiono AB, Diallo D, Sanogo E, Theisen M, et al. Natural antibody response to *Plasmodium falciparum* Exp-1, MSP-3 and GLURP long synthetic peptides and association with protection. Parasite Immunol. 2004;26:265–72. DOI: 10.1111/j. 0141-9838.2004.00705.x

[155]   Aidoo M, Lalvani A, Gilbert SC, Hu JT, Daubersies P, Hurt N, et al. Cytotoxic T-lymphocyte epitopes for HLA-B53 and other HLA types in the malaria vaccine candidate liver-stage antigen 3. Infect Immun. 2000;68:227–32.

[156]   Lyke KE, Burges RB, Cissoko Y, Sangare L, Kone A, Dao M, et al. HLA-A2 supertype-restricted cell-mediated immunity by peripheral blood mononuclear cells derived from

Malian children with severe or uncomplicated *Plasmodium falciparum* malaria and healthy controls. Infect Immun. 2005;73:5799–808. DOI: 10.1128/iai.73.9.5799-5808.2005

[157] Caspers P, Etlinger H, Matile H, Pink JR, Stuber D, Takacs B. A *Plasmodium falciparum* malaria vaccine candidate which contains epitopes from the circumsporozoite protein and a blood stage antigen, 5.1. Mol Biochem Parasitol. 1991;47:143–50.

[158] Reber-Liske R, Salako LA, Matile H, Sowunmi A, Sturchler D. [NANP]19-5.1. A malaria vaccine field trial in Nigerian children. Trop Geogr Med. 1995;47:61–3.

[159] Meis JF, Rijntjes PJ, Verhave JP, Ponnudurai T, Hollingdale MR, Smith JE, et al. Fine structure of the malaria parasite *Plasmodium falciparum* in human hepatocytes in vitro. Cell Tissue Res. 1986;244:345–50.

[160] Hill AV, Allsopp CE, Kwiatkowski D, Anstey NM, Twumasi P, Rowe PA, et al. Common west African HLA antigens are associated with protection from severe malaria. Nature. 1991;352:595–600. DOI: 10.1038/352595a0

[161] Hill AV, Elvin J, Willis AC, Aidoo M, Allsopp CE, Gotch FM, et al. Molecular analysis of the association of HLA-B53 and resistance to severe malaria. Nature. 1992;360:434–9. DOI: 10.1038/360434a0

[162] Zhu J, Hollingdale MR. Structure of *Plasmodium falciparum* liver stage antigen-1. Mol Biochem Parasitol. 1991;48:223–6.

[163] Walliker D, Quakyi IA, Wellems TE, McCutchan TF, Szarfman A, London WT, et al. Genetic analysis of the human malaria parasite *Plasmodium falciparum*. Science. 1987;236:1661–6.

[164] Joshi SK, Bharadwaj A, Chatterjee S, Chauhan VS. Analysis of immune responses against T- and B-cell epitopes from *Plasmodium falciparum* liver-stage antigen 1 in rodent malaria models and malaria-exposed human subjects in India. Infect Immun. 2000;68:141–50.

[165] Bucci K, Kastens W, Hollingdale MR, Shankar A, Alpers MP, King CL, et al. Influence of age and HLA type on interferon-gamma (IFN-gamma) responses to a naturally occurring polymorphic epitope of *Plasmodium falciparum* liver stage antigen-1 (LSA-1). Clin Exp Immunol. 2000;122:94–100.

[166] Connelly M, King CL, Bucci K, Walters S, Genton B, Alpers MP, et al. T-cell immunity to peptide epitopes of liver-stage antigen 1 in an area of Papua New Guinea in which malaria is holoendemic. Infect Immun. 1997;65:5082–7.

[167] John CC, Moormann AM, Sumba PO, Ofulla AV, Pregibon DC, Kazura JW. Gamma interferon responses to *Plasmodium falciparum* liver-stage antigen 1 and thrombospondin-related adhesive protein and their relationship to age, transmission intensity, and protection against malaria. Infect Immun. 2004;72:5135–42. DOI: 10.1128/iai.72.9.5135-5142.2004

[168] John CC, Sumba PO, Ouma JH, Nahlen BL, King CL, Kazura JW. Cytokine responses to *Plasmodium falciparum* liver-stage antigen 1 vary in rainy and dry seasons in highland Kenya. Infect Immun. 2000;68:5198–204.

[169] Luty AJ, Lell B, Schmidt-Ott R, Lehman LG, Luckner D, Greve B, et al. Interferon-gamma responses are associated with resistance to reinfection with *Plasmodium falciparum* in young African children. J Infect Dis. 1999;179:980–8. DOI: 10.1086/314689

[170] Fidock DA, Gras-Masse H, Lepers JP, Brahimi K, Benmohamed L, Mellouk S, et al. *Plasmodium falciparum* liver stage antigen-1 is well conserved and contains potent B and T cell determinants. J Immunol. 1994;153:190–204.

[171] Crompton PD, Kayala MA, Traore B, Kayentao K, Ongoiba A, Weiss GE, et al. A prospective analysis of the Ab response to *Plasmodium falciparum* before and after a malaria season by protein microarray. Proc Natl Acad Sci U S A. 2010;107:6958–63. DOI: 10.1073/pnas.1001323107

[172] John CC, Moormann AM, Pregibon DC, Sumba PO, McHugh MM, Narum DL, et al. Correlation of high levels of antibodies to multiple pre-erythrocytic *Plasmodium falciparum* antigens and protection from infection. Am J Trop Med Hyg. 2005;73:222–8.

[173] John CC, Tande AJ, Moormann AM, Sumba PO, Lanar DE, Min XM, et al. Antibodies to pre-erythrocytic *Plasmodium falciparum* antigens and risk of clinical malaria in Kenyan children. J Infect Dis. 2008;197:519–26. DOI: 10.1086/526787

[174] Krzych U, Lyon JA, Jareed T, Schneider I, Hollingdale MR, Gordon DM, et al. T lymphocytes from volunteers immunized with irradiated *Plasmodium falciparum* sporozoites recognize liver and blood stage malaria antigens. J Immunol. 1995;155:4072–7.

[175] Nahrendorf W, Scholzen A, Bijker EM, Teirlinck AC, Bastiaens GJ, Schats R, et al. Memory B-cell and antibody responses induced by *Plasmodium falciparum* sporozoite immunization. J Infect Dis. 2014;210:1981–90. DOI: 10.1093/infdis/jiu354

[176] Aurrecoechea C, Brestelli J, Brunk BP, Dommer J, Fischer S, Gajria B, et al. PlasmoDB: a functional genomic database for malaria parasites. Nucleic Acids Res. 2009;37:D539–43. DOI: 10.1093/nar/gkn814

[177] Benmohamed L, Thomas A, Bossus M, Brahimi K, Wubben J, Gras-Masse H, et al. High immunogenicity in chimpanzees of peptides and lipopeptides derived from four new *Plasmodium falciparum* pre-erythrocytic molecules. Vaccine. 2000;18:2843–55.

[178] Perlaza BL, Arevalo-Herrera M, Brahimi K, Quintero G, Palomino JC, Gras-Masse H, et al. Immunogenicity of four *Plasmodium falciparum* preerythrocytic antigens in Aotus lemurinus monkeys. Infect Immun. 1998;66:3423–8.

[179] Jiang G, Charoenvit Y, Moreno A, Baraceros MF, Banania G, Richie N, et al. Induction of multi-antigen multi-stage immune responses against *Plasmodium falciparum* in rhesus

monkeys, in the absence of antigen interference, with heterologous DNA prime/poxvirus boost immunization. Malar J. 2007;6:135. DOI: 10.1186/1475-2875-6-135

[180] Pichyangkul S, Kum-Arb U, Yongvanitchit K, Limsalakpetch A, Gettayacamin M, Lanar DE, et al. Preclinical evaluation of the safety and immunogenicity of a vaccine consisting of *Plasmodium falciparum* liver-stage antigen 1 with adjuvant AS01B administered alone or concurrently with the RTS,S/AS01B vaccine in rhesus primates. Infect Immun. 2008;76:229–38. DOI: 10.1128/iai.00977-07

[181] Hillier CJ, Ware LA, Barbosa A, Angov E, Lyon JA, Heppner DG, et al. Process development and analysis of liver-stage antigen 1, a preerythrocyte-stage protein-based vaccine for *Plasmodium falciparum*. Infect Immun. 2005;73:2109–15. DOI: 10.1128/iai.73.4.2109-2115.2005

[182] Brando C, Ware LA, Freyberger H, Kathcart A, Barbosa A, Cayphas S, et al. Murine immune responses to liver-stage antigen 1 protein FMP011, a malaria vaccine candidate, delivered with adjuvant AS01B or AS02A. Infect Immun. 2007;75:838–45. DOI: 10.1128/iai.01075-06

[183] Doolan DL, Mu Y, Unal B, Sundaresh S, Hirst S, Valdez C, et al. Profiling humoral immune responses to *P. falciparum* infection with protein microarrays. Proteomics. 2008;8:4680–94. DOI: 10.1002/pmic.200800194

[184] Prieur E, Druilhe P. The malaria candidate vaccine liver stage antigen-3 is highly conserved in *Plasmodium falciparum* isolates from diverse geographical areas. Malar J. 2009;8:247. DOI: 10.1186/1475-2875-8-247

[185] Toure-Balde A, Perlaza BL, Sauzet JP, Ndiaye M, Aribot G, Tall A, et al. Evidence for multiple B- and T-cell epitopes in *Plasmodium falciparum* liver-stage antigen 3. Infect Immun. 2009;77:1189–96. DOI: 10.1128/iai.00780-07

[186] Daubersies P, Ollomo B, Sauzet JP, Brahimi K, Perlaza BL, Eling W, et al. Genetic immunisation by liver stage antigen 3 protects chimpanzees against malaria despite low immune responses. PLoS One. 2008;3:e2659. DOI: 10.1371/journal.pone.0002659

[187] Perlaza BL, Valencia AZ, Zapata C, Castellanos A, Sauzet JP, Blanc C, et al. Protection against *Plasmodium falciparum* challenge induced in Aotus monkeys by liver-stage antigen-3-derived long synthetic peptides. Eur J Immunol. 2008;38:2610–15. DOI: 10.1002/eji.200738055

[188] Schwartz L, Brown GV, Genton B, Moorthy VS. A review of malaria vaccine clinical projects based on the WHO rainbow table. Malar J. 2012;11:11. DOI: 10.1186/1475-2875-11-11

[189] Fidock DA, Sallenave-Sales S, Sherwood JA, Gachihi GS, Ferreira-da-Cruz MF, Thomas AW, et al. Conservation of the *Plasmodium falciparum* sporozoite surface protein gene, STARP, in field isolates and distinct species of Plasmodium. Mol Biochem Parasitol. 1994;67:255–67.

[190] Ambrosino E, Dumoulin C, Orlandi-Pradines E, Remoue F, Toure-Balde A, Tall A, et al. A multiplex assay for the simultaneous detection of antibodies against 15 *Plasmodium falciparum* and *Anopheles gambiae* saliva antigens. Malar J. 2010;9:317. DOI: 10.1186/1475-2875-9-317

[191] Sarr JB, Orlandi-Pradines E, Fortin S, Sow C, Cornelie S, Rogerie F, et al. Assessment of exposure to *Plasmodium falciparum* transmission in a low endemicity area by using multiplex fluorescent microsphere-based serological assays. Parasit Vectors. 2011;4:212. DOI: 10.1186/1756-3305-4-212

[192] Suwancharoen C, Putaporntip C, Rungruang T, Jongwutiwes S. Naturally acquired IgG antibodies against the C-terminal part of *Plasmodium falciparum* sporozoite threonine-asparagine-rich protein in a low endemic area. Parasitol Res. 2011;109:315–20. DOI: 10.1007/s00436-011-2257-z

[193] Fidock DA, Pasquetto V, Gras H, Badell E, Eling W, Ballou WR, et al. *Plasmodium falciparum* sporozoite invasion is inhibited by naturally acquired or experimentally induced polyclonal antibodies to the STARP antigen. Eur J Immunol. 1997;27:2502–13. DOI: 10.1002/eji.1830271007

[194] Robson KJ, Hall JR, Jennings MW, Harris TJ, Marsh K, Newbold CI, et al. A highly conserved amino-acid sequence in thrombospondin, properdin and in proteins from sporozoites and blood stages of a human malaria parasite. Nature. 1988;335:79–82. DOI: 10.1038/335079a0

[195] Robson KJ, Frevert U, Reckmann I, Cowan G, Beier J, Scragg IG, et al. Thrombospondin-related adhesive protein (TRAP) of *Plasmodium falciparum*: expression during sporozoite ontogeny and binding to human hepatocytes. Embo j. 1995;14:3883–94.

[196] Rogers WO, Malik A, Mellouk S, Nakamura K, Rogers MD, Szarfman A, et al. Characterization of *Plasmodium falciparum* sporozoite surface protein 2. Proc Natl Acad Sci U S A. 1992;89:9176–80.

[197] Plebanski M, Aidoo M, Whittle HC, Hill AV. Precursor frequency analysis of cytotoxic T lymphocytes to pre-erythrocytic antigens of *Plasmodium falciparum* in West Africa. J Immunol. 1997;158:2849–55.

[198] Wizel B, Houghten RA, Parker KC, Coligan JE, Church P, Gordon DM, et al. Irradiated sporozoite vaccine induces HLA-B8-restricted cytotoxic T lymphocyte responses against two overlapping epitopes of the *Plasmodium falciparum* sporozoite surface protein 2. J Exp Med. 1995;182:1435–45.

[199] Bejon P, Mwacharo J, Kai O, Todryk S, Keating S, Lowe B, et al. The induction and persistence of T cell IFN-gamma responses after vaccination or natural exposure is suppressed by *Plasmodium falciparum*. J Immunol. 2007;179:4193–01.

[200] Todryk SM, Bejon P, Mwangi T, Plebanski M, Urban B, Marsh K, et al. Correlation of memory T cell responses against TRAP with protection from clinical malaria, and CD4

CD25 high T cells with susceptibility in Kenyans. PLoS One. 2008;3:e2027. DOI: 10.1371/journal.pone.0002027

[201] Muller HM, Reckmann I, Hollingdale MR, Bujard H, Robson KJ, Crisanti A. Thrombospondin related anonymous protein (TRAP) of *Plasmodium falciparum* binds specifically to sulfated glycoconjugates and to HepG2 hepatoma cells suggesting a role for this molecule in sporozoite invasion of hepatocytes. EMBO J. 1993;12:2881–9.

[202] Kester KE, Gray Heppner D Jr, Moris P, Ofori-Anyinam O, Krzych U, Tornieporth N, et al. Sequential Phase 1 and Phase 2 randomized, controlled trials of the safety, immunogenicity and efficacy of combined pre-erythrocytic vaccine antigens RTS,S and TRAP formulated with AS02 adjuvant system in healthy, malaria naive adults. Vaccine. 2014;32:6683-91. DOI: 10.1016/j.vaccine.2014.06.033

[203] WHO. Malaria Vaccine Rainbow Tables. 2016. Available from: http://www.who.int/vaccine_research/links/Rainbow/en/index.html. [Accessed: 2016-10-19]

[204] Prieur E, Gilbert SC, Schneider J, Moore AC, Sheu EG, Goonetilleke N, et al. A *Plasmodium falciparum* candidate vaccine based on a six-antigen polyprotein encoded by recombinant poxviruses. Proc Natl Acad Sci U S A. 2004;101:290–5. DOI: 10.1073/pnas.0307158101

[205] Porter DW, Thompson FM, Berthoud TK, Hutchings CL, Andrews L, Biswas S, et al. A human Phase I/IIa malaria challenge trial of a polyprotein malaria vaccine. Vaccine. 2011;29:7514–22. DOI: 10.1016/j.vaccine.2011.03.083

[206] Hill AV, Reyes-Sandoval A, O'Hara G, Ewer K, Lawrie A, Goodman A, et al. Prime-boost vectored malaria vaccines: progress and prospects. Hum Vaccin. 2010;6:78-83.

[207] Webster DP, Dunachie S, Vuola JM, Berthoud T, Keating S, Laidlaw SM, et al. Enhanced T cell-mediated protection against malaria in human challenges by using the recombinant poxviruses FP9 and modified vaccinia virus Ankara. Proc Natl Acad Sci U S A. 2005;102:4836–41. DOI: 10.1073/pnas.0406381102

[208] Bejon P, Kai OK, Mwacharo J, Keating S, Lang T, Gilbert SC, et al. Alternating vector immunizations encoding pre-erythrocytic malaria antigens enhance memory responses in a malaria endemic area. Eur J Immunol. 2006;36:2264–72. DOI: 10.1002/eji. 200636187

[209] Bejon P, Mwacharo J, Kai O, Mwangi T, Milligan P, Todryk S, et al. A phase 2b randomised trial of the candidate malaria vaccines FP9 ME-TRAP and MVA ME-TRAP among children in Kenya. PLoS Clin Trials. 2006;1:e29. DOI: 10.1371/journal.pctr. 0010029

[210] Bejon P, Mwacharo J, Kai OK, Todryk S, Keating S, Lang T, et al. Immunogenicity of the candidate malaria vaccines FP9 and modified vaccinia virus Ankara encoding the pre-erythrocytic antigen ME-TRAP in 1–6 year old children in a malaria endemic area. Vaccine. 2006;24:4709–15. DOI: 10.1016/j.vaccine.2006.03.029

[211] O'Hara GA, Duncan CJ, Ewer KJ, Collins KA, Elias SC, Halstead FD, et al. Clinical assessment of a recombinant simian adenovirus ChAd63: a potent new vaccine vector. J Infect Dis. 2012;205:772-81. DOI: 10.1093/infdis/jir850

[212] Ewer KJ, O'Hara GA, Duncan CJ, Collins KA, Sheehy SH, Reyes-Sandoval A, et al. Protective CD8+ T-cell immunity to human malaria induced by chimpanzee adenovirus-MVA immunisation. Nat Commun. 2013;4:2836. DOI: 10.1038/ncomms3836

[213] Hodgson SH, Ewer KJ, Bliss CM, Edwards NJ, Rampling T, Anagnostou NA, et al. Evaluation of the efficacy of ChAd63-MVA vectored vaccines expressing circumsporozoite protein and ME-TRAP against controlled human malaria infection in malaria-naive individuals. J Infect Dis. 2015;211:1076–86. DOI: 10.1093/infdis/jiu579

[214] Ogwang C, Kimani D, Edwards NJ, Roberts R, Mwacharo J, Bowyer G, et al. Prime-boost vaccination with chimpanzee adenovirus and modified vaccinia Ankara encoding TRAP provides partial protection against *Plasmodium falciparum* infection in Kenyan adults. Sci Transl Med. 2015;7:286re5. DOI: 10.1126/scitranslmed.aaa2373

[215] Richie TL, Charoenvit Y, Wang R, Epstein JE, Hedstrom RC, Kumar S, et al. Clinical trial in healthy malaria-naive adults to evaluate the safety, tolerability, immunogenicity and efficacy of MuStDO5, a five-gene, sporozoite/hepatic stage *Plasmodium falciparum* DNA vaccine combined with escalating dose human GM-CSF DNA. Hum Vaccin Immunother. 2012;8:1564-84. DOI: 10.4161/hv.22129

[216] Wang R, Richie TL, Baraceros MF, Rahardjo N, Gay T, Banania JG, et al. Boosting of DNA vaccine-elicited gamma interferon responses in humans by exposure to malaria parasites. Infect Immun. 2005;73:2863–72. DOI: 10.1128/iai.73.5.2863-2872.2005

[217] Tine JA, Lanar DE, Smith DM, Wellde BT, Schultheiss P, Ware LA, et al. NYVAC-Pf7: a poxvirus-vectored, multiantigen, multistage vaccine candidate for *Plasmodium falciparum* malaria. Infect Immun. 1996;64:3833–44.

[218] Ockenhouse CF, Sun PF, Lanar DE, Wellde BT, Hall BT, Kester K, et al. Phase I/IIa safety, immunogenicity, and efficacy trial of NYVAC-Pf7, a pox-vectored, multiantigen, multistage vaccine candidate for *Plasmodium falciparum* malaria. J Infect Dis. 1998;177:1664–73.

[219] Moorthy VS, Imoukhuede EB, Milligan P, Bojang K, Keating S, Kaye P, et al. A randomised, double-blind, controlled vaccine efficacy trial of DNA/MVA ME-TRAP against malaria infection in Gambian adults. PLoS Med. 2004;1:e33. DOI: 10.1371/journal.pmed.0010033

[220] Aly AS, Mikolajczak SA, Rivera HS, Camargo N, Jacobs-Lorena V, Labaied M, et al. Targeted deletion of SAP1 abolishes the expression of infectivity factors necessary for successful malaria parasite liver infection. Mol Microbiol. 2008;69:152–63. DOI: 10.1111/j.1365-2958.2008.06271.x

[221] Zhao J, Deng S, Liang J, Cao Y, Liu J, Du F, et al. Immunogenicity, protective efficacy and safety of a recombinant DNA vaccine encoding truncated Plasmodium yoelii

sporozoite asparagine-rich protein 1 (PySAP1). Hum Vaccin Immunother. 2013;9:1104–11. DOI: 10.4161/hv.23688

[222] Limbach K, Aguiar J, Gowda K, Patterson N, Abot E, Sedegah M, et al. Identification of two new protective pre-erythrocytic malaria vaccine antigen candidates. Malar J. 2011;10:65. DOI: 10.1186/1475-2875-10-65

2

Multiple Organ Dysfunction During Severe Malaria: The Role of the Inflammatory Response

Mariana Conceição de Souza,

Tatiana Almeida Pádua and

Maria das Graças Henriques

Abstract

Severe malaria is a systemic illness characterized by the dysfunction of one or more peripheral organs, such as the lungs [acute respiratory distress syndrome (ARDS)] and kidneys [acute kidney injury (AKI)]. Several clinical and experimental studies suggest that features of the inflammatory response are related to the multi-organ dysfunction observed in severe malaria. Our group has been dedicated to studying the roles of pro- and anti-inflammatory mediators in the multi-organ dysfunction observed in experimental severe malaria, especially in the lungs, kidneys, and brain. Herein, we explore severe malaria as a pathology derived from intense inflammatory responses in different organs and further distinguish and compare these organ-specific inflammatory responses. The pathophysiological mechanism of severe malaria is not fully elucidated; however, it is important to study it as a complex inflammatory response assembled by different actors, each one orchestrating a different mechanism.

Keywords: inflammation, cerebral malaria, acute respiratory distress syndrome, acute kidney injury, vascular permeability

1. Introduction

Severe malaria is a systemic illness characterized by one or more clinical manifestations, such as acute respiratory distress syndrome (ARDS), multiple convulsions, prostration, shock, abnormal bleeding, jaundice, and acute kidney injury (AKI) [1–3]. Severe malaria used to be exclusively attributed to *Plasmodium falciparum* infection. However, in the last 15–20 years, several reports of severe malaria attributed to *Plasmodium vivax* [4–6] and *Plasmodium knowlesi* [7–9] have been described, which led the World Health Organization (WHO) to add these species as causes of severe malaria [10]. According to the WHO, severe malaria evolves from an uncomplicated illness due to several factors, such as the host response, parasite virulence, comorbidities, and deficient health services for malaria patients. Beyond the three species cited above, *Plasmodium malariae* and *Plasmodium ovale* also affect multiple organs in children and adults, however with different intensity (**Table 1**). The multi-organ dysfunction observed during severe malaria is associated with a systemic inflammatory response triggered by, among other factors, leukocyte adhesion to organ microvasculature, parasitized erythrocytes and production of inflammatory mediators [11, 12]. Despite the morphological and biochemical differences among *Plasmodium* species, the mechanisms by which severe malaria develops appear to be similar. Herein, we discuss the inflammatory response underlying the Physiopathology of severe malaria in human and experimental data. We further discuss triggers of the inflammatory response and how chemical and cellular mediators of inflammation cause severe malaria-induced multi-organ damage [6, 7, 9, 13–36].

	Clinical manifestation			
	ARDS	CM	Jaundice	AKI
Species				
P. falciparum	[13, 14]	[13, 15–22]	[13, 14, 16, 17, 23]	[13, 14, 16, 18, 24]
P. vivax	[6, 23, 25–27]	[27]	[6, 23]	[6, 18, 27]
P. knowlesi	[9, 28, 29]	–	[32, 36]	[31, 32, 36]
P. malariae	[31]	[6, 18, 27]	[7, 28–30]	[31, 32, 36]
P. ovale	[31, 33, 34]	–	[33, 35]	[31, 35]

ARDS, acute respiratory distress syndrome; CM, cerebral malaria; AKI, acute kidney injury.

Table 1. Studies describing severe malaria clinical manifestation according *Plasmodium* species.

2. Molecular and cellular features of the malaria-induced inflammatory response

During severe malaria, leukocytes and lymphocytes produce soluble inflammatory mediators, such as pro-inflammatory cytokines, which activate endothelial cells [37]. Furthermore, proteins anchored on membranes of infected red blood cell (RBC) such as *P. falciparum* erythrocyte membrane protein 1 (PfEMP1), expressed by parasites, induce endothelium activation resulting in increased expression of adhesion molecules [38, 39] and the activation and adhesion of leukocytes to the microvasculature.

In both the pre-erythrocytic and erythrocytic phases, macrophages and monocytes are responsible for the cytokine storm during an acute malarial infection [40]. Activation of phagocytes is mediated by binding of the hemozoin/parasite DNA complex to TLR-9 and the consequent downstream activation of inflammasome signaling [41]. The hemozoin released into circulation during infected RBC lysis is taken up by circulating monocytes and tissue macrophages and activates inflammasome intracellular protein complexes, such as NOD-, LRR-, and pyrin domain-containing (NLRP)3 and NLRP12, resulting in caspase 1 activation and the subsequent release of interleukin (IL)-1β, which is involved in fever during malaria bursts [40, 42]. In addition to inducing pro-inflammatory cytokines, some studies demonstrate that hemozoin can also induce the expression of anti-inflammatory cytokines in monocytes, such as IL-10, which tightly regulates IL-12 and CCL5 production [43]. These cytokines and chemokines, respectively, are directly involved in the development of the immune response [44]. Mononuclear cell activation leads to the production of TNF-α and IL-12 by neutrophils. These cytokines stimulate innate immune cells, such as natural killer (NK) cells and γδ T cells (including γδ NKT cells), to rapidly produce IFN-γ. As a consequence, IL-12 and IFN-γ activate monocytes and macrophages to enhance the phagocytosis of infected RBCs (reviewed in [45, 46]) and produce reactive oxygen and nitrogen radicals, which kill parasites [47].

The activation of the cellular components of the innate immune system, such as dendritic cells (DCs), is important for the establishment of acquired immunity [40]. In the spleen, DCs present their processed antigens to naïve T cells (Th0) and induce a pro-inflammatory response (Th1) with mainly CD4+ T cells that produce IFN-γ. This lymphocyte subtype is involved in the beginning of malarial infection by further stimulating Th1 differentiation and subsequently stimulating B cells to produce specific antibodies to eliminate malaria parasites [46]. In addition, CD8+ T cells act in the effector phase, contributing to permeability changes in the blood-brain barrier (BBB) through perforin-dependent mechanisms [48].

Beyond leukocytes and lymphocytes, endothelial cells also play a crucial role in the inflammatory response during severe malaria. In the erythrocytic phase, endothelial activation accounts for many factors involved in the development of severe malaria [49], such as increased adhesion of infected RBCs [50], increased expression of chemokines [51], and increased adhesion of leukocytes to peripheral organ microvasculature [52]. Several soluble proteins have been described such as inflammatory markers of endothelial activation during severe malaria. The angiopoietin (Ang)-Tie2 axis is a critical regulator of endothelial quiescence, activation and dysfunction in infectious and oncologic diseases, atherosclerosis, and pulmonary hypertension [53, 54]. Ang-1 signals through its cognate receptor Tie-2 (a tyrosine kinase with immunoglobulin and endothelial growth factor homology domains), which is expressed on endothelial cells [53]. In addition, Ang-2 (partial/weak agonist of Tie-2) is released by endothelial cells and acts as an Ang-1 antagonist [55]. During cerebral malaria (CM), Ang-1 exerts anti-inflammatory effects by decreasing adhesion molecule expression and maintaining the integrity of the BBB by reinforcing VE-cadherin tight junctions [53, 54]. In contrast, Ang-2 is stored in Weibel-Palade bodies (WPB) within endothelial cells and is involved in the response to inflammatory stimuli. High levels of Ang-2 are observed in children with severe malaria [56]. In healthy subjects, the basal Ang-1 level is higher than that of Ang-2, while the opposite ratio is observed in fatal cases of severe malaria [57]. Another inflammatory marker of endothelial activation during sever malaria is the activation of endothelial cell protein C receptor (EPCR). EPCR is widely expressed on endothelial cells and leukocytes, and its activation is associated with severe malaria [58, 59]. EPCR is referred to as the cell surface conductor of cytoprotective coagulation factor signaling because it enhances the conversion of protein C into its activated state, activated protein C (APC). The EPCR/APC complex has anti-inflammatory and endothelial cytoprotective activities that help maintain vascular integrity [60, 61]. The binding of infected RBCs to EPCR impairs the formation of the EPCR/APC complex, which may lead to sequestration, complement activation, and endothelial dysfunction, as reflected by Weibel-Palade (WP) body exocytosis, with the release of von Willebrand factor (vWF) and angiopoietin-2 and the increased expression of other endothelial receptors, such as ICAM-1 [60].

3. Organ-specific inflammatory responses

The inflammatory features described above occur in different organs and at different intensities. Although there are few examples of leukocyte adhesion in the brain vasculature in the development of human cerebral malaria [62], necropsy in fatal cases of severe malaria reveals marked inflammatory cell infiltration in lung tissue [11]. Endothelium/leukocyte interactions in the lung differ from their interactions in the brain, likely due to differences in the BBB and the blood-air barrier tight junction compositions of the brain and lung endothelium. However, the malaria-induced inflammatory response that is responsible for kidney dysfunction is not related to inflammatory cell accumulation in renal tissue but depends on immunocomplex deposition and infected RBC adhesion to the renal vasculature [63].

3.1. Inflammatory components in the development of cerebral malaria

Cerebral malaria is mainly attributed to *P. falciparum* infection, especially in children under five years [64]. Cerebral complications during malaria are triggered by the mechanisms described above; however, the inflammatory response observed in the brain is unique.

Taylor and coworkers have been studying the pathogenesis of cerebral malaria (CM) and have observed three different pathologies: (i) CM1—presence of sequestered parasitized erythrocytes in the cerebral microvasculature; (ii) CM2—presence of sequestered parasitized erythrocytes in the cerebral microvasculature and vascular pathology; and (iii) CM3—non-malarial components involved in cerebral damage. Inflammatory mediators are involved in CM1 and CM2. As described above, adhesion molecules and EPCR expressed in brain endothelial cells induce parasitized erythrocyte adhesion [58]. Likewise, during CM2, leukocytes are observed in the intravascular space, and plasmatic proteins are found in the brain tissue, suggesting edema formation [62]. The role of leukocytes in the pathogenesis of cerebral malaria is unclear. A main characteristic of brain anatomy is the presence of the BBB, which confers protection against circulating cell diapedesis into brain tissue. Nevertheless, the BBB composition of postcapillary venules allows leukocyte diapedesis during non-malarial brain injury [65, 66]. However, leukocytes are not observed within brain tissue during CM2 [62, 67], suggesting an indirect contribution of these cells to the development of cerebral malaria. Cytokine production by leukocytes during *P. falciparum* infection may contribute to brain endothelial cell activation, indicating that leukocyte involvement in cerebral malaria does not depend on cell-cell contact [68, 69]. Wassmer and colleagues hypothesized that higher endothelial responses to TNF-α increase the probability of a patient developing cerebral malaria. The authors suggest that endothelial activation by TNF-α increases the expression of adhesion molecules, which facilitates the binding of parasitized erythrocytes, leading to CM1/CM2. Thus, CM1/CM2 is a pathogenesis triggered by parasitized erythrocytes but sustained by a local inflammatory response (**Figure 1**).

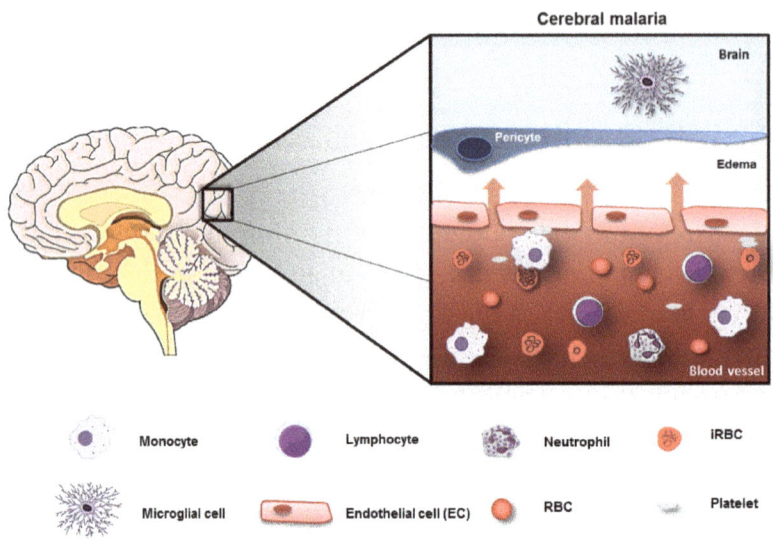

Figure 1. Inflammatory response during cerebral malaria—during cerebral malaria, it is possible to observe the presence of sequestered parasitized erythrocytes in the cerebral microvasculature, vascular pathology, leukocytes in the intravascular space and plasmatic proteins in brain tissue, suggesting edema formation. Figure created in the Mind the Graph platform (www.mindthegraph.com).

Although experimental models of severe malaria could not be used to predict human pathology, they have been extensively used to elucidate cellular and molecular pathophysiological processes. Several findings observed in human cerebral malaria are also observed in experimental models, including cytokine activity [70], endothelial activation [71], and edema formation [72]; however, the sequestration of parasitized erythrocytes during experimental cerebral malaria (ECM) is not well understood. Recent evidence showed that *Plasmodium berghei*-ANKA infected RBCs adhere to brain microvascular endothelial cells in a VCAM-1-dependent manner [73]. In addition, another study suggests transient contact between infected RBCs and the endothelium [74]. The expression of Pf-erythrocyte membrane protein (EMP)s and their ability to adhere to host adhesion molecules depends on the expression of structural proteins, such as knob-associated histidine-rich protein (KAHRP), that allow the formation of knobs on erythrocyte membranes [75]. *Plasmodium* species incapable of forming knobs in infected erythrocytes (knobless *Plasmodium*) show a passive adhesion of infected RBCs to activated endothelial cells [75]. Thus, knobless *Plasmodium* activates endothelial cells to the same extent as knob-forming *Plasmodium* [66, 73], which suggests that ECM may also be induced by parasitized erythrocytes.

The participation of leukocytes and lymphocytes in ECM has been extensively described [76]. Different from that observed in humans, during ECM, the adhesion of leukocytes and lymphocytes in the brain vasculature is well described [71, 74, 77]. In fact, monocytes, CD4+ T cells, CD8+ T cells and platelets adhere in brain post capillary venules but do not transmigrate to the brain tissue of *P. berghei* infected mice, supporting the idea that the brain disorder is due to leukocyte induced-endothelial dysfunction. Thus, strategies targeting endothelial stabilization revert ECM and prolong survival in mice [71, 78].

3.2. The inflammatory response in severe malaria-induced ARDS

Beyond the brain, the lungs are the most affected organ in severe malaria. Lung dysfunction occurs in 20% of all cases of adults with falciparum [3] or vivax [27] severe malaria. In knowlesi severe malaria, more than 50% of patients develop acute respiratory distress syndrome (ARDS) (reviewed in [3]). Recently, the methods for ARDS diagnosis are redefined, and ARDS is now classified as mild, moderate, or severe according to chest imaging, the origin of edema, oxygenation, and respiratory dysfunction timing [79], which supports the idea that the epidemiological data regarding malaria-induced ARDS may be underestimated. Nevertheless, ARDS can be caused by direct lung injury (pulmonary infection, aspiration, lung contusion, etc.) or by indirect lung injury (systemic inflammation, transfusion, burn injury, etc.) (reviewed in [80]). Thus, during severe malaria, lung dysfunction can be triggered directly by adhesion of infected RBCs to the lung vasculature or indirectly as a consequence of the activity of endothelial activators (**Figure 2**).

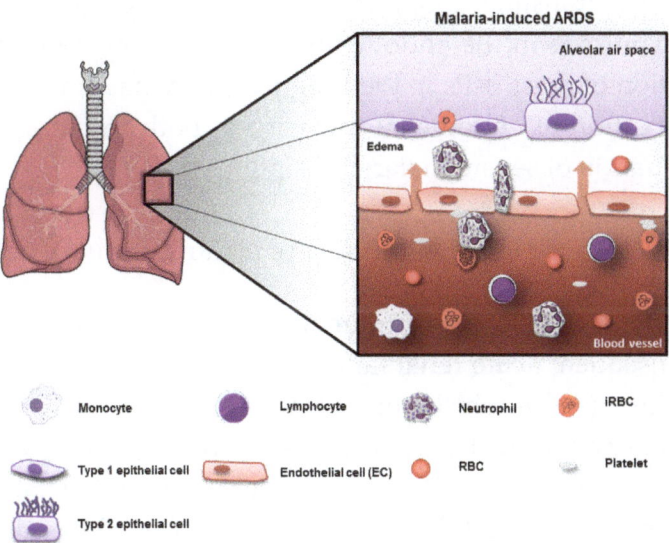

Figure 2. Inflammatory components observed in severe malaria-induced ARDS—in the lungs of patients with severe malaria who develop ARDS, increases in vascular permeability, infected erythrocytes, and intense neutrophil infiltration are often observed. Figure created in the Mind the Graph platform (www.mindthegraph.com).

Although CM is common in children, ARDS is often observed in adults [81]. In fact, the pathology observed in the lung tissue differs between adults and children. In children, few cases of pneumonia are observed [11], while an intense inflammatory cell infiltration is frequently noted [11, 82]. Milner and coworkers hypothesize that ARDS in children is an indirect effect of the inflammatory response induced by CM because non-specific lung dysfunction is observed. In fact, it has already been demonstrated that the inflammatory response triggered by brain injury directly affects the respiratory system by altering vascular permeability and allowing leukocyte influx into the lung parenchyma [83]. However, in adults, the presence of infected RBCs likely induces a local inflammatory response. Gillrie and coworkers proposed that merozoite-derived histones bind to pathogens-associated molecular patterns (PAMPs) expressed on endothelial cell membranes, leading to MAPK activation and the consequent production of pro-inflammatory mediators. In addition to the production of inflammatory mediators, *Plasmodium* also induces cell death and alterations in the expression of junctional proteins, which facilitates the influx of leukocytes to pulmonary tissue [84, 85].

Experimental models of severe malaria have revealed that ARDS begins when merosomes activate endothelial cells within pulmonary capillary beds [86, 87]. Thus, some authors suggest that the erythrocytic cycle starts in the lung capillaries [86]. In addition to merosomes, hemozoin and the close contact between infected erythrocytes and pulmonary endothelial cells trigger an inflammatory response 24 h after infection. This is characterized by intense leukocyte infiltration, as well as the production of proinflammatory mediators in the lung tissue, which persists for at least five days after infection [88–91]. Different from that observed in brain pathology, the inflammatory cellular infiltration in the lungs is mainly composed of neutrophils [90]. In fact, depletion of neutrophils impairs experimental severe malaria-induced ARDS and prolongs survival in mice [92, 93]. The participation of leukocytes in lung dysfunction during malaria may be explained, in part, by their interaction with the endothelium. In the brain, there is no leukocyte transmigration, while in the lung, tight junctional constitution and adhesion molecules expressed in the endothelium allow leukocyte transmigration and the consequent accumulation of these cells in the lung parenchyma. Thus, despite constitutional differences, the preservation of endothelial integrity in both the lungs and the brain may contribute to the attenuation of severe malaria symptoms.

3.3. The inflammatory response observed in severe malaria-induced acute kidney injury

Systemic disorders often result in secondary damage, such as functional and structural changes in the kidneys and consequent acute renal failure (ARF). The term ARF was replaced by the term acute kidney injury (AKI), which represents more than renal failure characteristics, according to the risk, injury, failure, loss, and end-stage renal failure (RIFLE) criteria [94, 95]. At present, the RIFLE criteria are widely used to diagnose AKI [96]. Severe malaria-derived AKI (smAKI) is more common in adults than in children [81]. Beyond the AKI reported in severe cases of *P. falciparum* and *P. vivax* malaria [97, 98], there have previously been reports of AKI in conjunction with the rare complications derived from infection with *P. ovale*, *P. malariae*, or *P. knowlesi* [35, 99, 100]. AKI is diagnosed in almost 50% of severe malaria cases. Currently, smAKI is diagnosed according to the WHO 2006 criteria; however, Thanachartwet and colleagues suggest that, according the RIFLE criteria, these numbers are underestimated. Instead, according the RIFLE criteria, almost 75% of severe malaria patients are developing AKI [96].

The pathophysiology of smAKI is still unclear. Because AKI can develop as a secondary effect of a systemic disease, some authors suggest that the systemic inflammatory response induced in peripheral organs during severe malaria contributes to smAKI development [101]. However, ultra-structural and histological studies of renal tissue in fatal cases of severe malaria reveal an intense inflammatory cell accumulation, indicating that smAKI can also be locally induced [18, 102].

In general, endothelial cell swelling, hypertrophy, and cytoplasmatic vacuolation suggest endothelial activation and are characteristic of smAKI [18, 102]. Such characteristics are similar between affected organs [3, 62]; however, unlike brain endothelial cells [103], kidney endothelial cells do not phagocytose infected RBCs. Regarding leukocytes, smAKI is characterized by the intense presence of mononuclear cells in peritubular capillaries, but not neutrophils, platelets, or eosinophils (**Figure 3**). Increased levels of plasmatic TNF-α [104], soluble urokinase-type plasminogen activator receptor (suPAR) expression [105], and mononuclear activation markers correlate with AKI in patients with severe malaria, suggesting that mononuclear activation induces tissue damage. Furthermore, mononuclear cells do not infiltrate the renal tissue interstitium as they do in the lungs [3], likely because, despite the activation of the renal endothelium, the tight junctions in renal tissue are not fully disrupted during severe malaria [106]. Another inflammatory characteristic that is mainly attributed to AKI is the deposition of immune complexes in the kidneys. The nephropathy associated with the deposition of immunoglobulin (Ig) isotypes G and M in the kidneys has previously been described in patients with severe malaria; however, the pathological events that result in immune complex deposition depend on the *Plasmodium* species and the time of patient death [107, 108].

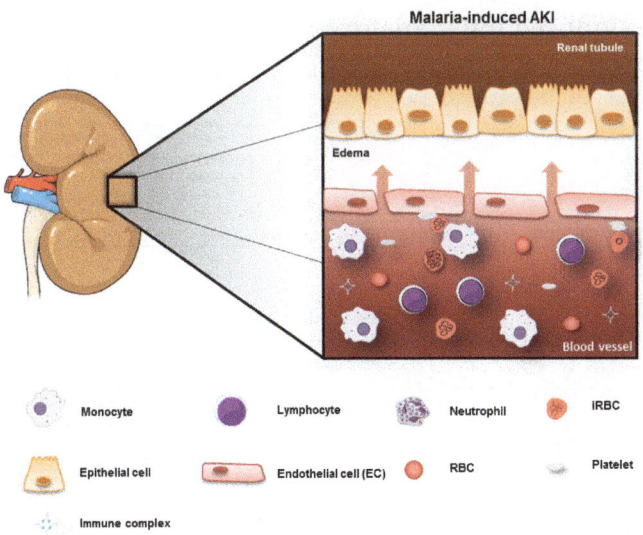

Figure 3. Severe malaria-induced AKI—during severe malaria-induced AKI, there is an intense mononuclear cell accumulation in renal tissue, endothelial cell swelling, hypertrophy, and cytoplasmatic vacuolation, suggesting endothelial activation. Different from that observed in the lungs and brain, this suggests that AKI results from deposition of immunoglobulins in the kidneys. Figure created in the Mind the Graph platform (www.mindthegraph.com).

Inflammatory components of AKI are also observed in experimental models of severe malaria. Endothelial dysfunction assessed through the evaluation of increased vascular permeability [109] and the expression of adhesion molecules [110] is also observed in experimental models of severe malaria. The activation of the glomerular endothelium may be involved in the accumulation of inflammatory cells and infected erythrocytes in glomeruli [111]. Furthermore, inflammatory cells present in the kidneys produce pro-inflammatory cytokines that perpetuate renal damage [111]. In fact, studies in which mice were rescued from severe malaria, i.e., were cured of *P. berghei* infection, showed that renal dysfunction persists for at least 14 days after cure, suggesting that severe malaria-induced AKI is mainly sustained by inflammatory components [112].

Overall, further studies are required to unveil the pathophysiology of smAKI. To date, it is not clear how kidney tissue damage begins. SmAKI may be a secondary effect of the systemic inflammatory response, may begin locally, or may be the sum of both of these processes; however, once established, smAKI persists even after parasite clearance by antimalarial drugs [24], which raise the possibility for new therapeutic approaches that target the inflammatory response in the kidney.

4. Conclusions

The findings presented above show the influence of the inflammatory response in the development and perpetuation of severe malaria. It has been shown that *Plasmodium*-associated molecular patterns such as homozoin/parasite DNA and proteins expressed on membrane of infected red blood cells trigger inflammatory response including macrophage activation, T cell differentiation, endothelial cell activation, and the production of several pro-inflammatory mediators. *Plasmodium*-induced inflammatory response occurs systemically, however, due to different anatomical and physiological characteristics, each organ develops a particular

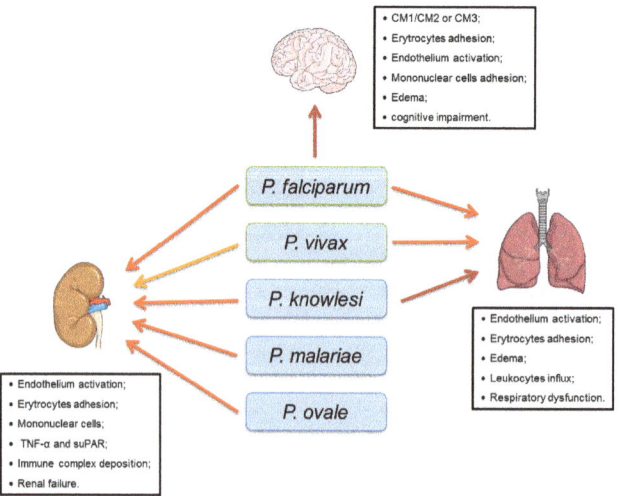

Figure 4. According to the WHO, severe malaria can be caused by *P. falciparum, P. vivax,* and *P. knowlesi.* However, the five *Plasmodium* species that infect humans are able to induce organ dysfunction due to a particular inflammatory response. Figure created in the Mind the Graph platform (www.mindthegraph.com).

inflammatory response that may lead to organ dysfunction (**Figure 4**). Although brain dysfunction is associated with activation of endothelial cells by the cytoadhesion of infected erythrocytes, severe malaria-induced ARDS is correlated with inflammatory cell accumulation in lung parenchyma.

Even though artemisinin derivatives are the treatment of choice for severe malaria, it accounts only for antimalarial purpose. In the last few years, host-directed therapies for malaria and other infectious diseases have been studied [113]. Several approaches aiming the inflammatory response have been studied in patients diagnosed with uncomplicated malaria [114, 115]; however, the treatment of severe malaria includes only supportive treatment. On the other hand, the use of experimental models of severe malaria suggested that the induction of cytoprotective pathways in brain as well the administration of anti-inflammatory drugs improve the survival of *P. berghei*-infected mice, especially when administrated as adjunctive treatment to antimalarial drugs [71, 76, 116, 117]. Indeed, a robust clinical evidence is yet necessary to provide the effectiveness of the treatment with inflammatory modulators as an adjunctive therapy to antimalarial drugs to improve patient outcomes.

Acknowledgements

This work was supported by grants from the Brazilian Council for Scientific and Technological Development (CNPq), Carlos Chagas Filho, the Rio de Janeiro State Research Supporting Foundation (FAPERJ), the Coordination for the Improvement of Higher Education Personnel (CAPES), and Fundação Oswaldo Cruz (FIOCRUZ).

Author details

Mariana Conceição de Souza[1,2], Tatiana Almeida Pádua[1,2] and Maria das Graças Henriques[1,2*]

*Address all correspondence to: gracahenriques@fiocruz.br

1 Laboratory of Applied Pharmacology, Farmanguinhos, Oswaldo Cruz Foundation, Rio de Janeiro, RJ, Brazil

2 National Institute of Science and Technology of Innovation on Diseases of Neglected Populations (INCT-IDPN), Rio de Janeiro, RJ, Brazil

References

[1] Mohan, A., Sharma, S. K., Bollineni, S. (2008) Acute lung injury and acute respiratory distress syndrome in malaria. J Vector Borne Dis 45, 179–93.

[2] Abdul Manan, J., Ali, H., Lal, M. (2006) Acute renal failure associated with malaria. J Ayub Med Coll Abbottabad 18, 47–52.

[3] Taylor, W. R., Hanson, J., Turner, G. D., White, N. J., Dondorp, A. M. (2012) Respiratory manifestations of malaria. Chest 142, 492–505.

[4] Rodriguez-Morales, A. J., Benitez, J. A., Arria, M. (2008) Malaria mortality in Venezuela: focus on deaths due to *Plasmodium vivax* in children. J Trop Pediatr 54, 94–101.

[5] Andrade, B. B., Reis-Filho, A., Souza-Neto, S. M., Clarencio, J., Camargo, L. M., Barral, A., Barral-Netto, M. (2010) Severe *Plasmodium vivax* malaria exhibits marked inflammatory imbalance. Malar J 9, 13.

[6] Lacerda, M. V., Fragoso, S. C., Alecrim, M. G., Alexandre, M. A., Magalhaes, B. M., Siqueira, A. M., Ferreira, L. C., Araujo, J. R., Mourao, M. P., Ferrer, M., Castillo, P., Martin-Jaular, L., Fernandez-Becerra, C., del Portillo, H., Ordi, J., Alonso, P. L., Bassat, Q. (2012) Postmortem characterization of patients with clinical diagnosis of *Plasmodium vivax* malaria: to what extent does this parasite kill? Clin Infect Dis 55, e67–74.

[7] Cox-Singh, J., Hiu, J., Lucas, S. B., Divis, P. C., Zulkarnaen, M., Chandran, P., Wong, K. T., Adem, P., Zaki, S. R., Singh, B., Krishna, S. (2010) Severe malaria —a case of fatal *Plasmodium knowlesi* infection with post-mortem findings: a case report. Malar J 9, 10.

[8] Cox-Singh, J., Davis, T. M., Lee, K. S., Shamsul, S. S., Matusop, A., Ratnam, S., Rahman, H. A., Conway, D. J., Singh, B. (2008) *Plasmodium knowlesi* malaria in humans is widely distributed and potentially life threatening. Clin Infect Dis 46, 165–71.

[9] William, T., Menon, J., Rajahram, G., Chan, L., Ma, G., Donaldson, S., Khoo, S., Frederick, C., Jelip, J., Anstey, N. M., Yeo, T. W. (2011) Severe *Plasmodium knowlesi* malaria in a tertiary care hospital, Sabah, Malaysia. Emerg Infect Dis 17, 1248–55.

[10] WHO (2014) Severe malaria. Trop Med Int Health 19, 7–131.

[11] Milner, D., Jr., Factor, R., Whitten, R., Carr, R. A., Kamiza, S., Pinkus, G., Molyneux, M., Taylor, T. (2013) Pulmonary pathology in pediatric cerebral malaria. Hum Pathol 44, 2719–26.

[12] Milner, D. A., Jr., Whitten, R. O., Kamiza, S., Carr, R., Liomba, G., Dzamalala, C., Seydel, K. B., Molyneux, M. E., Taylor, T. E. (2014) The systemic pathology of cerebral malaria in African children. Front Cell Infect Microbiol 4, 104.

[13] Mohapatra, B. N., Jangid, S. K., Mohanty, R. (2014) GCRBS score: a new scoring system for predicting outcome in severe falciparum malaria. J Assoc Physicians India 62, 14–7.

[14] Sulaiman, H., Ismail, M. D., Jalalonmuhali, M., Atiya, N., Ponnampalavanar, S. (2014) Severe *Plasmodium falciparum* infection mimicking acute myocardial infarction. Malar J 13, 341.

[15] Kariuki, S. M., Abubakar, A., Newton, C. R., Kihara, M. (2014) Impairment of executive function in Kenyan children exposed to severe falciparum malaria with neurological involvement. Malar J 13, 365.

[16] Asma, U. E., Taufiq, F., Khan, W. (2014) Prevalence and clinical manifestations of malaria in Aligarh, India. Korean J Parasitol 52, 621-9.

[17] Khan, W., Zakai, H. A., Umm, E. A. (2014) Clinico-pathological studies of Plasmodium falciparum and Plasmodium vivax - malaria in India and Saudi Arabia. Acta Parasitol 59, 206-12.

[18] Nayak, K. C., Kumar, S., Gupta, B. K., Gupta, A., Prakash, P., Kochar, D. K. (2014) Clinical and histopathological profile of acute renal failure caused by falciparum and vivax monoinfection: an observational study from Bikaner, northwest zone of Rajasthan, India. J Vector Borne Dis 51, 40-6.

[19] Milner, D. A., Jr., Lee, J. J., Frantzreb, C., Whitten, R. O., Kamiza, S., Carr, R. A., Pradham, A., Factor, R. E., Playforth, K., Liomba, G., Dzamalala, C., Seydel, K. B., Molyneux, M. E., Taylor, T. E. (2015) Quantitative assessment of multiorgan sequestration of parasites in fatal pediatric cerebral malaria. J Infect Dis 212, 1317–21.

[20] Milner, D. A., Jr., Vareta, J., Valim, C., Montgomery, J., Daniels, R. F., Volkman, S. K., Neafsey, D. E., Park, D. J., Schaffner, S. F., Mahesh, N. C., Barnes, K. G., Rosen, D. M., Lukens, A. K., Van Tyne, D., Wiegand, R. C., Sabeti, P. C., Seydel, K. B., Glover, S. J., Kamiza, S., Molyneux, M. E., Taylor, T. E., Wirth, D. F. (2012) Human cerebral malaria and Plasmodium falciparum genotypes in Malawi. Malar J 11, 35.

[21] Beare, N. A., Lewallen, S., Taylor, T. E., Molyneux, M. E. (2011) Redefining cerebral malaria by including malaria retinopathy. Future Microbiol 6, 349–55.

[22] Montgomery, J., Milner, D. A., Jr., Tse, M. T., Njobvu, A., Kayira, K., Dzamalala, C. P., Taylor, T. E., Rogerson, S. J., Craig, A. G., Molyneux, M. E. (2006) Genetic analysis of circulating and sequestered populations of *Plasmodium falciparum* in fatal pediatric malaria. J Infect Dis 194, 115–22.

[23] Saravu, K., Rishikesh, K., Kamath, A., Shastry, A. B. (2014) Severity in *Plasmodium vivax* malaria claiming global vigilance and exploration—a tertiary care centre-based cohort study. Malar J 13, 304.

[24] Plewes, K., Haider, M. S., Kingston, H. W., Yeo, T. W., Ghose, A., Hossain, M. A., Dondorp, A. M., Turner, G. D., Anstey, N. M. (2015) Severe falciparum malaria treated with artesunate complicated by delayed onset haemolysis and acute kidney injury. Malar J 14, 246.

[25] Londhe, C., Ganeriwal, A., deSouza, R. (2014) Study of clinical profile of acute respiratory distress syndrome and acute lung injury in *Plasmodium vivax* malaria. J Vector Borne Dis 51, 339–42.

[26] Kumari, M., Ghildiyal, R. (2014) Clinical profile of *Plasmodium vivax* malaria in children and study of severity parameters in relation to mortality: a tertiary care centre perspective in Mumbai, India. Malar Res Treat 2014, 765657.

[27] Quispe, A. M., Pozo, E., Guerrero, E., Durand, S., Baldeviano, G. C., Edgel, K. A., Graf, P. C., Lescano, A. G. (2014) *Plasmodium vivax* hospitalizations in a monoendemic malaria region: severe vivax malaria? Am J Trop Med Hyg 91, 11–7.

[28] Seilmaier, M., Hartmann, W., Beissner, M., Fenzl, T., Haller, C., Guggemos, W., Hesse, J., Harle, A., Bretzel, G., Sack, S., Wendtner, C., Loscher, T., Berens-Riha, N. (2014) Severe *Plasmodium knowlesi* infection with multi-organ failure imported to Germany from Thailand/Myanmar. Malar J 13, 422.

[29] Azidah, A. K., Mohd Faizal, M. A., Lili, H. Y., Zeehaida, M. (2014) Severe *Plasmodium knowlesi* infection with multiorgan involvement in north east peninsular Malaysia. Trop Biomed 31, 31–5.

[30] Nakaviroj, S., Kobasa, T., Teeranaipong, P., Putaporntip, C., Jongwutiwes, S. (2015) An autochthonous case of severe *Plasmodium knowlesi* malaria in Thailand. Am J Trop Med Hyg 92, 569–72.

[31] Hwang, J., Cullen, K. A., Kachur, S. P., Arguin, P. M., Baird, J. K. (2014) Severe morbidity and mortality risk from malaria in the United States, 1985–2011. Open Forum Infect Dis 1, ofu034.

[32] Bellanger, A. P., Bruneel, F., Barbot, O., Mira, J. P., Millon, L., Houze, P., Faucher, J. F., Houze, S. (2010) Severe *Plasmodium malariae* malaria in a patient with multiple susceptibility genes. J Travel Med 17, 201–2.

[33] Strydom, K. A., Ismail, F., Frean, J. (2014) *Plasmodium ovale*: a case of not-so-benign tertian malaria. Malar J 13, 85.

[34] Haydoura, S., Mazboudi, O., Charafeddine, K., Bouakl, I., Baban, T. A., Taher, A. T., Kanj, S. S. (2011) Transfusion-related *Plasmodium ovale* malaria complicated by acute respiratory distress syndrome (ARDS) in a non-endemic country. Parasitol Int 60, 114–6.

[35] Tomar, L. R., Giri, S., Bauddh, N. K., Jhamb, R. (2015) Complicated malaria: a rare presentation of *Plasmodium ovale*. Trop Doct 45, 140–2.

[36] Neri, S., Pulvirenti, D., Patamia, I., Zoccolo, A., Castellino, P. (2008) Acute renal failure in *Plasmodium malariae* infection. Neth J Med 66, 166–8.

[37] Odeh, M. (2001) The role of tumour necrosis factor-alpha in the pathogenesis of complicated falciparum malaria. Cytokine 14, 11–8.

[38] De las Salas, B., Segura, C., Pabon, A., Lopes, S. C., Costa, F. T., Blair, S. (2013) Adherence to human lung microvascular endothelial cells (HMVEC-L) of *Plasmodium vivax* isolates from Colombia. Malar J 12, 347.

[39] Tripathi, A. K., Sullivan, D. J., Stins, M. F. (2006) *Plasmodium falciparum*-infected erythrocytes increase intercellular adhesion molecule 1 expression on brain endothelium through NF-kappaB. Infect Immun 74, 3262–70.

[40] Gazzinelli, R. T., Kalantari, P., Fitzgerald, K. A., Golenbock, D. T. (2014) Innate sensing of malaria parasites. In Nat Rev Immunol 14, 744–57.

[41] Mac-Daniel, L., Menard, R. (2015) Plasmodium and mononuclear phagocytes. Microb Pathog 78, 43–51.

[42] Shio, M. T., Kassa, F. A., Bellemare, M. J., Olivier, M. (2010) Innate inflammatory response to the malarial pigment hemozoin. Microbes Infect 122010, 889–99.

[43] Keller, C. C., Yamo, O., Ouma, C., Ong'echa, J. M., Ounah, D., Hittner, J. B., Vulule, J. M., Perkins, D. J. (2006) Acquisition of hemozoin by monocytes down-regulates interleukin-12 p40 (IL-12p40) transcripts and circulating IL-12p70 through an IL-10-dependent mechanism: in vivo and in vitro findings in severe malarial anemia. Infect Immun 74, 5249–60.

[44] Were, T., Davenport, G. C., Yamo, E. O., Hittner, J. B., Awandare, G. A., Otieno, M. F., Ouma, C., Orago, A. S., Vulule, J. M., Ong'echa, J. M., Perkins, D. J. (2009) Naturally acquired hemozoin by monocytes promotes suppression of RANTES in children with malarial anemia through an IL-10-dependent mechanism. Microbes Infect 11, 811–9.

[45] Gazzinelli, R. T., Ropert, C., Campos, M. A. (2004) Role of the Toll/interleukin-1 receptor signaling pathway in host resistance and pathogenesis during infection with protozoan parasites. Immunol Rev 201, 9–25.

[46] Deroost, K., Pham, T. T., Opdenakker, G., Van den Steen, P. E. (2015) The immunological balance between host and parasite in malaria. FEMS Microbiol Rev 40, 208–57.

[47] Gowda, D. C. (2007) TLR-mediated cell signaling by malaria GPIs. Trends Parasitol 23, 596–604.

[48] Schofield, L., Grau, G. E. (2005) Immunological processes in malaria pathogenesis. Nat Rev Immunol 5, 722–35.

[49] Storm, J., Craig, A. G. (2014) Pathogenesis of cerebral malaria—inflammation and cytoadherence. Front Cell Infect Microbiol 4, 100.

[50] Wu, Y., Szestak, T., Stins, M., Craig, A. G. (2011) Amplification of *P. falciparum* cytoadherence through induction of a pro-adhesive state in host endothelium. PLoS One 6, e24784.

[51] Chakravorty, S. J., Carret, C., Nash, G. B., Ivens, A., Szestak, T., Craig, A. G. (2007) Altered phenotype and gene transcription in endothelial cells, induced by *Plasmodium falciparum*-infected red blood cells: pathogenic or protective? Int J Parasitol 37, 975–87.

[52] Maguire, G. P., Handojo, T., Pain, M. C., Kenangalem, E., Price, R. N., Tjitra, E., Anstey, N. M. (2005) Lung injury in uncomplicated and severe falciparum malaria: a longitudinal study in papua, Indonesia. J Infect Dis 192, 1966–74.

[53] Kim, H., Higgins, S., Liles, W. C., Kain, K. C. (2011) Endothelial activation and dysregulation in malaria: a potential target for novel therapeutics. Curr Opin Hematol 18, 177–85.

[54] Carvalho, L. J., Moreira, A. D., Daniel-Ribeiro, C. T., Martins, Y. C. (2014) Vascular dysfunction as a target for adjuvant therapy in cerebral malaria. Mem Inst Oswaldo Cruz 109(5), 577–588.

[55] Miller, L. H., Ackerman, H. C., Su, X. Z., Wellems, T. E. (2013) Malaria biology and disease pathogenesis: insights for new treatments. Nat Med 19, 156–67.

[56] Conroy, A. L., Glover, S. J., Hawkes, M., Erdman, L. K., Seydel, K. B., Taylor, T. E., Molyneux, M. E., Kain, K. C. (2012) Angiopoietin-2 levels are associated with retinopathy and predict mortality in Malawian children with cerebral malaria: a retrospective case-control study. Crit Care Med 40, 952–9.

[57] Jain, V., Lucchi, N. W., Wilson, N. O., Blackstock, A. J., Nagpal, A. C., Joel, P. K., Singh, M. P., Udhayakumar, V., Stiles, J. K., Singh, N. (2011) Plasma levels of angiopoietin-1 and -2 predict cerebral malaria outcome in Central India. Malar J 10, 383.

[58] Turner, L., Lavstsen, T., Berger, S. S., Wang, C. W., Petersen, J. E., Avril, M., Brazier, A. J., Freeth, J., Jespersen, J. S., Nielsen, M. A., Magistrado, P., Lusingu, J., Smith, J. D., Higgins, M. K., Theander, T. G. (2013) Severe malaria is associated with parasite binding to endothelial protein C receptor. Nature 498, 502–5.

[59] Smith, J. D., Rowe, J. A., Higgins, M. K., Lavstsen, T. (2013) Malaria's deadly grip: cytoadhesion of *Plasmodium falciparum*-infected erythrocytes. Cell Microbiol 15, 1976–83.

[60] Gleeson, E. M., O'Donnell, J. S., Preston, R. J. (2012) The endothelial cell protein C receptor: cell surface conductor of cytoprotective coagulation factor signaling. Cell Mol Life Sci 69, 717–26.

[61] Moxon, C. A., Wassmer, S. C., Milner, D. A., Jr., Chisala, N. V., Taylor, T. E., Seydel, K. B., Molyneux, M. E., Faragher, B., Esmon, C. T., Downey, C., Toh, C. H., Craig, A. G., Heyderman, R. S. (2013) Loss of endothelial protein C receptors links coagulation and inflammation to parasite sequestration in cerebral malaria in African children. Blood 122, 842–51.

[62] Dorovini-Zis, K., Schmidt, K., Huynh, H., Fu, W., Whitten, R. O., Milner, D., Kamiza, S., Molyneux, M., Taylor, T. E. (2011) The neuropathology of fatal cerebral malaria in malawian children. Am J Pathol, 1782011, 2146–58.

[63] Das, B. S. (2008) Renal failure in malaria. J Vector Borne Dis 45, 83–97.

[64] Taylor, T. E., Molyneux, M. E. (2015) The pathogenesis of pediatric cerebral malaria: eye exams, autopsies, and neuroimaging. Ann N Y Acad Sci 1342, 44–52.

[65] Alfieri, A., Srivastava, S., Siow, R. C., Cash, D., Modo, M., Duchen, M. R., Fraser, P. A., Williams, S. C., Mann, G. E. (2013) Sulforaphane preconditioning of the Nrf2/HO-1 defense pathway protects the cerebral vasculature against blood-brain barrier disruption and neurological deficits in stroke. Free Radic Biol Med 65, 1012–22.

[66] Silva, N. M., Manzan, R. M., Carneiro, W. P., Milanezi, C. M., Silva, J. S., Ferro, E. A., Mineo, J. R. (2010) Toxoplasma gondii: the severity of toxoplasmic encephalitis in C57BL/6 mice is associated with increased ALCAM and VCAM-1 expression in the central nervous system and higher blood-brain barrier permeability. Exp Parasitol 126, 167–77.

[67] Milner, D. A., Jr., Valim, C., Carr, R. A., Chandak, P. B., Fosiko, N. G., Whitten, R., Playforth, K. B., Seydel, K. B., Kamiza, S., Molyneux, M. E., Taylor, T. E. (2013) A histological method for quantifying *Plasmodium falciparum* in the brain in fatal paediatric cerebral malaria. Malar J 12, 191.

[68] Stanisic, D. I., Cutts, J., Eriksson, E., Fowkes, F. J., Rosanas-Urgell, A., Siba, P., Laman, M., Davis, T. M., Manning, L., Mueller, I., Schofield, L. (2014) gammadelta T cells and CD14+ monocytes are predominant cellular sources of cytokines and chemokines associated with severe malaria. J Infect Dis 210, 295–305.

[69] Kinra, P., Dutta, V. (2013) Serum TNF alpha levels: a prognostic marker for assessment of severity of malaria. Trop Biomed 30, 645–53.

[70] Togbe, D., de Sousa, P. L., Fauconnier, M., Boissay, V., Fick, L., Scheu, S., Pfeffer, K., Menard, R., Grau, G. E., Doan, B. T., Beloeil, J. C., Renia, L., Hansen, A. M., Ball, H. J., Hunt, N. H., Ryffel, B., Quesniaux, V. F. (2008) Both functional LTbeta receptor and TNF receptor 2 are required for the development of experimental cerebral malaria. PLoS One 3, e2608.

[71] Souza, M. C., Pádua, T. A., Torres, N. D., Souza Costa, M. F., Candéa, A. P., Maramaldo, T., Seito, L. N., Penido, C., Estato, V., Antunes, B., Silva, L., Pinheiro, A. A., Caruso-Neves, C., Tibiriçá, E., Carvalho, L., Henriques, M. G. (2015) Lipoxin A4 attenuates endothelial dysfunction during experimental cerebral malaria. Int Immunopharmacol 24, 400–407.

[72] Pamplona, A., Ferreira, A., Balla, J., Jeney, V., Balla, G., Epiphanio, S., Chora, A., Rodrigues, C. D., Gregoire, I. P., Cunha-Rodrigues, M., Portugal, S., Soares, M. P., Mota, M. M. (2007) Heme oxygenase-1 and carbon monoxide suppress the pathogenesis of experimental cerebral malaria. Nat Med 13, 703–10.

[73] El-Assaad, F., Wheway, J., Mitchell, A. J., Lou, J., Hunt, N. H., Combes, V., Grau, G. E. (2013) Cytoadherence of *Plasmodium berghei*-infected red blood cells to murine brain and lung microvascular endothelial cells in vitro. Infect Immun 81, 3984–91.

[74] Frevert, U., Nacer, A., Cabrera, M., Movila, A., Leberl, M. (2014) Imaging Plasmodium immunobiology in the liver, brain, and lung. Parasitol Int 63, 171–86.

[75] Horrocks, P., Pinches, R. A., Chakravorty, S. J., Papakrivos, J., Christodoulou, Z., Kyes, S. A., Urban, B. C., Ferguson, D. J., Newbold, C. I. (2005) PfEMP1 expression is reduced on the surface of knobless *Plasmodium falciparum* infected erythrocytes. In J Cell Sci 118, 2507–18.

[76] Souza, M. C., Padua, T. A., Henriques, M. G. (2015) Endothelial-leukocyte interaction in severe malaria: beyond the brain. Mediators Inflamm 2015, 168937.

[77] Nacer, A., Movila, A., Sohet, F., Girgis, N. M., Gundra, U. M., Loke, P., Daneman, R., Frevert, U. (2014) Experimental cerebral malaria pathogenesis—hemodynamics at the blood brain barrier. PLoS Pathog 10, e1004528.

[78] Nacer, A., Movila, A., Baer, K., Mikolajczak, S. A., Kappe, S. H. I., Frevert, U. (2012) Neuroimmunological blood brain barrier opening in experimental cerebral malaria. PLoS Pathog 8, e1002982.

[79] Barbas, C. S., Isola, A. M., Caser, E. B. (2014) What is the future of acute respiratory distress syndrome after the Berlin definition? Curr Opin Crit Care 20, 10–6.

[80] Shaver, C. M., Bastarache, J. A. (2014) Clinical and biological heterogeneity in acute respiratory distress syndrome: direct versus indirect lung injury. Clin Chest Med 35, 639–53.

[81] White, N. J., Pukrittayakamee, S., Hien, T. T., Faiz, M. A., Mokuolu, O. A., Dondorp, A. M. (2014) Malaria. Lancet 383, 723-35.

[82] Nayak, K. C., Mohini, Kumar, S., Tanwar, R. S., Kulkarni, V., Gupta, A., Sharma, P., Sirohi, P., Ratan, P. (2011) A study on pulmonary manifestations in patients with malaria from northwestern India (Bikaner). J Vector Borne Dis 48, 219–23.

[83] Mascia, L. (2009) Acute lung injury in patients with severe brain injury: a double hit model. Neurocrit Care 11, 417–26.

[84] Gillrie, M. R., Lee, K., Gowda, D. C., Davis, S. P., Monestier, M., Cui, L., Hien, T. T., Day, N. P., Ho, M. (2012) *Plasmodium falciparum* histones induce endothelial proinflammatory response and barrier dysfunction. Am J Pathol 180, 1028–39.

[85] Gillrie, M. R., Krishnegowda, G., Lee, K., Buret, A. G., Robbins, S. M., Looareesuwan, S., Gowda, D. C., Ho, M. (2007) Src-family kinase dependent disruption of endothelial barrier function by *Plasmodium falciparum* merozoite proteins. Blood 110, 3426–35.

[86] Baer, K., Klotz, C., Kappe, S. H., Schnieder, T., Frevert, U. (2007) Release of hepatic *Plasmodium yoelii* merozoites into the pulmonary microvasculature. PLoS Pathog 3, e171.

[87] Thiberge, S., Blazquez, S., Baldacci, P., Renaud, O., Shorte, S., Menard, R., Amino, R. (2007) In vivo imaging of malaria parasites in the murine liver. Nat Protoc 2, 1811–8.

[88] Deroost, K., Tyberghein, A., Lays, N., Noppen, S., Schwarzer, E., Vanstreels, E., Komuta, M., Prato, M., Lin, J. W., Pamplona, A., Janse, C. J., Arese, P., Roskams, T., Daelemans, D., Opdenakker, G., Van den Steen, P. E. (2013) Hemozoin induces lung inflammation and correlates with malaria-associated acute respiratory distress syndrome. Am J Respir Cell Mol Biol 48, 589–600.

[89] Souza, M. C., Silva, J. D., Pádua, T. A., Capelozzi, V. L., Rocco, P. R., Henriques, M. (2013) Early and late acute lung injury and their association with distal organ damage in murine malaria. Respir Physiol Neurobiol 186, 65–72.

[90] Aitken, E. H., Negri, E. M., Barboza, R., Lima, M. R., Alvarez, J. M., Marinho, C. R., Caldini, E. G., Epiphanio, S. (2014) Ultrastructure of the lung in a murine model of malaria-associated acute lung injury/acute respiratory distress syndrome. Malar J 13, 230.

[91] Epiphanio, S., Campos, M. G., Pamplona, A., Carapau, D., Pena, A. C., Ataide, R., Monteiro, C. A., Felix, N., Costa-Silva, A., Marinho, C. R., Dias, S., Mota, M. M. (2010) VEGF promotes malaria-associated acute lung injury in mice. PLoS Pathog 6, e1000916.

[92] Senaldi, G., Vesin, C., Chang, R., Grau, G. E., Piguet, P. F. (1994) Role of polymorpho-nuclear neutrophil leukocytes and their integrin CD11a (LFA-1) in the pathogenesis of severe murine malaria. Infect Immun 62, 1144–9.

[93] Belnoue, E., Potter, S. M., Rosa, D. S., Mauduit, M., Gruner, A. C., Kayibanda, M., Mitchell, A. J., Hunt, N. H., Renia, L. (2008) Control of pathogenic CD8+ T cell migration to the brain by IFN-gamma during experimental cerebral malaria. Parasite Immunol 30, 544–53.

[94] Thompson, B. T., Cox, P. N., Antonelli, M., Carlet, J. M., Cassell, J., Hill, N. S., Hinds, C. J., Pimentel, J. M., Reinhart, K., Thijs, L. G. (2004) Challenges in end-of-life care in the ICU: statement of the 5th International Consensus Conference in Critical Care: Brussels, Belgium, April 2003: executive summary. Crit Care Med 32, 1781–4.

[95] Bellomo, R., Ronco, C., Kellum, J. A., Mehta, R. L., Palevsky, P. (2004) Acute renal failure —definition, outcome measures, animal models, fluid therapy and information technology needs: the Second International Consensus Conference of the Acute Dialysis Quality Initiative (ADQI) Group. Crit Care 8, R204–12.

[96] Thanachartwet, V., Desakorn, V., Sahassananda, D., Kyaw Win, K. K., Supaporn, T. (2013) Acute renal failure in patients with severe falciparum malaria: using the WHO 2006 and RIFLE criteria. Int J Nephrol 2013, 841518.

[97] Saravu, K., Rishikesh, K., Parikh, C. R. (2014) Risk factors and outcomes stratified by severity of acute kidney injury in malaria. PLoS One 9, e90419.

[98] Kaushik, R., Kaushik, R. M., Kakkar, R., Sharma, A., Chandra, H. (2013) *Plasmodium vivax* malaria complicated by acute kidney injury: experience at a referral hospital in Uttarakhand, India. Trans R Soc Trop Med Hyg 107, 188–94.

[99] Badiane, A. S., Diongue, K., Diallo, S., Ndongo, A. A., Diedhiou, C. K., Deme, A. B., Ma, D., Ndiaye, M., Seck, M. C., Dieng, T., Ndir, O., Mboup, S., Ndiaye, D. (2014) Acute kidney injury associated with *Plasmodium malariae* infection. Malar J 13, 226.

[100] Barber, B. E., William, T., Grigg, M. J., Menon, J., Auburn, S., Marfurt, J., Anstey, N. M., Yeo, T. W. (2013) A prospective comparative study of knowlesi, falciparum, and vivax malaria in Sabah, Malaysia: high proportion with severe disease from *Plasmodium knowlesi* and *Plasmodium vivax* but no mortality with early referral and artesunate therapy. Clin Infect Dis 56, 383–97.

[101] Nacher, M., Treeprasertsuk, S., Singhasivanon, P., Silachamroon, U., Vannaphan, S., Gay, F., Looareesuwan, S., Wilairatana, P. (2001) Association of hepatomegaly and jaundice with acute renal failure but not with cerebral malaria in severe falciparum malaria in Thailand. Am J Trop Med Hyg 65, 828–33.

[102] Nguansangiam, S., Day, N. P., Hien, T. T., Mai, N. T., Chaisri, U., Riganti, M., Dondorp, A. M., Lee, S. J., Phu, N. H., Turner, G. D., White, N. J., Ferguson, D. J., Pongponratn, E. (2007) A quantitative ultrastructural study of renal pathology in fatal *Plasmodium falciparum* malaria. Trop Med Int Health 12, 1037–50.

[103] Howland, S. W., Poh, C. M., Renia, L. (2015) Activated brain endothelial cells cross-present malaria antigen. PLoS Pathog 11, e1004963.

[104] Day, N. P., Hien, T. T., Schollaardt, T., Loc, P. P., Chuong, L. V., Chau, T. T., Mai, N. T., Phu, N. H., Sinh, D. X., White, N. J., Ho, M. (1999) The prognostic and pathophysiologic role of pro- and antiinflammatory cytokines in severe malaria. J Infect Dis 180, 1288–97.

[105] Plewes, K., Royakkers, A. A., Hanson, J., Hasan, M. M., Alam, S., Ghose, A., Maude, R. J., Stassen, P. M., Charunwatthana, P., Lee, S. J., Turner, G. D., Dondorp, A. M., Schultz, M. J. (2014) Correlation of biomarkers for parasite burden and immune activation with acute kidney injury in severe falciparum malaria. Malar J 13, 91.

[106] Wichapoon, B., Punsawad, C., Chaisri, U., Viriyavejakul, P. (2014) Glomerular changes and alterations of zonula occludens-1 in the kidneys of *Plasmodium falciparum* malaria patients. Malar J 13, 176.

[107] Ward, P. A. and Kibukamusoke, J. W. (1969) Evidence for soluble immune complexes in the pathogenesis of the glomerulonephritis of quartan malaria. Lancet 1, 283–5.

[108] Houba, V., Allison, A. C., Adeniyi, A., Houba, J. E. (1971) Immunoglobulin classes and complement in biopsies of Nigerian children with the nephrotic syndrome. Clin Exp Immunol 8, 761–74.

[109] van der Heyde, H. C., Bauer, P., Sun, G., Chang, W. L., Yin, L., Fuseler, J., Granger, D. N. (2001) Assessing vascular permeability during experimental cerebral malaria by a radiolabeled monoclonal antibody technique. Infect Immun 69, 3460–5.

[110] Rui-Mei, L., Kara, A. U., Sinniah, R. (1998) In situ analysis of adhesion molecule expression in kidneys infected with murine malaria. J Pathol 185, 219–25.

[111] Sinniah, R., Rui-Mei, L., Kara, A. (1999) Up-regulation of cytokines in glomerulonephritis associated with murine malaria infection. Int J Exp Pathol 80, 87–95.

[112] Abreu, T. P., Silva, L. S., Takiya, C. M., Souza, M. C., Henriques, M. G., Pinheiro, A. A., Caruso-Neves, C. (2014) Mice rescued from severe malaria are protected against renal injury during a second kidney insult. PLoS One 9, e93634.

[113] Zumla, A., Rao, M., Wallis, R. S., Kaufmann, S. H., Rustomjee, R., Mwaba, P., Vilaplana, C., Yeboah-Manu, D., Chakaya, J., Ippolito, G., Azhar, E., Hoelscher, M., Maeurer, M. (2016) Host-directed therapies for infectious diseases: current status, recent progress, and future prospects. Lancet Infect Dis 16, e47–63.

[114] Yeo, T. W., Lampah, D. A., Gitawati, R., Tjitra, E., Kenangalem, E., McNeil, Y. R., Darcy, C. J., Granger, D. L., Weinberg, J. B., Lopansri, B. K., Price, R. N., Duffull, S. B., Celermajer, D. S., Anstey, N. M. (2007) Impaired nitric oxide bioavailability and l-arginine reversible endothelial dysfunction in adults with falciparum malaria. J Exp Med 204, 2693–704.

[115] Yeo, T. W., Lampah, D. A., Rooslamiati, I., Gitawati, R., Tjitra, E., Kenangalem, E., Price, R. N., Duffull, S. B., Anstey, N. M. (2013) A randomized pilot study of l-arginine infusion in severe falciparum malaria: preliminary safety, efficacy and pharmacokinetics. PLoS One 8, e69587.

[116] Souza, M. C., Silva, J. D., Padua, T. A., Torres, N. D., Antunes, M. A., Xisto, D. G., Abreu, T. P., Capelozzi, V. L., Morales, M. M., Pinheiro, A. A., Caruso-Neves, C., Henriques, M. G., Rocco, P. R. (2015) Mesenchymal stromal cell therapy attenuated lung and kidney injury but not brain damage in experimental cerebral malaria. Stem Cell Res Ther 6, 102.

[117] Reis, P. A., Estato, V., da Silva, T. I., d'Avila, J. C., Siqueira, L. D., Assis, E. F., Bozza, P. T., Bozza, F. A., Tibirica, E. V., Zimmerman, G. A., Castro-Faria-Neto, H. C. (2012) Statins decrease neuroinflammation and prevent cognitive impairment after cerebral malaria. PLoS Pathog 8, e1003099.

3

Structure and Functional Differentiation of PfCRT Mutation in Chloroquine Resistance (CQR) in *Plasmodium falciparum* Malaria

Pratap Parida, Kishore Sarma,
Biswajyoti Borkakoty and
Pradyumna Kishore Mohapatra

Abstract

Approximately one million deaths are attributed to malaria every year. Latest reports of multi-drug treatment failure of falciparum malaria underscore the desideratum to understand the molecular substratum of drug resistance. The mutations in the digestive vacuole transmembrane protein *Plasmodium falciparum* chloroquine resistance transporter (PfCRT) are mainly responsible for chloroquine resistance (CQR) in *Plasmodium falciparum*. Multiple mutations in the PfCRT are concerned in chloroquine resistance, but the evolution of intricate haplotypes is not yet well understood. *P. falciparum* resistance to chloroquine is the standard antimalarial drug and is mediated primarily by mutant forms of the PfCRT. In this chapter, we present the mechanism of action of the chloroquine, the structural changes of the gene after the mutations as well as different haplotypes of the PfCRT.

Keywords: antimalarial resistance, haplotype, homology modeling, mutations, PfCRT

1. Introduction

The rapid advancement and spread of malaria parasite along with antimalarial resistance is becoming a critical disaster to the world health. Chloroquine resistance (CQR) originated in Southeast Asia and South America, more or less simultaneously, in late 1950s and subsequently spread to several other malaria-endemic countries [1]. PfCRT, a candidate gene for

CQR, is present at the digestive vacuole membrane and it holds 10 putative transmembrane domains [2, 3]. Mutations in two genes, namely, the *Plasmodium falciparum* CQ resistance transporter (PfCRT) and multidrug resistance transporter-1 (pfmdr1), have been reported as responsible for CQR in *P. falciparum*. In addition, the polymorphisms of the PfCRT gene produce two different forms of PfCRT based on the drug response class, such as Chloroquine Sensitive (CQS) and CQR. The point mutations of the PfCRT codons are 72–76, 271, 326, 356, and 371, whereas two codons responsible for pfmdr1 are 86 and 1246 as molecular markers of CQ resistance [4]. The position of 72–76 of the PfCRT are considered as molecular markers used for detecting CQR malaria parasites due to the mutations in the positions 72–76 of the PfCRT, which were observed as a majority of *P. falciparum* endemic areas. There are five polymorphisms that form different haplotypes vary among the *P. falciparum* endemic regions. There are three major haplotypes based on specific mutations such as CVIETIHSESI, CVIETIHSESTI, and SVMNTIHSQDLR [2, 5–7].

Chloroquine was used as a synthetic drug in the early 1950s and 1970s [8]. The resistance to this drug was reported in Palian area of Cambodia nearer to Thai-Cambodia border as well as in Latin America. Subsequently the reported resistance to chloroquine in South Asia moved westward and during 1973, it was found to be present in North East region of India. Subsequently it spread to rest of India and beyond [9]. In 1950s, before the chloroquine resistance became widespread, it was the main drug which was cheap and having least toxicity as well as highly effective schizonticidal drug and also was effective against all the types of parasite species affecting human. But appearance of widespread resistance to chloroquine has contributed to resurgence of malaria in many countries of Asia including India [10].

By late 1980s, chloroquine became more or less obsolete for treating *P. falciparum* infections globally. However, due to high economical burden in introducing alternate treatment such as artesunate combination therapy, etc. for treatment of *Plasmodium vivax* restricted many countries like India to continue only with chloroquine for treatment of *P. vivax* [11]. This dual drug policy for the treatment of *P. falciparum* and *P. vivax* resulted in further consolidation of *P. falciparum*-resistant population in various southeastern regions of the Asia, especially in India [10].

In this chapter, we estimated certain scores of mutations such as (limbo, tango, and waltz score) to understand the changes that occur to the PfCRT protein after mutation with the help of homology modeling and single-nucleotide polymorphism (SNP).

2. *P. falciparum* CRT as a target for antimalarial drug design

Earlier, the parasite proteins involved in the resistance mechanism of malaria were unknown, but currently, it is well understood that the mutations in the PfCRT gene are causally involved in various methods such as *in vitro* and *in vivo* resistance as well as altered drug accumulation [2, 3, 12]. Identification of PfCRT gene, which encodes a putative transporter or channel protein, was a major achievement in the search for the genetic basis of CQR in *P. falciparum* [2]. PfCRT is a 48-kDa protein having 424 amino acids, 13 exon gene spanning 36 kb of chromosome 7 and 10 predicted transmembrane-spanning domains and is confined in a small area to the Digestive Vacuole (DV) membrane in erythrocytic stage parasites [2, 3]. The polymorphisms of PfCRT segregate precisely with two distinct drug response, which is considered either CQS or CQR. Fifteen polymorphic amino acid positions in PfCRT are associated with CQR in field isolates. These vary significantly depending on the geographic location and selection history, while CQS strains maintain an invariable wild-type allele [5–6, 13, 14]. K76T and S163R mutations in PfCRT[CQR] are primary and necessary for the resistance phenotype, which is the most reliable molecular marker of resistance among the various PfCRT mutations [10, 15, 16]. The endogenous role of PfCRT in the malaria parasite has not been clear yet despite the wealth of epidemiological and *in vitro* drug response data demonstrating the critical role of PfCRT mutations in producing CQR. An understanding of the natural role of PfCRT in a normally functioning cell is indeed needed to provide a clearer picture of how drug resistance works in the malaria parasite. Muhamad et al. studied the polymorphic pattern of PfCRT, which may be applied surveillance of chloroquine [17].

3. Mechanism of PfCRT

The mechanism involved in resistance against quinoline containing compound CQ in *P. falciparum* is still unclear [18, 19] and indeed the mode of action of this antimalarial chemotherapeutic agent is not beyond the debate. Chloroquine is thought to accumulate in high levels in the food vacuole of the asexual erythrocytic malaria parasites, where it acts by interfering with the polymerization of heme (hematin) into the hemozoin. The malaria parasite feeds by degrading hemoglobin of host cell, producing free ferriprotoporphyrin IX (FP) as a by-product. Ferriprotoporphyrin IX (FP) is highly toxic to the parasite and is neutralized via a process of biomineralization (polymerization) to form innocuous hemozoin crystals (β-hematin) known as malaria pigment. Chloroquine is thought to inhibit parasite growth by inhibiting the detoxification of ferriprotoporphyrin IX (FP) [20–23]. Chloroquine (CQ) appears to trap FP in a μ-oxodimeric form and prevents the formation of the β-hematin dimers that are required for hemozoin formation [24]. Thus, CQ causes a buildup of toxic FP molecules that eventually destroy the integrity of malaria parasite protein and membranes [25].

Current studies highlight an important gene connected to the resistance, *P. falciparum* chloroquine resistance transporter (PfCRT). It encodes a new transporter and also differentiates between the global selective sweeps of different haplotypes having the mutation, K76T [26]. The PfCRT gene which produces the transport proteins on the plasma membrane of the parasite's food vacuole, have been confirmed of involving with the resistance of the parasite to antimalarial drugs [27].

The mechanisms involved in the development of CQ resistance are also unclear. It is postulated that CQ resistance could arise as a consequence of any phenotypic and genotypic alteration(s), which reduces the concentration of the drug in the food vacuole of the parasite. This leads to a change in parasite biology and can lead to reduced uptake of the drug or enhanced CQ efflux from the cell or a combination of both resulting in reduced accumulation of drug inside the digestive vacuole of the parasite. It has been established that in CQ-resistant parasites, the accumulation of chloroquine inside the vacuole is significantly less than that in CQ-sensitive parasites [28, 29]. It was originally thought that this lack of accumulation was due to the result of an efflux mechanism, and P-glycoprotein was implicated as the pump responsible for the efflux. However subsequent studies have suggested that efflux rates of CQ-resistant and CQ-sensitive strains are similar. So it appears that CQ resistance involves a diminished level of drug uptake rather than, or as well as, enhanced efflux. Chloroquine-resistant parasites are known to get rid themselves of the drugs 40–50 times faster than sensitive parasites [30] but the biochemical basis of this efflux is not clear. The efflux of chloroquine and in fact the entire chloroquine-resistant phenotype can be reversed with Ca^+ channel blockers such as verapamil and diltiazem [31]. This phenomenon is biologically very similar to multi-drug resistance (MDR) phenotype of mammalian tumor cells, where a wide spectrum of chemotherapeutic agents is expelled from the cells by a verapamil-sensitive pump [32–35]. Verapamil (VPL), which inhibits P-glycoprotein (encoded by mdr gene) mediated multi-drug resistance (MDR) in mammalian tumor cells, also partly reverses chloroquine resistance in malaria parasites grown *in vitro* [31]. Because this reversal phenomenon is in some ways analogous to the reversal of MDR in mammalian tumor cell lines, CQ resistance has been postulated to involve an energy driven P-glycoprotein pump similar to that encoded by the mammalian mdr gene [31]. Two *P. falciparum* genes, which are homolog to mammalian mdr, have been identified and mapped to chromosome 5 and named pfmdr1 and pfmdr2 [36–38]. Associations have been reported between chloroquine resistance and mutations or amplification of the mdr-like gene pfmdr1, which encodes P-glycoprotein homolog-1 (Pgh1) [36, 39], which has been found to be located in the food vacuole membrane of the erythrocytic stages of the parasite [40], suggesting that it could be involved in drug transport across this membrane [41]. DNA sequencing of the pfmdr1 gene from reference strains and field isolates has revealed several point mutations that correlated with CQ resistance [39]. In earlier studies, several point mutations or nucleotide changes at position 754, 1049, 3598, 3622, and 4234 in pfmdr1 gene resulting in amino acid change at codons 86, 184, 1034, 1042, and 1246, respectively, have been shown to be associated with CQ resistance [42, 43]. But the role of these mutations in pfmdr1 in CQ resistance is controversial [44–51]. It has been observed that most of the southeast Asian CQ-resistant isolates (K1 genotype, on the basis of 3' polymorphism in pfmdr1) have the mutation at nucleotide 754 resulting in amino acid change at codon 86 from asparagines to tyrosine (N86Y) while CQ-resistant South American isolates (7G8 genotype based on 3' polymorphism in pfmdr1) have not shown mutation at codon 86 but mutational change at codon 184, 1034, 1042, and 1246 have been shown. Out of these several mutations described, the mutation at codon 86 appears to be an important, as this may be involved in substrate specificity of the gene product (P-glycoprotein) and may alter the transport activity of the protein [52]. Moreover, mutation at codon 86 has also been correlated to CQ resistance in parasites selected *in vitro* for CQ resistance [53]. However, studies from different geographical areas of the world have given the controversial picture of this mutation. Some field studies have confirmed the presence of this mutation in chloroquine-resistant isolates from Malaysia [42], Nigeria [54] Guinea-Bissau [55], and sub-Saharan Africa [56]. No association with this mutation, however, was found in isolates from Sudan [44], Thailand [45], and Cambodia [46]. Moreover, genetic studies found no linkage between chloroquine resistance and the pfmdr1 gene [57]. In India, Bhattacharya and Pillai have found strong association between chloroquine resistance and certain mutations in the pfmdr1 gene of *P. falciparum* isolates [58]. However, that study was conducted in small number *P. falciparum* strains. Gómez-Saladín et al. found the involvement of tyr86 mutation of pfmdr1 gene in CQ resistance but no significant association between tyr86 mutation and level of resistance with chloroquine [59]. Majority of pfmdr1 studies reported till date have indicated conflicting pieces of evidence, which suggest that CQ resistance in *P. falciparum* involves multiple transport mechanisms and multiple genes.

Another locus governing chloroquine resistance in a *P. falciparum* genetic cross has been mapped on chromosome 7 and has been named as cg2 (candidate gene) [57, 60]. A protein specified by this gene has size variation in three repeat regions (k, φ, and ω) several non-silent point mutations and size variation in a central poly-Asn tract. Recently, field studies have identified a series of mutations in cg2 gene in chloroquine-resistant *P. falciparum* strains suggesting that polymorphism in cg2 gene was highly associated with CQ resistance [61, 62]. Chloroquine-resistant strains have been found to consist of 16 tandem repeat units in omega repeat region (Dd2 type) of cg2 gene, while the chloroquine-sensitive strains have either ≤15 or ≥17 repeat units [54]. A significant but incomplete association has been found between the presence of the cg2 Dd2-like omega repeat length polymorphism and *in vitro* resistance and between the tyr86 allele of pfmdr1 and *in vitro* resistance [49]. Adagu and Warhurst have reported the ala281 mutation in cg2 gene and Dd2-type kappa (k) repeats in CQ-resistant isolates of northern Nigeria [62]. They have also reported the significant association between tyr86 mutation in pfmdr1 and Dd2-type kappa (k) repeat and ala 281 mutation of cg2 gene.

Recently PfCRT, a gene with 13 exons, has been identified near cg2 on chromosome 7 [2]. This gene encodes, a transmembrane protein "PfCRT" in the digestive vacuole of malaria parasites. Sets of point mutations in PfCRT were associated with *in vitro* chloroquine resistance in clinical isolates and laboratory lines of *P. falciparum* from Africa, South America, and southeast Asia [7, 12, 14, 63–66]. One mutation, the substitution of lysine (K76) by threonine (T76) at position 76 (K76T), was present in all resistant isolates and absent in all sensitive isolates tested *in vitro* [12, 14, 64, 66–69]. A significant association was found between an allele of the *P. falciparum* chloroquine resistance transporter gene (PfCRT-T76) with both *in vitro* and *in vivo* resistance and a significant association between pfmdr1-tyr86 and PfCRT-T76 has also been observed among resistant isolates, which suggests a joint action of the two genes in high-level CQ resistance [65]. Furthermore, it has also been observed that although the PfCRT-K76T mutation was present in all CQ-resistant isolates, yet this mutation was also present in patients who recovered clinically after CQ therapy [68, 70]. Hence, it has been suggested that other mechanism(s) might be involved in modulating outcome of therapy in such cases [64].

The nature of these genetic polymorphisms and their relationship with drug-resistant strains has not been studied in Indian strains of *P. falciparum*. Further, a specific marker capable of diagnosing a chloroquine resistance is yet not available. It was therefore, important to investigate whether the CQ-resistant *P. falciparum* parasites could be identified directly from a blood sample by a rapid, sensitive, and specific method like PCR, which may be of great help in prompt treatment of falciparum malaria, particularly the severe and complicated one.

Therefore, the present study was undertaken to investigate the mutation(s) and genetic polymorphism(s) in the gene PfCRT.

There is a divergence in the literature for the exact mechanism of PfCRT-producing CQR. One theory is that by using energy to transport CQ out of the DV, the protein mediates active drug efflux (similar to that of HuMDR1), which makes it away of its targets [71]. Mutations in the protein may alter its substrate specificity by using this model, which leads to greater CQ affinity for mutant isoforms.

One more hypothesis is that PfCRT facilitates the diffusion of the charged drug species (which is also known as "charged drug leak" hypothesis; [72, 73]). Inside the acidic DV, the drug molecules present are charged as compared to the outside of the DV, which neglects the drug binding. The charged molecules require some kind of carrier as they cannot pass through the hydrophobic environment of a membrane. A benefit of this suggestion is that it provides an explanation for the significance of the K76T mutation. In this mutation, the lysine in wild-type CQS isoforms has a basic side group having positive charge that repels protonated CQ, while the neutral threonine allows for an open pore through which charged CQ may pass.

Another mechanism is there based on the pH alterations of the DV, which may be influenced by PfCRT. It has been shown that CQR parasites have a more acidic DV than CQS parasites by calculating the pH of the DV [74], which is very surprising because at low pH weak base partitioning would predict increased drug accumulation. However, the rates of hematin aggregation and hemozoin formation are increased at acidic pH; as a result, it would reduce the quantity of target available for CQ binding [2]. The amount of surplus unbound drug may alter the equilibrium of passive drug accumulation [73] or may be transported out of the DV by mutant PfCRT [75].

4. Structure of *P. falciparum* CRT and its mutants

The PfCRT gene identified as the determinant gene for CQR gene since the genetic cross between a CQR clone of Indochina (Dd2) and a CQS clone of Honduras (HB3) [57]. The PfCRT protein is of 48.6 kDa, which contains 424 amino acids encoded by a 13 exon gene in the chromosome having 36-kb segment (**Figure 1**) [2]. It may catalyze chloroquine quinine flux

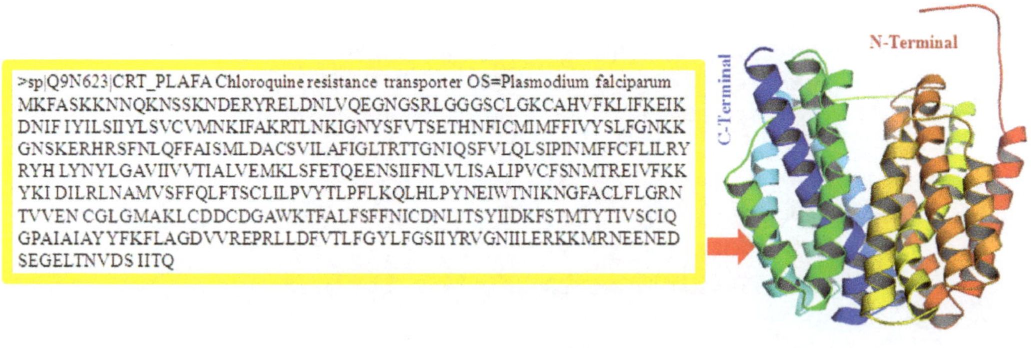

>sp|Q9N623|CRT_PLAFA Chloroquine resistance transporter OS=Plasmodium falciparum
MKFASKKNNQKNSSKNDERYRELDNLVQEGNGSRLGGGSCLGKCAHVFKLIFKEIK
DNIF IYILSIIYLSVCVMNKIFAKRTLNKIGNYSFVTSETHNFICMIMFFIVYSLFGNKK
GNSKERHRSFNLQFFAISMLDACSVILAFIGLTRTTGNIQSFVLQLSIPINMFFCFLILRY
RYH LYNYLGAVIIVVTIALVEMKLSFETQEENSIIFNLVLISALIPVCFSNMTREIVFKK
YKI DILRLNAMVSFFQLFTSCLILPVYTLPFLKQLHLPYNEIWTNIKNGFACLFLGRN
TVVEN CGLGMAKLCDDCDGAWKTFALFSFFNICDNLITSYIIDKFSTMTYTIVSCIQ
GPAIAIAYYFKFLAGDVVREPRLLDFVTLFGYLFGSIIYRVGNIILERKKMRNEENED
SEGELTNVDS IITQ

Figure 1. The homology model of the protein using the genebank sequence.

with H$^+$ across the digestive vacuole membrane having with 10 putative TMSs [76]. Nessler et al. observed activate various endogenous transporters in frog oocytes, which helps in transporting quinoline drugs including quinine and quinidine [77]. The drug specificity that determines levels of accumulation is because of the mutations in TMSs 1, 4, and 9 alter, which builds an idea of these TMSs play a role in substrate binding [78]. The substrates responsible for PfCRT mutants are chloroquine-resistant reversers [79].

Rapid progressions of chloroquine resistance (CQR) have activated the identification of some other genetic target(s) in genome of *P. falciparum* such as the mutation in K76T of PfCRT gene including three other positions 72, 74, and 75 [80]. The three mutations may present high resistance to CQ than the K76T mutant [81].

The protein is a member of the drug metabolite transporter (DMT) superfamily (TC #2.A.7) [82]. PfCRT contains drug/metabolite transporter domain. This domain is found in protein which is engaged in pectinase, cellulase, and blue pigment regulation. In plasmodium species, the PfCRT is situated at the intra-erythrocytic digestive vacuole. Mutations in this protein present verapamil-reversible chloroquine resistance to *P. falciparum*. The mutations in PfCRT result in increased compartment acidification. PfCRT-cognate vicissitudes in chloroquine replication involve altered drug flux across the parasite digestive vacuole membrane. Bray et al., concluded that PfCRT is mediated by the efflux of chloroquine from the digestive vacuole [72].

5. Analysis of single nucleotide variants scores

Three parameters have been considered for the estimation of structural changes of the PfCRT gene such as aggregation prediction (TANGO), amyloid prediction (WALTZ), and chaperone-binding prediction (LIMBO). SNPeffect 4.0: online prediction of molecular and structural effects of protein-coding variants was used for the study [83]. The three different positions of PfCRT gene were mutated manually in the protein sequence, that is, at 74, 75, and 76 positions. The mutated and the wild-type proteins were further processed using the SNPeffect software to calculate the difference in TANGO, WALTZ, and LIMBO score. The TANGO score obtained for the mutation of M74I, N75E, and K76T is given in **Figure 2**. The WALTZ scores of the wild type and the mutants are given in **Figure 3**. The LIMBO scores are given in **Figure 4**.

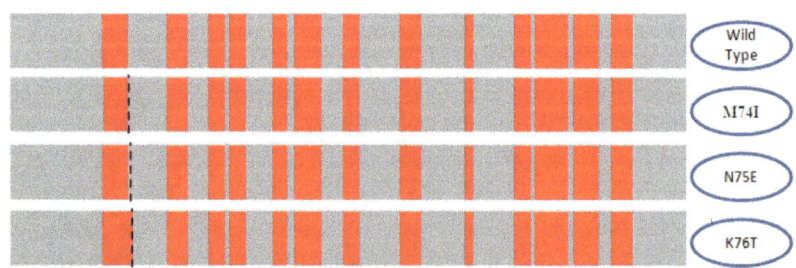

Figure 2. The aggregation prediction showing the differences of LIMBO scores of the wild-type PfCRT with the mutants.

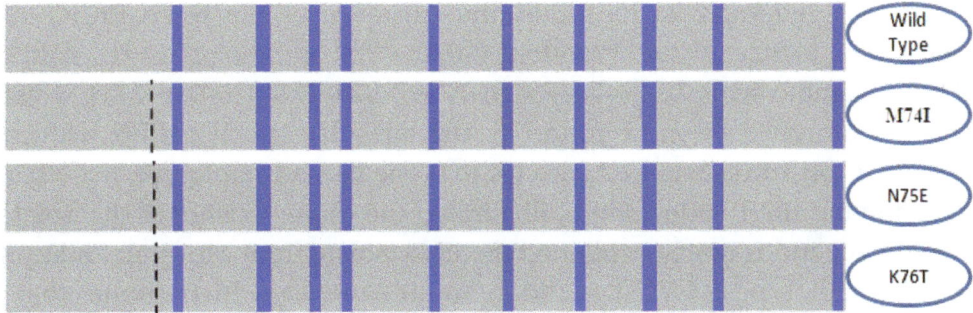

Figure 3. The amyloid prediction showing the differences of LIMBO scores of the wild-type PfCRT with the mutants.

Figure 4. The chaperone-binding prediction showing the differences of LIMBO scores of the wild-type PfCRT with the mutants.

6. The multiple haplotypes of PfCRT

In South America and southeast Asia, the CQR *P. falciparum* was first came into sight in the late 1950s and early 1960s, leading to the suggestion of Su et al., that resistance rises from two independent basic events [61]. Further studies have been done to analyze a huge number of geographically diversed PfCRT alleles and microsatellite genotypes from parasite isolates have identified at least three additional independent foci of resistance [5, 6]. CQR creation has been discovered in the Thai-Cambodian border region still now (eventually spreading westward into Africa), Papua New Guinea, the Philippines, Colombia, and Peru [84].

Cooper et al. revealed that 21 exclusive CQR PfCRT protein sequences are identified from field isolates and two additional haplotypes have been created using CQ selective pressure on the 106/1 parasite line in laboratory [3]. It is impossible to differentiate the CQR foci or the genetic variations of the subsequent involved in one origin without understanding performing the whole analysis of the PfCRT sequence and its surrounding loci by means of microsatellite typing. Johnson et al. developed four unique CQS haplotypes using the drug selection procedures of a laboratory [85].

Based on different geographical locations, the existence of the three PfCRT haplotypes revealed. According to Su et al. and Wootton et al. the first and the oldest resistant haplotype is CVIETIHSESII (amino acids 72–73–74–75–76–77–97–220–271–326–356–371), which exists in the FCB line of southeast Asia and is found in African isolates such as RB8, with consistency of spreading the CQR from Asia to Africa [5, 61]. The second haplotype is CVIETIHSESTI, which is found in the 102/1 Sudan strain, illustrated the characteristics of the isolates such as Dd2 from Thailand, and is newly explained the PH4 isolate from Morong, Philippines [2, 6]. An older PfCRT haplotype is CVIET found in South America, which implies that it may be because of the traveler who recently traveled to the location [86]. The third haplotype is detected in the INDO19, FCQ22, and 7G8 isolate line from Thailand, Papua New Guinea, and Brazil, respectively, and is reported as SVMNTIHSQDLR [2, 6, 7].

Different mutations in the PfCRT gene which change the nucleotide sequence into different genes and form different haplotypes are very general with the incidence of chloroquine resistant (CQR) [87].

7. Conclusion

The haplotype variations of PfCRT broadly classified into three groups, namely southeast Asian, Latin America, and Papua new guinea. This is used as a marker in the study of *P. falciparum* population diversity along with other markers. It is noteworthy to point out that PfCRT plays an important role in CQ transport and intracellular pH (pHi) regulation in parasite and the problem of drug resistance to antimalarials. In order to study the functions of wild-type PfCRT and mutants of PfCRT, calculation of different structural estimation score were generated where it showed that there is a notable variation in LIMBO, TANGO, and WALTZ scores.

Conflicts

The authors declared that there is no conflict of interest.

Author details

Pratap Parida, Kishore Sarma, Biswajyoti Borkakoty and Pradyumna Kishore Mohapatra[*]

*Address all correspondence to: Mohapatrapk@icmr.org.in

Regional Medical Research Centre, NE Region, Indian Council of Medical Research, Dibrugarh, Assam, India

References

[1] R.G. Ridley, "Medical need, scientific opportunity and the drive for anti-malarial drugs," *Nature*, Vol. 415, pp. 686–93, 2002.

[2] D.A. Fidock, T. Nomura, A.K. Talley, R.A. Cooper, S.M. Dzekunov, M.T. Ferdig, L.M. Ursos, A.B. Sidhu, B. Naudé, K.W. Deitsch, X.Z. Su, J.C. Wootton, P.D. Roepe and T.E. Wellems, "Mutations in the *P. falciparum* digestive vacuole transmembrane protein PfCRT and evidence for their role in chloroquine resistance," *Mol Cell*, Vol. 6, pp. 861–71, 2000.

[3] R.A. Cooper, M.T. Ferdig, X.Z. Su, L.M. Ursos, J. Mu, T. Nomura, H. Fujioka, D.A. Fidock, P.D. Roepe and T.E. Wellems, "Alternative mutations at position 76 of the vacuolar transmembrane protein PfCRT are associated with chloroquine resistance and unique stereospecific quinine and quinidine responses in *Plasmodium falciparum*," *Mol Pharmacol*, Vol. 61, pp. 35–42, 2002.

[4] W.M. Atroosh, H.M. Al-Mekhlafi, M.A. Mahdy and J. Surin, "The detection of pfcrt and pfmdr1 point mutations as molecular markers of chloroquine drug resistance, Pahang, Malaysia," *Malar J*, Vol. 11, pp. 251, 2012.

[5] J.C. Wootton, X. Feng, M.T. Ferdig, R.A. Cooper, J. Mu, D.I. Baruch, A.J. Magill and X.Z. Su, "Genetic diversity and chloroquine selective sweeps in *Plasmodium falciparum*," *Nature*, Vol. 418, pp. 320–323, 2002.

[6] N. Chen, D.E. Kyle, C. Pasay, E.V. Fowler, J. Baker, J.M. Peters and Q. Cheng, "pfcrt Allelic types with two novel amino acid mutations in chloroquine-resistant *Plasmodium falciparum* isolates from the Philippines, *Antimicrob Agents Chemother*, Vol. 47, pp. 3500–3505, 2003.

[7] N. Chen, B. Russell, J. Staley, B. Kotecka, P. Nasveld and Q. Cheng, "Sequence polymorphisms in pfcrt are strongly associated with chloroquine resistance in *Plasmodium falciparum*," *J Infect Dis*, Vol. 183, pp. 1543–1545, 2001.

[8] R.M. Packard, "The origins of antimalarial-drug resistance," *N Engl J Med*, Vol. 371, pp. 397–399, 2014.

[9] U. Arora, G.S. Sonal, G.P. Dhillon, H.G. Thakor, "Emergence of drug resistance in India," *J Indian Med Assoc*, Vol. 106, pp. 678–681, 2008.

[10] N.K. Shah, G.P. Dhillon, A.P. Dash, U. Arora, S.R. Meshnick, N. Valecha, "Antimalarial drug resistance of *Plasmodium falciparum* in India: changes over time and space," *Lancet Infect Dis*, Vol. 11, pp. 57–64, 2011.

[11] N.M. Douglas, N.M. Anstey, B.J. Angus, F. Nosten, R.N. Price, "Artemisinin combination therapy for vivax malaria," *Lancet Infect Dis*, Vol. 10, pp. 405–416, 2010.

[12]   A. Djimdé, O.K. Doumbo, R.W. Steketee and C.V. Plowe, "Application of a molecular marker for surveillance of chloroquine-resistant falciparum malaria," *Lancet*, Vol. 358, pp. 890–891, 2001.

[13]   W. Plummer, L.M. Pereira and C.V. Carrington, "Pfcrt and pfmdr1 alleles associated with chloroquine resistance in *Plasmodium falciparum* from Guyana, South America," *Mem Inst Oswaldo Cruz*, Vol, 99, pp. 389–392, 2004.

[14]   V. Durrand, A. Berry, R. Sem, P. Glaziou, J. Beaudou and T. Fandeur, "Variations in the sequence and expression of the *Plasmodium falciparum* chloroquine resistance transporter (Pfcrt) and their relationship to chloroquine resistance in vitro," *Mol Biochem Parasitol*, Vol. 136, pp. 273–85, 2004.

[15]   V. Lakshmanan, P.G. Bray, D. Verdier-Pinard, D.J. Johnson, P. Horrocks, R.A. Muhle, G.E. Alakpa, R.H. Hughes, S.A. Ward, D.J. Krogstad, A.B. Sidhu and D.A. Fidock, "A critical role for PfCRT K76T in *Plasmodium falciparum* verapamil-reversible chloroquine resistance," *EMBO J*, Vol. 24, pp. 2294–2305, 2005.

[16]   C.V. Plowe, "Monitoring antimalarial drug resistance: making the most of the tools at hand," *J Exp Biol*, Vol. 206, pp. 3745–3752, 2003.

[17]   P. Muhamad, W. Chaijaroenkul, P. Phompradit, R. Rueangweerayut, P. Tippawangkosol and K. Na-Bangchang, "Polymorphic patterns of pfcrt and pfmdr1 in *Plasmodium falciparum* isolates along the Thai-Myanmar border," *Asian Pac J Trop Biomed*, Vol. 3, 931–935, 2013.

[18]   S. Karcz and A.F. Cowman, "Similarities and differences between the multidrug resistance phenotype of mammalian tumor cells and chloroquine resistance in *Plasmodium falciparum*," *Exp Parasitol*, Vol. 73, pp. 233–240, 1991.

[19]   P.G. Bray and S.A. Ward, "Malaria chemotherapy: resistance to quinoline containing drugs in *Plasmodium falciparum*," *FEMS Microbiol Lett*, Vol. 113, pp. 1–7, 1993.

[20]   A.F. Slater and A. Cerami, "Inhibition by chloroquine of a novel haem polymerase enzyme activity in malaria trophozoites," *Nature*, Vol. 355, pp. 167–169, 1992.

[21]   A. Dorn, R. Stoffel, H. Matile, A. Bubendorf and R.G. Ridley, "Malarial haemozoin/beta-haematin supports haem polymerization in the absence of protein," *Nature*, Vol. 374, pp. 269–71, 1995.

[22]   K. Raynes, M. Foley, L. Tilley and L.W. Deady, "Novel bisquinoline antimalarials. Synthesis, antimalarial activity, and inhibition of haem polymerization," *Biochem Pharmacol*, Vol. 52, pp. 551–559, 1996.

[23]   D.J. Sullivan, "Theories on malarial pigment formation and quinoline action," *Int J Parasitol*, Vol. 32, pp. 1645–1653, 2002.

[24]   L.M. Ursos and P.D. Roepe, "Chloroquine resistance in the malarial parasite, *Plasmodium falciparum*," *Med Res Rev*, Vol. 22, pp. 465–491, 2002.

[25] N. Campanale, C. Nickel, C.A. Daubenberger, D.A. Wehlan, J.J. Gorman, N. Klonis, K. Becker and L. Tilley, "Identification and characterization of heme-interacting proteins in the malaria parasite, *Plasmodium falciparum*," *J Biol Chem*, Vol. 278, pp. 27354–27361, 2003.

[26] R.A. Cooper, C.L. Hartwig and M.T. Ferdig, "pfcrt is more than the *Plasmodium falciparum* chloroquine resistance gene: a functional and evolutionary perspective," *Acta Trop*, Vol. 94, pp. 170–180, 2005.

[27] J. Marfurt, I. Müller, A. Sie, O. Oa, J.C. Reeder, T.A. Smith, Beck HP, Genton B, "The usefulness of twenty-four molecular markers in predicting treatment outcome with combination therapy of amodiaquine plus sulphadoxine-pyrimethamine against falciparum malaria in Papua New Guinea," Malar J, Vol. 7, pp. 61, 2008.

[28] C.D. Fitch, "*Plasmodium falciparum* in owl monkeys: drug resistance and chloroquine binding capacity," *Science*, Vol. 169, pp. 289–290, 1970.

[29] P.G. Bray, M. Mungthin, R.G. Ridley and S.A. Ward, "Access to hematin: the basis of chloroquine resistance," *Mol Pharmacol*, Vol. 54, pp. 170–179, 1998.

[30] D.J. Krogstad, I.Y. Gluzman, D.E. Kyle, A.M. Oduola, S.K. Martin, W.K. Milhous and P.H. Schlesinger, "Efflux of chloroquine from *Plasmodium falciparum*: mechanism of chloroquine resistance," *Science*, Vol. 238, pp. 1283–1285, 1987.

[31] S.K. Martin, A.M. Oduola and W.K. Milhous, "Reversal of chloroquine resistance in *Plasmodium falciparum* by verapamil," *Science*, Vol. 235, pp. 899–901, 1987.

[32] J.L. Biedler and H. Riehm, "Cellular resistance to actinomycin D in Chinese hamster cells in vitro: cross-resistance, radioautographic, and cytogenetic studies," *Cancer Res*, Vol. 30, pp. 1174–1184, 1970.

[33] V. Ling and L.H. Thompson, "Reduced permeability in CHO cells as a mechanism of resistance to colchicines," *J Cell Physiol*, Vol. 83, pp. 103–116, 1974.

[34] T. Skovsgaard, "Mechanisms of resistance to daunorubicin in Ehrlich ascites tumor cells," *Cancer Res*, Vol. 38, pp. 1785–1791, 1978.

[35] T. Tsuruo, H. Iida, K. Naganuma, S. Tsukagoshi and Y. Sakurai, "Promotion by verapamil of vincristine responsiveness in tumor cell lines inherently resistant to the drug," *Cancer Res*, Vol. 43, 808–813, 1983.

[36] S.J. Foote, J.K. Thompson, A.F. Cowman and D.J. Kemp, "Amplification of the multi-drug resistance gene in some chloroquine-resistant isolates of *P. falciparum*," *Cell*, Vol. 57, pp. 921–930, 1989.

[37] C.M. Wilson, A.E. Serrano, A. Wasley, M.P. Bogenschutz, A.H. Shankar and D.F. Wirth, "Amplification of a gene related to mammalian mdr genes in drug-resistant *Plasmodium falciparum*," *Science*, Vol. 244, pp. 1184–1186, 1989.

[38] M.G. Zalis, C.M. Wilson, Y. Zhang and D.F. Wirth, "Characterization of the pfmdr2 gene for *Plasmodium falciparum*," *Mol Biochem Parasitol*, Vol. 63, pp. 311, 1994.

[39] S.J. Foote, D.E. Kyle, R.K. Martin, A.M. Oduola, K. Forsyth, D.J. Kemp and A.F. Cowman, "Several alleles of the multidrug-resistance gene are closely linked to chloroquine resistance in *Plasmodium falciparum*," *Nature*, Vol. 345, pp. 255–258, 1990.

[40] A.F. Cowman, S. Karcz, D. Galatis and J.G. Culvenor, "A P-glycoprotein homologue of *Plasmodium falciparum* is localized on the digestive vacuole," *J Cell Biol*, Vol. 113, pp. 1033–1042, 1991.

[41] S.R. Karcz, D. Galatis and A.F. Cowman, "Nucleotide binding properties of a P-glycoprotein homologue from *Plasmodium falciparum*," *Mol Biochem Parasitol*, Vol. 58, 269–276, 1993.

[42] J. Cox-Singh, B. Singh, A. Alias and M.S. Abdullah, "Assessment of the association between three pfmdr1 point mutations and chloroquine resistance in vitro of Malaysian *Plasmodium falciparum* isolates," *Trans R Soc Trop Med Hyg*, Vol. 89, pp. 436–437, 1995.

[43] M.T. Duraisingh, C.J. Drakeley, O. Muller, R. Bailey, G. Snounou, G.A. Targett, B.M. Greenwood and D.C. Warhurst, "Evidence for selection for the tyrosine-86 allele of the pfmdr 1 gene of *Plasmodium falciparum* by chloroquine and amodiaquine," *Parasitology*, Vol. 114, pp. 205–211, 1997.

[44] F.M. Awad-el-Kariem, M.A. Miles and D.C. Warhurst, "Chloroquine-resistant *Plasmodium falciparum* isolates from the Sudan lack two mutations in the pfmdr1 gene thought to be associated with chloroquine resistance," *Trans R Soc Trop Med Hyg*, Vol. 86, 587–589, 1992.

[45] C.M. Wilson, S.K. Volkman, S. Thaithong, R.K. Martin, D.E. Kyle, W.K. Milhous and D.F. Wirth, "Amplification of pfmdr1 associated with mefloquine and halofantrine resistance in *Plasmodium falciparum* from Thailand," *Mol Biochem Parasitol*, Vol. 57, pp. 151–160, 1993.

[46] L.K. Basco, P.E. de Pecoulas, J. Le Bras, C.M. Wilson, "*Plasmodium falciparum*: molecular characterization of multidrug-resistant Cambodian isolates," *Exp Parasitol*, Vol. 82, pp. 97–103, 1996.

[47] M.T. Duraisingh, P. Jones, I. Sambou, L. von Seidlein, M. Pinder and D.C. Warhurst, "The tyrosine-86 allele of the pfmdr1 gene of *Plasmodium falciparum* is associated with increased sensitivity to the anti-malarials mefloquine and artemisinin," *Mol Biochem Parasitol*, Vol. 108, pp. 13–23, 2000.

[48] M.T. Duraisingh, C. Roper, D. Walliker and D.C. Warhurst, "Increased sensitivity to the antimalarials mefloquine and artemisinin is conferred by mutations in the pfmdr1 gene of *Plasmodium falciparum*," *Mol Microbiol*, Vol. 36, pp. 955–961, 2000.

[49] M.T. Duraisingh, L.V. von Seidlein, A. Jepson, P. Jones, I. Sambou, M. Pinder and D.C. Warhurst, "Linkage disequilibrium between two chromosomally distinct loci associ-

ated with increased resistance to chloroquine in *Plasmodium falciparum*," *Parasitology*, Vol. 121, pp. 1–7, 2000.

[50] R.N. Price, A.C. Uhlemann, A. Brockman, R. McGready, E. Ashley, L. Phaipun, R. Patel, K. Laing, S. Looareesuwan, N.J. White, F. Nosten and S. Krishna, "Mefloquine resistance in *Plasmodium falciparum* and increased pfmdr1 gene copy number," *Lancet*, Vol. 364, pp. 438–447, 2004.

[51] M.T. Duraisingh and A.F. Cowman, "Contribution of the pfmdr1 gene to antimalarial drug-resistance" *Acta Trop*, Vol. 94, pp. 181–190, 2005.

[52] K.H. Choi, C.J. Chen, M. Kriegler and I.B. Roninson, "An altered pattern of cross resistance in multidrug resistant cells results from spontaneous mutation in mdr1 (p-glycoprotein) gene," *Cell*, Vol. 53, pp. 519–529, 1988.

[53] S.A. Peel, P. Bright, B. Yount, J. Handy and R.S. Baric, "A strong association between mefloquine and halofantrine resistance and amplification, overexpression, and mutation in the P-glycoprotein gene homolog (pfmdr) of *Plasmodium falciparum* in vitro, *Am J Trop Med Hyg*, Vol. 51, pp. 648–658, 1994.

[54] I.S. Adagu, D.C. Warhurst, W.N. Ogala, I. Abdu-Aguye, L.I. Audu, F.O. Bamgbola and U.B. Ovwigho, "Antimalarial drug response of *Plasmodium falciparum* from Zaria, Nigeria," *Trans R Soc Trop Med Hyg*, Vol. 89, pp. 422–425, 1995.

[55] I.S. Adagu, F. Dias, L. Pinheiro, L. Rombo, V. do Rosario and D.C. Warhurst, "Guinea Bissau: association of chloroquine resistance of *Plasmodium falciparum* with the Tyr86 allele of the multiple drug-resistance gene Pfmdr1," *Trans R Soc Trop Med Hyg*, Vol. 90, pp. 90–91, 1996.

[56] L.K. Basco, P. Ringwald, R. Thor, J.C. Doury and J. Le Bras, "Activity in vitro of chloroquine, cycloguanil, and mefloquine against African isolates of *Plasmodium falciparum*: presumptive evidence for chemoprophylactic efficacy in Central and West Africa," *Trans R Soc Trop Med Hyg*, Vol. 89, pp. 657–658, 1995.

[57] T.E. Wellems, L.J. Panton, I.Y. Gluzman, V.E. do Rosario, R.W. Gwadz, A. Walker-Jonah and D.J. Krogstad, "Chloroquine resistance not linked to mdr-like genes in a *Plasmodium falciparum* cross," *Nature*, Vol. 345, pp. 253–255, 1990.

[58] P.R. Bhattacharya and C.R. Pillai, "Strong association, but incomplete correlation, between chloroquine resistance and allelic variation in the pfmdr-1 gene of *Plasmodium falciparum* isolates from India," *Ann Trop Med Parasitol*, Vol. 93, pp. 679–84, 1999.

[59] E. Gómez-Saladín, D.J. Fryauff, W.R. Taylor, B.S. Laksana, A.I. Susanti, Purnomo, B. Subianto, and T.L. Richie, "*Plasmodium falciparum* mdr1 mutations and in vivo chloroquine resistance in Indonesia," *Am J Trop Med Hyg*, Vol. 61, 240–244, 1999.

[60] T.E. Wellems, A. Walker-Jonah and L.J. Panton, "Genetic mapping of the chloroquine-resistance locus on *Plasmodium falciparum* chromosome 7," *Proc Natl Acad Sci U S A*, Vol. 88, pp. 3382–3386, 1991.

[61] X. Su, L.A. Kirkman, H. Fujioka and T.E. Wellems, "Complex polymorphisms in an approximately 330 kDa protein are linked to chloroquine-resistant *P. falciparum* in Southeast Asia and Africa," *Cell*, Vol. 91, pp. 593–603, 1997.

[62] I.S. Adagu and D.C. Warhurs, "Association of cg2 and pfmdr1 genotype with chloroquine resistance in field samples of *Plasmodium falciparum* from Nigeria," *Parasitology*, Vol. 119, pp. 343–348, 1999.

[63] L.K. Basco and P. Ringwald, "Molecular epidemiology of malaria in Yaounde, Cameroon V. analysis of the omega repetitive region of the *plasmodium falciparum* CG2 gene and chloroquine resistance," *Am J Trop Med Hyg*, Vol. 61, pp. 807–813, 1999.

[64] L.K. Basco and P. Ringwald, "Point mutations in the *Plasmodium falciparum* cg2 gene, polymorphism of the kappa repeat region, and their relationship with chloroquine resistance," *Trans R Soc Trop Med Hyg*, Vol. 95, pp. 309–314, 2001.

[65] P.P. Vieira, M. Das Gracas Alecrim, L.H. DA Silva, I. Gonzalez-Jimenez and M.G. Zalis, "Analysis of the PfCRT K76T mutation in *Plasmodium falciparum* isolates from the Amazon region of Brazil," *J Infect Dis*, Vol. 183, pp. 1832–33, 2001.

[66] P. Lim, S. Chy, F. Ariey, S. Incardona, P. Chim, R. Sem, M.B. Denis, S. Hewitt, S. Hoyer, D. Socheat, M.P. Odile and F. Thierry, "Pfcrt polymorphism and chloroquine resistance in *Plasmodium falciparum* strains isolated in Cambodia," *Antimicrob Agents Chemother*, Vol. 47, pp. 87–94, 2003.

[67] H.A. Babiker, S.J. Pringle, A. Abdel-Muhsin, M. Mackinnon, P. Hunt and D. Walliker, "High-level chloroquine resistance in Sudanese isolates of *Plasmodium falciparum* is associated with mutations in the chloroquine resistance transporter gene pfcrt and the multidrug resistance Gene pfmdr1," *J Infect Dis*, Vol. 183, pp. 1535–1538, 2001.

[68] G. Dorsey, M.R. Kamya, A. Singh and P.J. Rosenthal, "Polymorphisms in the *Plasmodium falciparum* pfcrt and pfmdr-1 genes and clinical response to chloroquine in Kampala, Uganda," *J Infect Dis*, Vol. 183, pp. 1417–1420, 2001.

[69] R. Durand, S. Jafari, J. Vauzelle, J. Delabre, Z. Jesic and J. Le Bras, "Analysis of pfcrt point mutations and chloroquine susceptibility in isolates of *Plasmodium falciparum*," *Mol Biochem parasitol*, Vol. 114, pp. 95–102, 2001.

[70] A.G. Mayor, X. Gómez-Olivé, J.J. Aponte, S. Casimiro, S. Mabunda, M. Dgedge, A. Barreto and P.L. Alonso, "Prevalence of the K76T mutation in the putative *Plasmodium falciparum* chloroquine resistance transporter (pfcrt) gene and its relation to chloroquine resistance in Mozambique," *J Infect Dis*, Vol. 183, pp. 1413–1416, 2001.

[71] C.P. Sanchez, J.E. McLean, P. Rohrbach, D.A. Fidock, W.D. Stein and M. Lanzer, "Evidence for a pfcrt-associated chloroquine efflux system in the human malarial parasite *Plasmodium falciparum*," *Biochemistry*, Vol. 44, pp. 9862–9870, 2005.

[72] P.G. Bray, R.E. Martin, L. Tilley, S.A. Ward, K. Kirk and D.A. Fidock, "Defining the role of PfCRT in Plasmodium falciparum chloroquine resistance," *Mol Microbiol*, Vol. 56, pp. 323–333, 2005.

[73] H Zhang, M Paguio and P.D. Roepe, "The antimalarial drug resistance protein *Plasmodium falciparum* chloroquine resistance transporter binds chloroquine," *Biochemistry*, Vol. 43, pp. 8290–8296, 2004.

[74] T.N. Bennett, A.D. Kosar, L.M. Ursos, S. Dzekunov, A.B. Singh Sidhu, D.A. Fidock and P.D. Roepe, "Drug resistance-associated pfCRT mutations confer decreased *Plasmodium falciparum* digestive vacuolar pH," *Mol Biochem Parasitol*, Vol. 133, 99–114, 2004.

[75] E.M. Howard, H. Zhang and P.D. Roepe, "A novel transporter, Pfcrt, confers antimalarial drug resistance," *J Membr Biol*, Vol. 190, pp. 1–8, 2002.

[76] T.E. Wellems, "Plasmodium chloroquine resistance and the search for a replacement antimalarial drug," *Science*, Vol. 298, pp. 124–126, 2002.

[77] S. Nessler, O. Friedrich, N. Bakouh, R.H. Fink, C.P. Sanchez, G. Planelles and M. Lanzer, "Evidence for activation of endogenous transporters in Xenopus laevis oocytes expressing the *Plasmodium falciparum* chloroquine resistance transporter, PfCRT," *J Biol Chem*, Vol. 279, pp. 39438–39446, 2004.

[78] R.A. Cooper, K.D. Lane, B. Deng, J. Mu, J.J. Patel, T.E. Wellems, X. Su and M.T. Ferdig, "Mutations in transmembrane domains 1, 4 and 9 of the *Plasmodium falciparum* chloroquine resistance transporter alter susceptibility to chloroquine, quinine and quinidine," *Mol Microbiol*, Vol. 63, pp. 270–282, 2007.

[79] A.M. Lehane and K. Kirk, "Efflux of a range of antimalarial drugs and 'chloroquine resistance reversers' from the digestive vacuole in malaria parasites with mutant PfCRT," *Mol Microbiol*, Vol. 77, pp. 1039–1051, 2010.

[80] G. Awasthi and A. Das, "Genetics of chloroquine-resistant malaria: a haplotypic view," *Mem Inst Oswaldo Cruz*, Vol. 108, pp. 947–961, 2013.

[81] N. Takahashi, K. Tanabe, T. Tsukahara, M. Dzodzomenyo, L. Dysoley, B. Khamlome, J. Sattabongkot, M. Nakamura, M. Sakurai, J. Kobayashi, A. Kaneko, H. Endo, F. Hombhanje, T. Tsuboi and T. Mita, "Large-scale survey for novel genotypes of *Plasmodium falciparum* chloroquine-resistance gene pfcrt," *Malar J*, 11, pp. 92, 2012.

[82] C.V. Tran and M.H. Saier Jr, "The principal chloroquine resistance protein of *Plasmodium falciparum* is a member of the drug/metabolite transporter superfamily," *Microbiology*, Vol. 150, pp. 1–3, 2004.

[83] G. De Baets, J. Van Durme, J. Reumers, S. Maurer-Stroh, P. Vanhee, J. Dopazo, J. Schymkowitz and F. Rousseau, "SNPeffect 4.0: on-line prediction of molecular and structural effects of protein-coding variants," *Nucleic Acids Res*, Vol. 40, pp. D935–D939, 2012.

[84] K. Hayton and X.Z. Su, "Genetic and biochemical aspects of drug resistance in malaria parasites," *Curr Drug Targets Infect Disord*, Vol. 4, pp. 1–10, 2004.

[85] D.J. Johnson, D.A. Fidock, M. Mungthin, V. Lakshmanan, A.B. Sidhu, P.G. Bray and S.A. Ward, "Evidence for a central role for PfCRT in conferring *Plasmodium falciparum* resistance to diverse antimalarial agents," *Mol Cell*, Vol. 15, pp. 867–877, 2004.

[86] P.P. Vieira, M.U. Ferreira, Md. Alecrim, W.D. Alecrim, L.H. da Silva, M.M. Sihuincha, D.A. Joy, J. Mu, X.Z. Su and M.G. Zalis, "pfcrt Polymorphism and the spread of chloroquine resistance in *Plasmodium falciparum* populations across the Amazon Basin." *J Infect Dis*, Vol. 190, pp. 417–424, 2004.

[87] G. Awasthi, G.B. Satya Prasad and A. Das, "Pfcrt haplotypes and the evolutionary history of chloroquine-resistant *Plasmodium falciparum*," *Mem Inst Oswaldo Cruz*, Vol. 107, pp. 129–134, 2012.

4

Identification and Validation of Novel Drug Targets for the Treatment of *Plasmodium falciparum* Malaria

Sergey Lunev, Fernando A. Batista, Soraya S. Bosch,

Carsten Wrenger and Matthew R. Groves

Abstract

In order to counter the malarial parasite's striking ability to rapidly develop drug resistance, a constant supply of novel antimalarial drugs and potential drug targets must be available. The so-called Harlow-Knapp effect, or "searching under the lamp post," in which scientists tend to further explore only the areas that are already well illuminated, significantly limits the availability of novel drugs and drug targets. This chapter summarizes the pool of electron transport chain (ETC) and carbon metabolism antimalarial targets that have been "under the lamp post" in recent years, as well as suggest a promising new avenue for the validation of novel drug targets. The interplay between the pathways crucial for the parasite, such as pyrimidine biosynthesis, aspartate metabolism, and mitochondrial tricarboxylic acid (TCA) cycle, is described in order to create a "road map" of novel antimalarial avenues.

Keywords: malaria, *Plasmodium falciparum*, drug design, drug target validation, protein interference, metabolic map, oligomerization

1. Introduction

"Portrait of a serial killer," a commentary published in 2002 in Nature Journal states: "Malaria may have killed half of all the people that ever lived" [1]. Despite the effort and funds spent on malaria eradication, it continues to infect approximately 200 million people worldwide every year and kill one in every four infected [2]. While effective in the past, current antimalarials are becoming less and less reliable as the parasite rapidly develops drug resistance [3]. There have been a number of extensive reviews covering the recent status of antimalarial research and parasite's resistance [3–11]. The shared message highlighted in these articles is that a constant supply of novel antimalarials is urgently required. Similarly to the Harlow-Knapp effect described for human kinase research [12], the majority of the antimalarial research is currently aimed at optimization of existing drugs targeting the known and validated pathways.

The currently used antimalarial drugs can be classified into few classes based on the mode of action [3, 7]. Briefly, the groups that receive the most attention of the researchers include the artemisinins and chloroquine-like compounds, which target the food vacuole and heme processing and detoxification [13, 14], antifolates targeting the mitochondrial dihydrofolate reductase (DHFR) and dihydropteroate synthase (DHPS), such as proguanil [15, 16], and mitochondrial inhibitors targeting the electron transport chain and consequently the pyrimidine biosynthesis. Unfortunately, resistance has been reported for nearly all available treatments [3, 7]. Unsurprisingly, compounds such as artemisinin and quinolines that target a broad range of essential pathways within the parasite have successfully been used for nearly 40 years before the widespread of resistance had been reported. In contrast, single-target drugs, such as antifolates and atovaquone, have lost their efficacy within few years of clinical use [11, 17]. A number of promising approaches to counter the fast emerging drug resistance suggested by Verlinden et al. include extension of combination therapy to three or more orthogonal drugs, development and use of multitargeting compounds interfering with unrelated targets, and deeper look into the unexplored alternative targets [3]. In all three cases, in order to successfully overcome the parasite's remarkable ability to develop resistance to nearly all drugs used against it, by far, a number of novel validated drug targets must be significantly expanded.

This chapter summarizes the pool of the mitochondrial and carbon metabolism targets that have been "under the spotlight" in recent years, as well as suggest a promising new avenue for the validation of novel drug targets. We will focus on the interplay between the pathways crucial for the parasite, such as pyrimidine biosynthesis, aspartate metabolism, and mitochondrial TCA cycle, in order to create a "road map" for further antimalarial drug development.

2. The Harlow-Knapp effect

A scientific analogue of biblical "The rich get richer and the poor get poorer" can be rephrased as "the propensity of the biomedical and pharmaceutical research communities to focus their activities, as quantified by the number of publications and patents, on a small fraction of the proteome" [12] or the "Harlow-Knapp effect." It was first noted by Harlow and colleagues [18] and further expanded by Knapp group [19], based on the analysis of the amount of publications and patents featuring human protein kinases. Kinases are known to regulate the majority of the cellular pathways including those involved in cancer and other diseases. It was observed that despite the availability of human kinome [20] more than three quarters of protein research was still focused on just 10 per cent of the kinases that were already known before the kinome publication [21]. Edwards and co-workers have also noticed that "the availability of research tools influences a protein's popularity." In other words, scientists tend to further explore the well-known systems, ignoring the less studied biomolecules where the probing tools are yet unavailable.

The availability of such tools for each system greatly limits the research opportunities and the attention to said system. Antimalarial research is not an exception to Harlow-Knapp effect: a limited opportunity for genetic manipulation [22] and complex life cycle of the parasite makes novel drug target validation highly challenging. Similarly to the human kinase research scientists tend to "keep looking under the spot light" among the few already validated targets, such as mitochondrial bc1 complex in malaria (target of the widely used Atovaquone), trying to optimize the existing compounds. Since first mentioned in the literature, there have been published more than 40 articles featuring plasmodial bc1 complex [23] and to the date it remains one of the most cited plasmodial enzyme.

Dihydroorotate dehydrogenase from *Plasmodium falciparum* (*Pf*DHODH) is another clear example of the Harlow-Knapp effect in antimalarial research. Since first proposed as a potential drug target more than a decade ago [24] and first inhibitors reported few years later [25], the major part of the research effort was focused on the optimization of the initial scaffold. In addition to the recent achievements in *Pf*DHODH inhibitor discovery by Phillips et al. [26], orthogonal methods, such as fragment-based drug design and virtual screening, have already yielded a number of very potent chemical scaffolds for this enzyme [27].

This divergent approach should be further exploited for other targets in order to yield novel and more potent scaffolds and support the antimalarial research.

3. Combinational therapy

The compound artemisinin and its derivatives have long been considered the most active and potent antimalarials for their efficacy against nearly all parasite stages [9, 14]. Artemisinins are believed to cause alkylation of proteins and heme and lead to oxidative damage within the parasite as well as affect the heme-related detoxification, although the exact mode of action is still a subject of debate [9, 14, 28]. Artemisinin-based combination therapy (ACT) is still recommended by World Health Organisation (WHO) for the treatment of uncomplicated falciparum and non-falciparum malaria in nearly all areas [7]. ACT implies the use of the fast acting artemisinin component, responsible for the rapid parasitemia clearance, in combination with another long-acting drug partner to eliminate the remaining parasites and suppress the selection of artemisinin resistance [29]. Despite the recent widespread of artemisinin-resistant falciparum malaria in Southeast Asia [30], the proven efficacy of combination therapy suggests that there is a pressing need for greater variety of highly effective antimalarial compounds. Combination of two or more drugs with different mode of action and resistance mechanisms significantly lowers the chances of the parasites to develop resistance to such treatment [31]. Thus, the research focus should be extended from optimization of existing compounds to development of novel research tools in order to explore and dissect other potentially druggable pathways of the parasite and thus bypass of the Harlow-Knapp effect. As stated by Verlinden et al.: "History has clearly indicated that new antimalarials must be continually developed in the ensuing event of resistance development to the current antimalarial arsenal." The occurrence of drug resistance in malaria is significantly faster than the development of antimalarials [3]. Thus, a constant supply of novel unrelated antimalarial compounds with orthogonal modes of action is urgently required.

4. The mitochondria as drug target for *P. falciparum* malaria

Mitochondria are organelles that act as the power plants of the cell, as they produce energy for all cellular activities. There are several molecular and functional differences between the mitochondria of *Plasmodium* species and those from the host. It is also known that the plasmodial mitochondria play a critical and essential role in the parasite's life cycle [5, 32, 33]. Previous studies have suggested that oxidative phosphorylation is not an essential pathway for parasite's survival during blood stage [34, 35]. In this stage, the parasite depends mainly on glycolysis as an energy source [36–38]. The observed glucose consumption in *P. falciparum*-infected red blood cells (RBC) was 75- to100-fold higher than in uninfected RBC [39]. Extraordinary glucose uptake during the infection leads to hypoglycemia, which together with an increased production of lactate and resulting lactic acidosis, are the major causes of mortality during severe malaria [40]. Thus, it is generally believed that the role of mitochondria in the parasite is not oxidative phosphorylation but the maintenance of the inner mitochondrial potential. Currently, the chemotherapeutic Malarone, a combination of mitochondrial *bc1* complex inhibitor Atovaquone and the dihydrofolate reductase inhibitor Proguanil, collapses the inner mitochondrial potential and induces parasite's growth arrest, confirming the mitochondrial metabolism to be crucial for the viability of the parasite. The importance of mitochondria for *Plasmodium* development in asexual stage is reinforced by the validation of another component of mitochondrial electron transport chain (ETC), dihydroorotate dehydrogenase (DHODH), as drug target [41, 42].

5. Electron transport chain (ETC)

The plasmodial mitochondrial electron transport chain (ETC) is composed of non-proton motive quinone reductases, such as dihydroorotate dehydrogenase (DHODH), malate-quinone oxidoreductase (MQO), glycerol 3-phosphate dehydrogenase (G3PDH), type II NADH dehydrogenase (NDH2, Alternative Complex I), and succinate dehydrogenase (SDH, Complex II), and proton motive respiratory complexes, including bc1 complex (Complex III), cytochrome *c* oxidase (Complex IV), and ATP synthase (Complex V) (**Figure 1**). The ETC requires ubiquinone (coenzyme Q) and *cytochrome c1* that function as electron carriers between the complexes [33, 44–47]. The (possible) roles of the ETC enzymes and their known inhibitors will be discussed in the following topics.

5.1. Dihydroorotate dehydrogenase (DHODH)

The *P. falciparum* enzyme dihydroorotate dehydrogenase (*Pf*DHODH) bridges the ETC and the pyrimidine biosynthesis; *Pf*DHODH catalyzes the key step of oxidation of dihydroorotate to orotate (a precursor for the biosynthesis of pyrimidine bases). The flavin mononucleotide (FMN)-dependent oxidation reaction catalyzed by DHODH can be divided in two half reactions: firstly, the oxidation of dihydroorotate through reduction of FMN and, secondly, the reoxidation of FMNH2 to regenerate the active enzyme. Two electrons resulting from this oxidation reaction are fed into the ETC through Flavin mononucleotide cofactor to

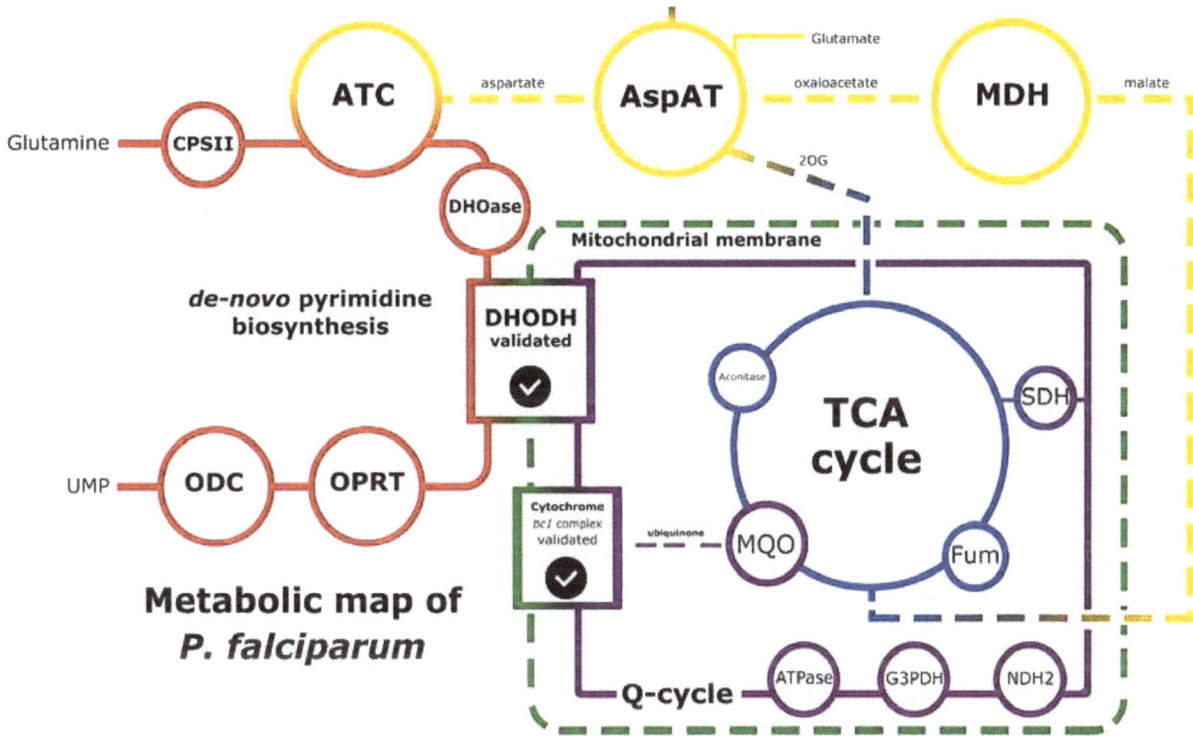

Figure 1. Suggested "roadmap" of essential metabolic processes of *Plasmodium falciparum* **such as pyrimidine biosynthesis, aspartate metabolism, and mitochondrial TCA cycle. The map includes already-validated drug targets** *Pf*DHODH **[24] and cytochrome** *bc1* **complex [23, 43], as well as other promising targets.**

ubiquinone, generated at the cytochrome bc1 complex, bridging pyrimidine metabolism and ETC [24, 48, 49]. Inhibition of *Pf*DHODH results in disruption of *de novo* biosynthesis of pyrimidines [48]. During the blood stage, the parasite depends strictly on this pathway for pyrimidine availability, which is essential for the formation of DNA, RNA, glycoproteins, and phospholipids [44].

Given the essential role of the *Pf*DHODH in the survivability of blood stage parasite and the significant differences to human DHODH [24], it is reasonable that the malarial enzyme has emerged as a novel validated drug target [26, 48, 50]. Inhibition of human DHODH was shown to be effective in treatment of autoimmune diseases, such as rheumatoid arthritis [51, 52]. The development of potent *h*DHODH inhibitors, such leflunomide and brequinar, led to the search of analogues with potential to inhibit plasmodial DHODH. These analogues were found to be poorly effective [53], potentially due to the differences in leflunomide and brequinar binding sites between human and plasmodial DHODH. These differences make *Pf*DHODH a potential species-specific drug target [24], which was extensively explored by a considerable number of studies. Although early research have not yielded effective results, the following studies have led to important achievements in the discovery of *Pf*DHODH inhibitors, such as benzimidazolyl thiophene-2-carboxamides [54–56], s-benzyltriazolopyrimidines [57], N-substituted salicylamides [58], trifluoromethyl phenyl butenamide derivatives [59], and triazolopyrimidine-based inhibitors [25, 60–64]. The triazolopyrimidine-based compound DSM265 was shown to be a potent inhibitor of the *Pf*DHODH and *Plasmodium vivax* DHODH

(*Pv*DHODH) with excellent selectivity versus *h*DHODH [48]. DSM265 has become the first DHODH inhibitor to enter the human antimalarial clinical trials, and preclinical development description was recently published, showing significant differences in DSM265 inhibitory activity between mammalian and plasmodial DHODHs. The kill rate of DSM265 for *in vitro* blood stage activity has shown to be similar to atovaquone, but significantly lower than observed for artemisinin and chloroquine. In addition, DSM265 has shown favorable pharmacokinetic properties, predicted to provide therapeutic concentrations for more than 8 days after a single oral dose in the range of 200–400 mg, what represents an advantage over current treatment options that are dosed daily. DSM265 was well tolerated in repeat dose, showed cardiovascular safety studies in mice and dogs, was not mutagenic, and was inactive against panels of human enzymes/receptors. Together, these data suggest that DSM265 has a high potential to be validated as a drug combination partner for either single-dose treatment or once-weekly chemoprevention [26].

5.2. Cytochrome bc1 (complex III)

The cytochrome bc1, also known as ubiquinol:cytochrome c oxidoreductase or complex III, is the only enzyme complex common to almost all respiratory ETCs [65]. This complex is composed of 11 different polypeptides, and its catalytic core is composed of three subunits, namely cytochrome b, cytochrome c1, and Rieske protein, also known as iron-sulfur protein (ISP) [66–68]. Cytochrome bc1 is found in the inner mitochondrial membrane and functions as a transporter of protons into the intermembrane space through the oxidation and reduction of ubiquinone in the Q cycle [67–70]. This enzymatic complex contains two distinct binding sites for the reduction and oxidation of ubiquinol and ubiquinone, both located within cytochrome b. The Qo site acts to oxidize ubiquinol near the intermembrane space, whereas the Qi site binds and reduces ubiquinone near the mitochondrial matrix [71, 72].

Although the crystal structure of plasmodial bc1 complex has not been solved, the high degree of sequence homology with other organisms of which the X-ray crystal structure is known (e.g. *Saccharomyces cerevisiae* [73]), allowed the discovery of many inhibitors. Cytochrome bc1 of *Plasmodium* is in fact a major drug target for the treatment and prevention of malaria and, to date, is the only component of the ETC with a clinically used antimalarial drug association [23, 43]. The compound atovaquone, a hydroxynaphthoquinone, inhibits cytochrome bc1 by binding to the Qo site. This inhibition leads to parasite death through the collapse of the *Plasmodium* mitochondrial membrane potential with no effect on the mammalian host [42, 74, 75]. Although atovaquone is a potent plasmodial bc1 complex inhibitor, its clinical utility is limited by the rapid emergence of resistant parasites when used as monotherapy [76]. Resistance to atovaquone has been developed due to mutations in the codon 268 (Y268S/C/N). These mutations affect the binding of the atovaquone to the target [77]. Because of that, atovaquone is used together with proguanil (Malarone) for treating uncomplicated malaria or as chemoprophylaxis for preventing malaria in travellers.

Aside of atovaquone, other bc1 complex inhibitors were described, as acridones [78], quinolones [79–81], pyridones [82, 83], and benzene sulfonamides [84]. Although many compounds have presented inhibitory potential against bc1 complex, this target might be considered underexploited, since the majority of these compounds target the Qo site [85]. The Qi site of cytochrome bc1 has been far less explored and only the binding of a few compounds has been reported [86–89].

5.3. Type II NADH dehydrogenase (NDH2)

Instead of the canonical multimeric complex I, or NADH:dehydrogenase, found in mammalian mitochondria, the *Plasmodium* ETC possesses the type II NADH:quinone oxidoreductase (NDH2). This enzyme, also known as alternative complex I, is a five quinone-dependent oxidoreductase enzyme involved in the redox reaction of NADH oxidation with subsequent quinol production [90]. Although the activity of NDH2 is still not biochemically confirmed in *P. falciparum*, it has been described in some detail for other organisms that also possess the type II NADH:quinone oxidoreductase, such as plants, fungi, and bacteria [91–96]. Differently from complex I, NDH2 is not involved in the direct pumping of protons across the membrane. Instead of proton pumping, NDH2 enables the H+-unregulated generation of mitochondrial reducing power supplying the various respiratory chains with reducing equivalents from NAD(P)H [45, 90].

So far, no crystal structure of the *P. falciparum* NDH2 (*Pf*NDH2) is available, and prediction of *Pf*NDH2 is based on sequence and structural similarities to other redox enzymes [45, 91, 97]. Although reverse genetics of *Pf*NDH2 was shown to be not lethal [98], *Pf*NDH2 was described as a putative "choke point" in the mitochondrial ETC and has been highlighted as a potential target for antimalarial development [45, 90, 99]. Given the lack of structural data for *Pf*NDH2 and its poor homology to any other structure in PDB, the existing studies aiming to inhibit *Pf*NDH2 for "druggable" proposes have used chemoinformatics and virtual screening methods. *Pf*NDH2 (as other NDH2 analogues) has shown to be insensitive to rotenone, a well-known inhibitor of complex I [90, 100]. The compound 1-hydroxy-2-dodecyl-4(1H)quinolone (HDQ), initially identified as an inhibitor of yeast NDH2 [101], was reported to be a potent inhibitor of *P. falciparum* proliferation [102]. In fact, HDQ inhibits *Pf*NDH2 but, in addition, it disrupts mitochondrial function through the potent inhibition of the bc1 complex [103]. The compounds dibenziodolium chloride (DPI) and diphenyliodonium chloride (IDP) have also been reported to inhibit *Pf*NDH2 activity in crude lysate fractions and both have shown efficacy against whole parasite proliferation [90]. However, a further study put the potential of *Pf*NDH2 inhibition by these compounds into question, since the authors were unable to corroborate the previous findings through dose-effect profiles using purified recombinant *Pf*NDH2 [100]. These results suggest that DPI and IDP may not be effective inhibitors of *Pf*NDH2, but their antiparasitic effect might be attributed to other enzymes instead (*e.g. Pf*DHODH) [100]. Inhibition of *Pf*NDH2 by artemisinin has also been demonstrated, suggesting a dual role for mitochondria in the action of artemisinin [104]. More recently, Antoine et al. [105] demonstrated that the low degree of inhibition of this enzyme by artemisinin indicates a non-ETC mode of action.

In more recent efforts, Biagini et al. [81] undertook a high-throughput screen (HTS) against *Pf*NDH2 using HDQ in combination with a range of chemoinformatics as starting point. This approach led to the selection of the quinolone core as the key target for SAR, followed by the selection of CK-2-68 as a lead for further development [81, 106]. Structural alterations aiming to improve the inhibitory activity and aqueous solubility led to the compounds SL-2-64 and SL-2-25, the last presenting activity against *Pf*NDH2 and whole-cell *P. falciparum* at nanomolar range. *In vivo* experiments using *Plasmodium berghei*-infected mice demonstrated that SL-2-25 was able to clear parasitemia in the Peters' standard 4-day suppressive test when given orally a dose of 20 mg kg^{-1} [107]. SL-2-25, as other quinolones in this study, had the ability to inhibit both *Pf*NDH2 and cytochrome bc1 at low nanomolar range, the same dual inhibition previously observed for HDQ. This dual targeting of two key mitochondrial enzymes suggests that the quinolone pharmacophore is a privileged scaffold for inhibition of both drug targets.

Although the recent efforts to inhibit NDH2 with antimalarial purposes have been a good improvement in the knowledge of its potential as a drug target, the report of *Pf*NDH2 crystal structure would allow a deep investigation on both biochemical characterization and drug design targeting *Pf*NDH2.

5.4. Mitochondrial glycerol-3-phosphate dehydrogenase (mG3DH)

Mitochondrial glycerol 3-phosphate dehydrogenase (mG3DH) is a ubiquinone-linked flavo-protein embedded in the mitochondrial inner membrane that transfers reducing equivalents directly from glycerol 3-phosphate into the electron transport chain [108, 109]. The *P. falciparum* genome has homologues of both cytoplasmic and mitochondrial G3DH and assays indicate that the addition of glycerol-3-phosphate stimulates electron transport through the inner membrane [110–112]. Together with NDH2, mitochondrial G3DH from *P. falciparum* (*Pf*mG3DH) is also suggested to play an important role in the redox balance under conditions of low O$_2$. Further studies might clarify the essentiality of mG3PDH in *Plasmodium* survivability and also evaluate its potential as a drug target.

5.5. Succinate dehydrogenase (SDH)

The succinate dehydrogenase (SDH), also known as succinate: ubiquinone oxidoreductase (SQO) or complex II, is an enzymatic complex involved in both TCA cycle, functioning as a primary dehydrogenase, and in mitochondrial ETC, functioning as electron donor [113]. This dual role makes SDH a direct connection between major systems in aerobic energy metabolism. The enzyme has been isolated and characterized from prokaryotic [114–117] and eukaryotic organisms [118–121], including *P. falciparum* [122, 123]. SDH is located in the cytoplasmic membrane in bacteria [124] and in the mitochondrial inner membrane in eukaryotes [125]. The enzymatic complex is highly conserved and is basically composed of four subunits: a flavoprotein subunit (SDH1) and an iron-sulfur subunit (SDH2) together form a soluble heterodimer that binds to a membrane anchor b-type cytochrome (a CybL (SDH3)/CybS (SDH4) heterodimer). In *P. falciparum*, the two major subunits possess molecular masses of 55 kDa (Fp, flavoprotein subunit) and 35 kDa (Ip, iron-sulfur protein subunit) [122]. The SDH activity has shown to be essential for *Plasmodium* survivability, what makes this enzyme an attractive target for antimalarial development. The already reported differences in kinetic properties between *P. falciparum* SDH (*Pf*SDH) and human SDH increase the probability that *Pf*SDH inhibitors might represent potent and selective antimalarial compounds [122]. In fact, SDH has shown sensitivity to a number of inhibitors, such as 5-substituted 2,3-dimethoxy-6-phytyl-1,4-benzoquinone derivatives, plumbagin and licochalcone [125], but so far, inhibitors with potential for antimalarial development still have to be discovered.

5.6. Malate-quinone oxyreductase (MQO)

The malate-quinone oxidoreductase (MQO) is a peripheral membrane-bound flavoprotein, which catalyzes the oxidation of malate to oxaloacetate, reducing ubiquinone [126]. *Plasmodium* species possesses a group 2 MQO, in contrast to bacterial group 1 MQO [127]. *P. falciparum* MQO (*Pf*MQO) is part of both mitochondrial ETC and TCA cycle, substituting other mitochondrial malate dehydrogenases (MDH) [111, 112, 128]. To date, no crystal structure of the *Plasmodium* MQO or inhibition studies are available. However, recent experiments showed that while knockout of six enzymes of plasmodial TCA cycle did not cause any significant growth inhibition, no viable MQO-knockout strains of *P. falciparum* could be obtained yet [34]. These findings as well as the absence of MQO in the human host make the enzyme an interesting target for antimalarial drug discovery.

5.7. ATPase

Although malaria parasites generate most of their ATP through aerobic glycolysis during the blood stage of their life cycle, they appear to possess a complete ATP synthase complex [47]. *P. falciparum* ATP synthase (*Pf*ATP synthase) is not reported to generate ATP but is suggested to act as a proton leak for the ETC [46, 47]. The use of bedaquiline, TMC207, has been proven to be effective for the treatment of multidrug-resistant tuberculosis. This compound targets *Mycobacterium tuberculosis* ETC through inhibition of ATP synthase rising the hypothesis that this may also be a valid drug target for malaria in the future [129]. So far, only one *Pf*ATP synthase inhibitor was described. The compound almitrine, originally developed as a respiratory stimulant, has activity against *Pf*ATP synthase and at the cellular level [130]. Recently, a genetic study demonstrated that mitochondrial ATP synthase is dispensable in blood stage *P. berghei*, although is essential in the mosquito phase [131]. For *P. falciparum*, previous attempts to knock out the mitochondrial ATP synthase subunits were unsuccessful, suggesting an essential role played by this enzyme complex in blood stages of the parasite [47]. The difference in essentiality of ATP synthase between *P. falciparum* and *P. berghei* could be explained by a possible distinction in the requirements of the two species for ATP [131]. Still, more studies are needed to define whether or not ATP synthase is essential in *P. falciparum* blood stage and consequently evaluate its potential as antimalarial target.

6. Tricarboxylic acid (TCA) cycle

While *Plasmodium* relies mainly on glycolysis during the blood stage, the TCA metabolism does occur in asexual *Plasmodium*, but at low turnover [35]. The exact function of the plasmodial TCA cycle is still a subject of debate, as it does not seem to function like a conventional TCA cycle. In 2010, a branched TCA pathway has been suggested for the parasite [132] but further retracted [133]. It was proposed that plasmodial TCA enzymes function not only in the classical but also in the reverse direction, generating either reductive or an oxidative pathway, depending on the direction. Both pathways would result in the generation of malate, which is subsequently exported from the mitochondria, with α-ketoglutarate (2OG) being anti-ported to feed both the oxidative and reductive pathways [132]. Depending on the nutrient availability, *Plasmodium* species might not excrete malate as metabolic waste, utilizing it for metabolic purposes [134].

Further metabolomic studies suggest that *P. falciparum* utilizes conventional TCA cycle during both sexual and asexual blood stages [35]. Functional respiratory chain appears to be essential for the maintenance of inner mitochondrial membrane potential as well as protein and metab-olite transport within the mitochondrion. The authors have also reported an increased sensi-tivity of gametocyte stages to sodium fluoroacetate (NaFAc). NaFAc was previously reported to inhibit TCA cycle enzyme aconitase in *Leishmania* [135]. Both sexual and asexual cultures of *P. falciparum* treated with 1 mM NaFAc showed significant citrate accumulation in the para-site as well as decrease in downstream TCA metabolites, suggesting the specific inhibition of aconitase of *P. falciparum*. However, no significant growth inhibition of the asexual para-sites was observed, while gametocyte development was significantly reduced. These findings provide a potential for future transmission-blocking therapy.

Recently, Ke et al. [34] reported significant flexibility in TCA cycle metabolism of *P. falci-parum*. The knockout experiments with all TCA cycle enzymes showed altered substrate fluxes between mitochondrial and cytosolic pools in nearly all cases. Out of eight enzymes of the TCA cycle, knockout of six enzymes of the TCA cycle showed no detectable growth defects. However, the authors were unable to disrupt the genes encoding fumarate hydratase and malate-quinone oxyreductase, suggesting potentially essential role of these two enzymes in asexual parasite development.

Although the fully functional TCA cycle appears to be dispensable for parasite survival in asexual blood stages [34], the interplay of some TCA enzymes with other essential pathways still represents an interesting target for antimalarial drug development. Below, we describe the role of three enzymes (aspartate aminotransferase, malate dehydrogenase, and fumarate hydratase) in *Plasmodium* metabolism and also their potential for antimalarial drug discovery. Other enzymes involved in this pathway (e.g., *Pf*SDH, *Pf*MQO) were previously described within the ETC section (see above).

6.1. Aspartate aminotransferase

The enzyme aspartate aminotransferase (AspAT) catalyzes the reversible reaction of L-aspar-tate and α-ketoglutarate into oxaloacetate and L-glutamate. The AspAT from *P. falciparum* (*Pf*AspAT) was placed into the Ia subfamily, being the most divergent member of this group. The crystal structure of *Pf*AspAT reveals an architecture similar to that previously determined in the *Escherichia coli* (1B4X14–17) [136–139], yeast cytosolic [140], pig heart cyto-solic [141], and mitochondrial and cytosolic chicken [142–144] homologues. *Pf*AspAT is a homodimeric enzyme [145, 146], and each subunit consists of a large PLP (cofactor) binding domain, a smaller domain, that shifts the enzyme from "closed" to "open" form in order to provide substrate binding and N-terminal region that stabilizes the interaction between the two monomers into a dimer [142, 147, 148]. Two independent active sites are positioned near the oligomeric interface and are formed by residues from both subunits [146]. The active site is highly conserved between available AspATs, making the design of species-specific inhibitors very challenging. However, it is known that the active site requires the formation of a homodimer, and analysis of AspAT has highlighted the N-terminal region as being highly divergent from other AspAT family members in both sequence and structure [145, 146]. Such a divergence may allow a more specific interference with the parasitic AspAT oligomeric surfaces, which offers a unique opportunity to generate highly specific interference with protein function *in vivo*. Such an approach will be further discussed in this chapter.

6.2. Malate dehydrogenase

The enzyme malate dehydrogenase (MDH) catalyzes the reversible NAD(P)+-dependent oxidation of oxaloacetate to malate. Like other members of the NAD+-dependent dehydrogenase family, the MDHs possess two functional domains, the catalytic domain and the NAD+-binding domain. Protozoan MDHs are differentiated into two subdivisions: mitochondrial and cytosolic MDHs, the first being part of the TCA cycle, providing oxaloacetate for the generation of citrate and NADH to fuel the mitochondrial electron-transport chain. The mitochondrial MDH is absent in *P. falciparum*, being replaced by *Pf*MQO (described in ETC section). The cytosolic MDH is present in *P. falciparum* (*Pf*MDH) acting as a supplier of metabolites, such as malate, to the mitochondria and might be responsible for the generation of reducing equivalents to feed the respiratory chain [149].

The crystal structure of *Pf*MDH has recently been solved [150]. Analysis of *Pf*MDH structure revealed a tetrameric assembly, although isoforms of the enzyme from other species have been reported to be present as either dimers or tetramers. Similar to *Pf*AspAT, the oligomeric nature of *Pf*MDH and the low degree of evolutionally conservation of the oligomeric interface residues provide an opportunity for a highly specific protein interference approach (described further).

6.3. Fumarate hydratase

Fumarate hydratase (FH) is an enzyme that catalyzes the reversible conversion of fumarate to malate. Although *P. falciparum* contains a fumarate hydratase homologue (*Pf*FH), it differs substantially from the "class II" type enzyme found in yeast and mammalian cells [151, 152]. Instead, the *Pf*FH resembles the iron-sulfur-containing "class I"-type enzymes found in some bacteria and archaea [153]. *Pf*FH was shown to be essential to the asexual stages of the parasite [34]. *Pf*FH was initially suggested to be located within the mitochondrion [153], however, this localization is yet not entirely clear.

Fumarate is a side product of the purine salvage pathway and acts as metabolic intermediate of the TCA cycle. As previously mentioned, *P. falciparum* does not export fumarate as metabolic waste but converts the metabolite to aspartate through malate and oxaloacetate. Besides, *P. falciparum*-infected erythrocytes and free parasites incorporate labeled fumarate into the nucleic acid and protein fractions [153]. Taken together, these data provide a biosynthetic function for fumarate hydratase and suggest that this enzyme could therefore be targeted for the development of antimalarial chemotherapeutics.

7. Pyrimidine biosynthetic pathway

A key-step for spreading of malaria parasites in the human host is the extensive and rapid replication of parasite DNA, which depends on the availability of essential metabolites, such as pyrimidines [154, 155]. In the *Plasmodium* species, besides the DNA, the pyrimidine nucleotide is also involved in the biosynthesis of RNA, phospholipids, and glycoproteins [155–157]. Sequencing studies have revealed that, in malaria parasites, the genes encoding for the pyrimidine biosynthetic pathway enzymes have been conserved, whereas those responsible for pyrimidines salvage have not [158]. It means that, while human cells are able to acquire pyrimidines either through *de novo* synthesis or by salvaging, the malaria parasites lack pyrimidine salvage enzymes and depend exclusively on the *de novo* pathway as source of pyrimidines for their survival [5, 33]. *De novo* synthesis from carbamoyl phosphate and aspartic acid follows basically the same steps found in the human host and in other eukaryotes: orotic acid is formed by dihydroorotase (DHOase) and DHODH. The orotic acid is so turned into orotidine 5'-monophosphate (OMP) by addition to 5'-phospo-D-ribosyl-α-1-pyrophosphate, a step carried out by orotate phosphoribosyltransferase (OPRT). OMP is subsequently decarboxylated to uridine 5'-monophosphate (UMP), the precursor of all other pyrimidine nucleotides and deoxynucleotides needed for nucleic acid synthesis [159]. Excepting for *Pf*DHODH, which is discussed in the ETC topic, the enzymes involved in *de novo* pyrimidine biosynthesis pathway that could potentially be exploited for the discovery of novel antimalarials as discussed below.

7.1. Carbamoyl phosphate synthetase II

Carbamoyl phosphate synthetase II (CPSII) is responsible for the first step of the *de novo* pyrimidine biosynthesis, catalyzing the formation of carbamoyl phosphate in the cytosol from bicarbonate, glutamine, and ATP [160]. Differently from the human CPSII, CPSII from *P. falciparum* (*Pf*CPSII) is a monofunctional protein [155]. *Pf*CPSII also differs from its mammalian homologue by the presence of two inserted sequences, located between junctions of the glutamine aminotransferase and synthetase domains [161]. Although the absence of structural information and activity inhibitors, the druggable potential of this enzyme has already been demonstrated by the potent growth inhibitory effect of a synthetic ribozyme with specificity for the *Pf*CPSII gene over *P. falciparum* cultures [162]. The same synthetic ribozyme has shown no toxicity to mammalian cells. Other mini ribozymes were further redesigned to improve cleavage activities and metabolic stabilities [163]. These results suggest that the discover of compounds capable to inhibit *Pf*CPSII in a specific way might be promising antimalarial candidates, since ribozyme approaches have a significant more challenging application due to target accessibility, stability, specificity, and delivery efficiency [164].

7.2. Aspartate transcarbamoylase (ATC)

Aspartate transcarbamoylase (ATC, EC 2.1.3.2) catalyzes the condensation of aspartate and carbamoyl phosphate to form N-carbamoyl-L-aspartate and inorganic phosphate. Previous studies with human tumor tissues showed significantly elevated levels of ATC nearly in all samples [165]. In *P. falciparum*, ATC is also present as monofunctional protein, unlike its human homologue. Although a number of publications suggest ATC from *P. falciparum* to be a promising drug target [166–168], it has not been fully characterized and no inhibitors have yet been reported. Recently reported crystal structure of the truncated *Pf*ATC revealed high level of sequence conservation among homologous enzymes from other organisms, especially in the active site area [169].

7.3. Dihydroorotase

Similarly to CPSII, *P. falciparum* dihydroorotase (*Pf*DHOase) is a monofunctional protein and thus differs from the mammalian host, in which the 36.7 kDa enzyme is located on the central part of the 240 kDa CAD multifunctional protein [170]. This enzyme catalyzes the reversible cyclization of N-carbamoyl-L-aspartate (CA-asp) to L-dihydroorotate (L-DHO) [159]. Orotate and a series of 5-substituted derivatives were found to inhibit competitively the purified enzyme from *P. falciparum* culture. In mice infected with *P. berghei*, 5-fluoro orotate and 5-amino orotate at a dose of 25 µg/g body weight eliminated parasitemia after a 4-day treatment, an effect comparable to that of the same dose of chloroquine. The infected mice treated with 5-fluoro orotate at a lower dose of 2.5 µg/g had a 95% reduction in parasitemia [171]. The moderate inhibition of *Pf*DHOase by L-6-thiodihydroorotate (TDHO) in cultured parasites induced major accumulation of CP-asp and growth arrest, similar to atovaquone [172]. The analysis of physical, kinetic, and inhibitory properties of the recombinant *Pf*DHOase performed by Krungkrai et al. suggests that specific inhibitors may limit the pyrimidine nucleotide pool in the parasite, but have no significant adverse effect to human host [173]. Although the low amount of information about *Pf*DHOase does not allow to confirm it as a good candidate to antimalarial development, the report of its crystal structure and biochemical characterization could clarify whether this enzyme is essential or not to the parasite's survivability.

7.4. Orotate phosphoribosyl transferase and orotidine 5′-monophosphate decarboxylase

The last two steps of the pyrimidine biosynthesis in *P. falciparum* are catalyzed by a heteromeric complex that consists of two homodimers of *Pf*OPRT and *Pf*OPDC encoded by two separate genes [174, 175].

The enzyme orotate phosphoribosyl transferase (OPRT) catalyzes the formation of orotidine 5′-monophosphate (OMP) from α-D-phosphoribosyl pyrophosphate (PRPP) and orotate, the fifth step of the pyrimidine biosynthesis [155]. The OPRT inhibitors reported so far includes the compound 5′-Fluoroorotate, an alternative substrate for this enzyme that was shown to inhibit the *in vitro* growth of *P. falciparum* at nanomolar range [176, 177] and to clear parasitemia from *P. berghei*-infected mice [171]. This antimalarial activity is related to the inactivation of malarial thymidylate synthase by 5′-fluoro-2′-deoxy-UMP metabolite through covalent binding to methylene tetrahydrofolate at the active site. The compound pyrazofurin has also been described as a moderate inhibitor of *P. falciparum* OPRT (*Pf*OPRT), inhibiting its activity at micromolar range by blocking the maturation of trophozoites to schizonts [176, 178]. Interestingly, pyrazofurin does not affect the OPRT activity in mammalian cells [179].

A recent study of the transition state analogues of *Pf*OPRT also showed that despite the tight binding *in vitro*, the synthetized compounds failed to inhibit the parasite culture growth *in vivo* [180–182]. No growth inhibition was observed at high compound concentrations up to 100 μM, suggesting poor compound accessibility *in vivo*.

Recently, the crystal structure of *Pf*OPRT has been reported, which shows a homodimeric assembly, where each of two active sites include amino acids from both chains [183]. Despite the high level of homology with human OPRT, the active site of *Pf*OPRT has few amino acids that differ from *Hs*OPRT. The authors suggest that these differences might lead to the design of selective substrate-like inhibitors in the future.

Orotidine 5′-monophosphate decarboxylase (OPDC) catalyzes the final step of *de novo* pyrimidine biosynthesis pathway, the decarboxylation of orotidine 5′-monophosphate (OMP) to uridine 5′-monophosphate (UMP), with no need for the presence of a cofactor or metal ion [184]. Many inhibitors of plasmodial OPDC have been described so far, being the most promising inhibitor, the nucleotide 5′-monophosphate analogue xanthosine 5′-monophosphate (XMP) [185]. XMP acts as a competitive inhibitor with tighter binding than OMP. The *P. falciparum* OPDC inhibition by XMP is highly selective, having a 150-fold preference for the malarial enzyme compared to human OPDC. Other inhibitors include the 6-iodouridine 5′-monophosphate (6-iodo-UMP) [186], 6-azidouridine 5′-monophosphate (6-N3-UMP) [187], barbiturate 5′-monophosphate (BMP) [185], 6-N-methylamino uridine [187], and 6-N,N-dimethylamino uridine [187]. Although a considerable number of *Pf*ODC inhibitors have been described and a crystal structure of *Pf*OPDC is available [188], a deeper investigation is necessary to clarify *Pf*OPDC as validated drug target.

8. Protein interference assay (PIA) as drug validation tool

We have recently proposed a novel promising drug-target validation approach that relies on common feature of all biological systems—oligomerization [22]. Oligomerization is a self-assembly of two or more copies of one protein molecule (or different molecules) into one object. Recent analysis shows that majority (60%) of non-redundant protein structures available in the Protein Data Bank (PDB) represent dimerization or higher oligomerization order (Hashimoto *et al.*, 2011). In many cases, the biological activity of a protein complex is dependent on correct oligomeric order. Oligomerization may be required for a number of reasons, including the correct active site or cofactor binding site assembly on the oligomeric interface or allosteric regulation. Examples where dimerization is crucial for the formation of active sites on the oligomeric interface include previously mentioned aspartate aminotransferase (AspAT) [22], aspartate transcarbamoylase (ATC), and orotate phosphoribosyl transferase (*Pf*OPRT) [183] from *P. falciparum*. In addition, the physiological assembly of *Pf*OPRT/*Pf*OPDC heterotetramer was shown to be more effective compared to the monofunctional enzymes [189]. A number of recent publications also suggest that the protein oligomerization to be a key driving force in evolution [190–194].

Another important aspect of oligomerization is remarkable selectivity and binding affinity. Large surface area of the intraoligomeric interfaces and evolutionary diversity allow oligomeric partners selectively bind to each other with no cross-reactivity in the system. In majority of cases, purification of oligomeric proteins from both native and recombinant sources can be performed without any foreign protein incorporations in the assembly. Unlike the active sites and cofactor binding sites where evolutionary constraints restrict the sequence diversity to retain the function, oligomeric interfaces are significantly less conserved among homologous proteins [195, 196]. Thus, small molecule compounds reacting with the conserved active site of target enzyme of the parasite will likely interact with the host's homologous enzyme.

Direct interference with protein self-assembly would provide an opportunity for a highly selective modulation of protein activity or function both *in vitro* and *in vivo*.

9. Making (breaking) bad proteins

The recently proposed protein interference assay (PIA) [22] involves the utilization of structural knowledge (data) and mutagenic modification of one (or more) partner proteins in the assembly. These modifications may affect the binding site for a cofactor, catalytic activity, or disrupt the oligomeric interface of the target protein. Thus, recombinant and, most importantly, controlled co-expression of both wild type and its inactive (hyperactive) mutant would allow the formation of the complex with modified activity *in vitro*.

Previously mentioned homodimeric *Pf*OPRT, as part of the *Pf*OPRT/*Pf*ORDC heterotetramer, could also be a subject to PIA. The active sites of *Pf*OPRT were reported to contain the amino acids from both subunits, suggesting that introduction of the active site mutants with modified activity *in vivo* would also affect the native *Pf*OPRT. This assay would potentially bypass previously observed difficulties with poor inhibitor accessibility and aid in validation of the enzyme as antimalarial drug target.

Despite the obvious limitation of PIA approach to oligomeric proteins, this assay would still allow partial assessment of the system of interest, as many of the studied pathways are likely to involve at least one oligomeric assembly. We suggest that PIA would also allow re-evaluation of the previously studied promising targets where conventional validation approaches have failed.

10. Conclusion

In order to assess a gene's product role, one must possess a set of tools, such as genetic manipulations (e.g. knockout, silencing etc.), to modulate the target function *in vivo*. Sufficient specificity (with little or no cross-reactivity) is essential for correct interpretation of the data.

Although genetic manipulations have been proven to be highly effective in model and fully defined systems, less studied and complex systems remain highly challenging. In many pathogenic systems, including human malaria, conventional genetic manipulation techniques or small molecule inhibitor approaches do not always provide the desired efficacy [22]. In a number of human pathogens, multiple life cycle stages in different hosts and vectors make both *in vitro* and *in vivo* target characterization challenging to approach. A number of classic techniques such as silencing RNA [197, 198] have already been reported to be non-effective in certain cases [199–202].

In addition, the use of small molecule inhibitor approaches *in vivo* is associated with high costs and is often limited due to the variety of host-specific reasons that are difficult to predict, such as rapid metabolism, poor membrane transport, or localization. For example, while a number of compounds were reported to inhibit *Pf*OPRT activity *in vitro* as well as clear parasitemia in *P. berghei*-infected mice, *in vivo* trials with *P. falciparum* have failed [180]. Thus, potential drug targets may remain unexplored due to the inability to use the existing validation tool set.

Insufficient amount of effective target validation tools significantly limits the understanding of human pathogenic systems and hinders the rate of novel drug development. A constant supply of robust and effective techniques is needed in order to successfully dissect yet unexplored parasitic pathways, provide the basis for rational drug design, and counter-balance the ability of many human pathogens to rapidly develop drug resistance. We believe that protein interference assay (PIA) will enrich the currently available research toolset.

Authvor details

Sergey Lunev[1†], Fernando A. Batista[1†], Soraya S. Bosch[2], Carsten Wrenger[2] and Matthew R. Groves[1]*

* Corresponding author E-mail: m.r.groves@rug.nl

1 Department of Drug Design, Groningen Research Institute of Pharmacy, University of Groningen, Groningen, The Netherlands

2 Unit for Drug Discovery, Department of Parasitology, Institute of Biomedical Sciences, University of São Paulo, São Paulo, SP, Brazil

† These authors contributed equally

References

[1] Whitfield J. Portrait of a serial killer. Nature News (2002), http://www.nature.com/news/2002/021003/full/news021001-6.html.

[2] WHO. World Malaria Report. World Health Organisation. 2015 (Geneva, Switzerland).

[3] Verlinden BK, Louw A, Birkholtz LM. Resisting resistance: is there a solution for malaria? Expert Opin Drug Discov. 2016;11(4):395-406.

[4] Muller IB, Hyde JE. Antimalarial drugs: modes of action and mechanisms of parasite resistance. Future Microbiol. 2010;5(12):1857-1873.

[5] Rodrigues T, Lopes F, Moreira R. Inhibitors of the mitochondrial electron transport chain and de novo pyrimidine biosynthesis as antimalarials: The present status. Curr Med Chem. 2010;17(10):929-956.

[6] Biamonte MA, Wanner J, Le Roch KG. Recent advances in malaria drug discovery. Bioorg Med Chem Lett. 2013;23(10):2829-2843.

[7] Cui L, Mharakurwa S, Ndiaye D, Rathod PK, Rosenthal PJ. Antimalarial drug resistance: literature review and activities and findings of the ICEMR Network. Am J Trop Med Hyg (2015). Vol 93(3 Suppl): 57–68.

[8] Mbengue A, Bhattacharjee S, Pandharkar T, Liu H, Estiu G, Stahelin RV, et al. A molecular mechanism of artemisinin resistance in *Plasmodium falciparum* malaria. Nature. 2015;520(7549):683-687.

[9] Paloque L, Ramadani AP, Mercereau-Puijalon O, Augereau JM, Benoit-Vical F. *Plasmodium falciparum*: multifaceted resistance to artemisinins. Malar J. 2016;15(1):149.

[10] Avitia-Domínguez C, Sierra-Campos E, Betancourt-Conde I, Aguirre-Raudry M, Vázquez-Raygoza A, Luevano-De la Cruz A, et al. Targeting plasmodium metabolism to improve antimalarial drug design. Curr Protein Pept Sci. 2016;17(3):260-274.

[11] Wells TN, Hooft van Huijsduijnen R, VanVoorhis WC. Malaria medicines: a glass half full? Nat Rev Drug Discov. 2015;14(6):424-442.

[12] Isserlin R, Bader GD, Edwards A, Frye S, Willson T, Yu FH. The human genome and drug discovery after a decade. Roads (still) not taken. arXiv (2011) arXiv:1102.0448 [q-bio.OT].

[13] Fitch CD. Ferriprotoporphyrin IX, phospholipids, and the antimalarial actions of quinoline drugs. Life Sci. 2004;74(16):1957-1972.

[14] Cui L, Su XZ. Discovery, mechanisms of action and combination therapy of artemisinin. Expert Rev Anti Infect Ther. 2009;7(8):999-1013.

[15] Carrington HC, Crowther AF, Davey DG, Levi AA, Rose FL. A metabolite of paludrine with high antimalarial activity. Nature. 1951;168(4288):1080.

[16] Crowther AF, Levi AA. Proguanil, the isolation of a metabolite with high antimalarial activity. Br J Pharmacol Chemother. 1953;8(1):93-97.

[17] Muregi FW. Antimalarial drugs and their useful therapeutic lives: rational drug design lessons from pleiotropic action of quinolines and artemisinins. Curr Drug Discov Technol. 2010;7(4):280-316.

[18] Grueneberg DA, Degot S, Pearlberg J, Li W, Davies JE, Baldwin A, et al. Kinase requirements in human cells: I. Comparing kinase requirements across various cell types. Proc Natl Acad Sci U S A. 2008;105(43):16472-16477.

[19] Fedorov O, Müller S, Knapp S. The (un)targeted cancer kinome. Nat Chem Biol. 2010;6(3):166-169.

[20] Manning G, Whyte DB, Martinez R, Hunter T, Sudarsanam S. The protein kinase complement of the human genome. Science. 2002;298(5600):1912-1934.

[21] Edwards AM, Isserlin R, Bader GD, Frye SV, Willson TM, Yu FH. Too many roads not taken. Nature. 2011;470(7333):163-165.

[22] Meissner KA, Lunev S, Wang YZ, Linzke M, de Assis Batista F, Wrenger C, et al. Drug target validation methods in malaria—Protein interference assay (PIA) as a tool for highly specific drug target validation. Curr Drug Targets (2016). (in press).

[23] Fry M, Pudney M. Site of action of the antimalarial hydroxynaphthoquinone, 2-[trans-4-(4'-chlorophenyl) cyclohexyl]-3-hydroxy-1,4-naphthoquinone (566C80). Biochemical Pharmacology. 1992;43(7):1545-1553.

[24] Baldwin J, Farajallah AM, Malmquist NA, Rathod PK, Phillips MA. Malarial dihydroorotate dehydrogenase. Substrate and inhibitor specificity. J Biol Chem. 2002;277(44):41827-41834.

[25] Baldwin J, Michnoff CH, Malmquist NA, White J, Roth MG, Rathod PK, et al. High-throughput screening for potent and selective inhibitors of *Plasmodium falciparum* dihydroorotate dehydrogenase. J Biol Chem. 2005;280(23):21847-21853.

[26] Phillips MA, Lotharius J, Marsh K, White J, Dayan A, White KL, et al. A long-duration dihydroorotate dehydrogenase inhibitor (DSM265) for prevention and treatment of malaria. Sci Transl Med. 2015;7(296):296ra111.

[27] Pavadai E, El Mazouni F, Wittlin S, de Kock C, Phillips MA, Chibale K. Identification of new human malaria parasite Plasmodium falciparum dihydroorotate dehydrogenase inhibitors by pharmacophore and structure-based virtual screening. J Chem Inf Model. (2016). Vol 56(3):548-62.

[28] Robert A, Benoit-Vical F, Claparols C, Meunier B. The antimalarial drug artemisinin alkylates heme in infected mice. Proc Natl Acad Sci U S A. 2005;102(38):13676-13680.

[29] Nosten F, White NJ. Artemisinin-based combination treatment of falciparum malaria. Am J Trop Med Hyg. 2007;77(6 Suppl):181-192.

[30] Ashley EA, Dhorda M, Fairhurst RM, Amaratunga C, Lim P, Suon S, et al. Spread of artemisinin resistance in Plasmodium falciparum malaria. N Engl J Med. 2014;371(5):411-423.

[31] White N. Antimalarial drug resistance and combination chemotherapy. Philos Trans R Soc Lond B Biol Sci. 1999;354(1384):739-749.

[32] Ke H, Morrisey JM, Ganesan SM, Painter HJ, Mather MW, Vaidya AB. Variation among *Plasmodium falciparum* strains in their reliance on mitochondrial electron transport chain function. Eukaryotic cell. 2011;10(8):1053-1061.

[33] Vaidya AB, Mather MW. Mitochondrial evolution and functions in malaria parasites. Annu Rev Microbiol 2009;63:249-267.

[34] Ke H, Lewis IA, Morrisey JM, McLean KJ, Ganesan SM, Painter HJ, et al. Genetic investigation of tricarboxylic acid metabolism during the Plasmodium falciparum life cycle. Cell Rep. 2015;11(1):164-174.

[35] MacRae JI, Dixon MW, Dearnley MK, Chua HH, Chambers JM, Kenny S, et al. Mitochondrial metabolism of sexual and asexual blood stages of the malaria parasite *Plasmodium falciparum*. BMC biology. 2013;11:67.

[36] Bryant C, Voller A, Smith MJ. The incorporation of radioactivity from (14C) glucose into the soluble metabolic intermediates of malaria parasites. Am J Trop Med Hyg. 1964;13:515-519.

[37] Scheibel LW, Pflaum WK. Cytochrome oxidase activity in platelet-free preparations of *Plasmodium falciparum*. J Parasitol. 1970;56(6):1054.

[38] Roth EF, Calvin MC, Max-Audit I, Rosa J, Rosa R. The enzymes of the glycolytic pathway in erythrocytes infected with *Plasmodium falciparum* malaria parasites. Blood. 1988;72(6):1922-1925.

[39] Roth EF, Raventos-Suarez C, Perkins M, Nagel RL. Glutathione stability and oxidative stress in *P. falciparum* infection in vitro: responses of normal and G6PD deficient cells. Biochem Biophys Res Commun. 1982;109(2):355-362.

[40] Planche T, Krishna S. Severe malaria: metabolic complications. Curr Mol Med. 2006;6(2):141-153.

[41] Fleck SL, Pudney M, Sinden RE. The effect of atovaquone (566C80) on the maturation and viability of *Plasmodium falciparum* gametocytes in vitro. Trans R Soc Trop Med Hyg. 1996;90(3):309-312.

[42] Srivastava IK, Rottenberg H, Vaidya AB. Atovaquone, a broad spectrum antiparasitic drug, collapses mitochondrial membrane potential in a malarial parasite. J Biol Chem. 1997;272(7):3961-3966.

[43] Mather MW, Darrouzet E, Valkova-Valchanova M, Cooley JW, McIntosh MT, Daldal F, et al. Uncovering the molecular mode of action of the antimalarial drug atovaquone using a bacterial system. J Biol Chem. 2005;280(29):27458-27465.

[44] Nixon GL, Pidathala C, Shone AE, Antoine T, Fisher N, O'Neill PM, et al. Targeting the mitochondrial electron transport chain of Plasmodium falciparum: New strategies towards the development of improved antimalarials for the elimination era. Future Med Chem. 2013;5(13):1573-1591.

[45] Fisher N, Bray PG, Ward SA, Biagini GA. The malaria parasite type II NADH:quinone oxidoreductase: an alternative enzyme for an alternative lifestyle. Trends Parasitol. 2007;23(7):305-310.

[46] Fry M, Webb E, Pudney M. Effect of mitochondrial inhibitors on adenosinetriphosphate levels in *Plasmodium falciparum*. Comp Biochem Physiol B Comp Biochem. 1990;96(4):775-782.

[47] Balabaskaran Nina P, Morrisey JM, Ganesan SM, Ke H, Pershing AM, Mather MW, et al. ATP synthase complex of *Plasmodium falciparum*: dimeric assembly in mitochondrial membranes and resistance to genetic disruption. J Biol Chem. 2011;286(48):41312-41322.

[48] Phillips MA, Rathod PK. Plasmodium dihydroorotate dehydrogenase: a promising target for novel anti-malarial chemotherapy. Infect Disord Drug Targets. 2010;10(3): 226-239.

[49] Gutteridge WE, Dave D, Richards WH. Conversion of dihydroorotate to orotate in parasitic protozoa. Biochim et Biophys Acta. 1979;582(3):390-401.

[50] Stocks PA, Barton V, Antoine T, Biagini GA, Ward SA, O'Neill PM. Novel inhibitors of the *Plasmodium falciparum* electron transport chain. Parasitology. 2014;141(1):50-65.

[51] Herrmann ML, Schleyerbach R, Kirschbaum BJ. Leflunomide: an immunomodulatory drug for the treatment of rheumatoid arthritis and other autoimmune diseases. Immunopharmacology. 2000;47(2-3):273-289.

[52] Shannon PVRE, Eichholtz T., Linstead D, Masdin P, Skinner R, inventor. Condensed heterocyclic compounds as anti-inflammatory and immunomodulatory agents, 1999. Google Patents, WO1999045926B1.

[53] Boa AN, Canavan SP, Hirst PR, Ramsey C, Stead AM, McConkey GA. Synthesis of brequinar analogue inhibitors of malaria parasite dihydroorotate dehydrogenase. Bioorg Med Chem. 2005;13(6):1945-1967.

[54] Patel V, Booker M, Kramer M, Ross L, Celatka CA, Kennedy LM, et al. Identification and characterization of small molecule inhibitors of *Plasmodium falciparum* dihydroorotate dehydrogenase. J Biol Chem. 2008;283(50):35078-35085.

[55] Booker ML, Bastos CM, Kramer ML, Barker RH, Jr., Skerlj R, Sidhu AB, et al. Novel inhibitors of *Plasmodium falciparum* dihydroorotate dehydrogenase with anti-malarial activity in the mouse model. J Biol Chem. 2010;285(43):33054-33064.

[56] Skerlj RT, Bastos CM, Booker ML, Kramer ML, Barker RH, Jr., Celatka CA, et al. Optimization of potent inhibitors of *P. falciparum* dihydroorotate dehydrogenase for the treatment of malaria. ACS Med Chem Lett. 2011;2(9):708-713.

[57] Bedingfield PT, Cowen D, Acklam P, Cunningham F, Parsons MR, McConkey GA, et al. Factors influencing the specificity of inhibitor binding to the human and malaria parasite dihydroorotate dehydrogenases. J Med Chem. 2012;55(12):5841-5850.

[58] Fritzson I BP, Sundin AP, McConkey G, Nilsson UJ. N-substituted salicylamides as selective malaria parasite dihydroorotate dehydrogenase inhibitors. Med Chem Commun. 2011;2:3.

[59] Davies M, Heikkila T, McConkey GA, Fishwick CW, Parsons MR, Johnson AP. Structure-based design, synthesis, and characterization of inhibitors of human and *Plasmodium falciparum* dihydroorotate dehydrogenases. J Med Chem. 2009;52(9):2683-2693.

[60] Phillips MA, Gujjar R, Malmquist NA, White J, El Mazouni F, Baldwin J, et al. Triazolopyrimidine-based dihydroorotate dehydrogenase inhibitors with potent and selective activity against the malaria parasite *Plasmodium falciparum*. J Med Chem. 2008;51(12):3649-3653.

[61] Deng X, Gujjar R, El Mazouni F, Kaminsky W, Malmquist NA, Goldsmith EJ, et al. Structural plasticity of malaria dihydroorotate dehydrogenase allows selective binding of diverse chemical scaffolds. J Biol Chem. 2009;284(39):26999-27009.

[62] Gujjar R, Marwaha A, El Mazouni F, White J, White KL, Creason S, et al. Identification of a metabolically stable triazolopyrimidine-based dihydroorotate dehydrogenase inhibitor with antimalarial activity in mice. J Med Chem. 2009;52(7):1864-1872.

[63] Gujjar R, El Mazouni F, White KL, White J, Creason S, Shackleford DM, et al. Lead optimization of aryl and aralkyl amine-based triazolopyrimidine inhibitors of *Plasmodium falciparum* dihydroorotate dehydrogenase with antimalarial activity in mice. J Med Chem. 2011;54(11):3935-3949.

[64] Marwaha A, White J, El Mazouni F, Creason SA, Kokkonda S, Buckner FS, et al. Bioisosteric transformations and permutations in the triazolopyrimidine scaffold to identify the minimum pharmacophore required for inhibitory activity against *Plasmodium falciparum* dihydroorotate dehydrogenase. J Med Chem. 2012;55(17):7425-7436.

[65] Schutz M, Brugna M, Lebrun E, Baymann F, Huber R, Stetter KO, et al. Early evolution of cytochrome bc complexes. J Mol Biol. 2000;300(4):663-675.

[66] Gao X, Wen X, Yu C, Esser L, Tsao S, Quinn B, et al. The crystal structure of mitochondrial cytochrome bc1 in complex with famoxadone: the role of aromatic-aromatic interaction in inhibition. Biochemistry. 2002;41(39):11692-11702.

[67] Berry EA, Guergova-Kuras M, Huang LS, Crofts AR. Structure and function of cytochrome bc complexes. Annu Rev Biochem. 2000;69:1005-1075.

[68] Iwata S, Lee JW, Okada K, Lee JK, Iwata M, Rasmussen B, et al. Complete structure of the 11-subunit bovine mitochondrial cytochrome bc1 complex. Science. 1998;281(5373):64-71.

[69] Mitchell P. Possible molecular mechanisms of the protonmotive function of cytochrome systems. J Theor Biol. 1976;62(2):327-367.

[70] Rieske JS, Zaugg WS, Hansen RE. Studies on the electron transfer system. Lix. Distribution of iron and of the component giving an electron paramagnetic resonance signal at G = 1.90 in subfractions of complex 3. J Biol Chem. 1964;239:3023-3030.

[71] Berry EA, Huang LS. Conformationally linked interaction in the cytochrome bc[1] complex between inhibitors of the Q(o) site and the Rieske iron-sulfur protein. Biochim Biophys Acta. 2011;1807(10):1349-1363.

[72] Vaidya AB. Mitochondrial and plastid functions as antimalarial drug targets. Curr Drug Targets Infect Disord. 2004;4(1):11-23.

[73] Hunte C, Koepke J, Lange C, Rossmanith T, Michel H. Structure at 2.3 A resolution of the cytochrome bc(1) complex from the yeast Saccharomyces cerevisiae co-crystallized with an antibody Fv fragment. Structure. 2000;8(6):669-684.

[74] Srivastava IK, Vaidya AB. A mechanism for the synergistic antimalarial action of atovaquone and proguanil. Antimicrob Agents Chemother. 1999;43(6):1334-1339.

[75] Birth D, Kao WC, Hunte C. Structural analysis of atovaquone-inhibited cytochrome bc1 complex reveals the molecular basis of antimalarial drug action. Nature Commun 2014;5:4029.

[76] Looareesuwan S, Viravan C, Webster HK, Kyle DE, Hutchinson DB, Canfield CJ. Clinical studies of atovaquone, alone or in combination with other antimalarial drugs, for treatment of acute uncomplicated malaria in Thailand. Am J Trop Med Hyg. 1996;54(1):62-66.

[77] Brunton LL, Chabner BA, Knollman BC. Goodman and Gilman's The Pharmacological Basis of Therapeutics. 11th ed. New York: McGraw Hill; 2011.

[78] Winter RW, Kelly JX, Smilkstein MJ, Dodean R, Bagby GC, Rathbun RK, et al. Evaluation and lead optimization of anti-malarial acridones. Exp Parasitol. 2006;114(1):47-56.

[79] Nilsen A, Miley GP, Forquer IP, Mather MW, Katneni K, Li Y, et al. Discovery, synthesis, and optimization of antimalarial 4(1H)-quinolone-3-diarylethers. J Med Chem. 2014;57(9):3818-3834.

[80] Nilsen A, LaCrue AN, White KL, Forquer IP, Cross RM, Marfurt J, et al. Quinolone-3-diarylethers: a new class of antimalarial drug. Sci Transl Med. 2013;5(177):177ra37.

[81] Biagini GA, Fisher N, Shone AE, Mubaraki MA, Srivastava A, Hill A, et al. Generation of quinolone antimalarials targeting the *Plasmodium falciparum* mitochondrial respiratory chain for the treatment and prophylaxis of malaria. Proc Natl Acad Sci USA. 2012;109(21):8298-8303.

[82] Yeates CL, Batchelor JF, Capon EC, Cheesman NJ, Fry M, Hudson AT, et al. Synthesis and structure-activity relationships of 4-pyridones as potential antimalarials. J Med Chem. 2008;51(9):2845-2852.

[83] Bueno JM, Herreros E, Angulo-Barturen I, Ferrer S, Fiandor JM, Gamo FJ, et al. Exploration of 4(1H)-pyridones as a novel family of potent antimalarial inhibitors of the plasmodial cytochrome bc1. Future Med Chem. 2012;4(18):2311-2323.

[84] Lukens AK, Heidebrecht RW, Jr., Mulrooney C, Beaudoin JA, Comer E, Duvall JR, et al. Diversity-oriented synthesis probe targets *Plasmodium falciparum* cytochrome b ubiquinone reduction site and synergizes with oxidation site inhibitors. J Infect Dis. 2015;211(7):1097-1103.

[85] Esser L, Quinn B, Li YF, Zhang M, Elberry M, Yu L, et al. Crystallographic studies of quinol oxidation site inhibitors: a modified classification of inhibitors for the cytochrome bc(1) complex. J Mol Biol. 2004;341(1):281-302.

[86] Gao X, Wen X, Esser L, Quinn B, Yu L, Yu CA, et al. Structural basis for the quinone reduction in the bc1 complex: a comparative analysis of crystal structures of mitochondrial cytochrome bc1 with bound substrate and inhibitors at the Qi site. Biochemistry. 2003;42(30):9067-9080.

[87] Li H, Zhu XL, Yang WC, Yang GF. Comparative kinetics of Qi site inhibitors of cytochrome bc1 complex: picomolar antimycin and micromolar cyazofamid. Chem Biol Drug Design. 2014;83(1):71-80.

[88] Berry EA, Huang LS, Lee DW, Daldal F, Nagai K, Minagawa N. Ascochlorin is a novel, specific inhibitor of the mitochondrial cytochrome bc1 complex. Biochim Biophys Acta. 2010;1797(3):360-370.

[89] Capper MJ, O'Neill PM, Fisher N, Strange RW, Moss D, Ward SA, et al. Antimalarial 4(1H)-pyridones bind to the Qi site of cytochrome bc1. Proc Natl Acad Sci USA. 2015;112(3):755-760.

[90] Biagini GA, Viriyavejakul P, O'neill PM, Bray PG, Ward SA. Functional characterization and target validation of alternative complex I of Plasmodium falciparum mitochondria. Antimicrob Agents Chemother. 2006;50(5):1841-1851.

[91] Kerscher SJ. Diversity and origin of alternative NADH:ubiquinone oxidoreductases. Biochim Biophys Acta. 2000;1459(2-3):274-283.

[92] Luttik MA, Overkamp KM, Kotter P, de Vries S, van Dijken JP, Pronk JT. The Saccharomyces cerevisiae NDE1 and NDE2 genes encode separate mitochondrial NADH dehydrogenases catalyzing the oxidation of cytosolic NADH. J Biol Chem. 1998;273(38):24529-24534.

[93] Marres CA, de Vries S, Grivell LA. Isolation and inactivation of the nuclear gene encoding the rotenone-insensitive internal NADH: ubiquinone oxidoreductase of mitochondria from Saccharomyces cerevisiae. Eur J Biochem/FEBS. 1991;195(3):857-862.

[94] Melo AM, Bandeiras TM, Teixeira M. New insights into type II NAD(P)H:quinone oxidoreductases. Microbiol Mol Biol Rev: MMBR. 2004;68(4):603-616.

[95] Rasmusson AG, Soole KL, Elthon TE. Alternative NAD(P)H dehydrogenases of plant mitochondria. Annu Rev Plant Biol. 2004;55:23-39.

[96] Yagi T. Bacterial NADH-quinone oxidoreductases. J Bioenerg Biomembr. 1991;23(2):211-225.

[97] Mattevi A, Obmolova G, Sokatch JR, Betzel C, Hol WG. The refined crystal structure of Pseudomonas putida lipoamide dehydrogenase complexed with NAD+ at 2.45 A resolution. Proteins. 1992;13(4):336-351.

[98] Boysen KE, Matuschewski K. Arrested oocyst maturation in Plasmodium parasites lacking type II NADH:ubiquinone dehydrogenase. J Biol Chem. 2011;286(37):32661-32671.

[99] Yeh I, Hanekamp T, Tsoka S, Karp PD, Altman RB. Computational analysis of Plasmodium falciparum metabolism: organizing genomic information to facilitate drug discovery. Genome Res. 2004;14(5):917-924.

[100] Dong CK, Patel V, Yang JC, Dvorin JD, Duraisingh MT, Clardy J, et al. Type II NADH dehydrogenase of the respiratory chain of *Plasmodium falciparum* and its inhibitors. Bioorg Med Chem Lett. 2009;19(3):972-975.

[101] Eschemann A, Galkin A, Oettmeier W, Brandt U, Kerscher S. HDQ (1-hydroxy-2-dodecyl-4(1H)quinolone), a high affinity inhibitor for mitochondrial alternative NADH dehydrogenase: evidence for a ping-pong mechanism. J Biol Chem. 2005;280(5):3138-3142.

[102] Saleh A, Friesen J, Baumeister S, Gross U, Bohne W. Growth inhibition of Toxoplasma gondii and Plasmodium falciparum by nanomolar concentrations of 1-hydroxy-2-dodecyl-4(1H)quinolone, a high-affinity inhibitor of alternative (type II) NADH dehydrogenases. Antimicrob Agents Chemother. 2007;51(4):1217-1222.

[103] Vallieres C, Fisher N, Antoine T, Al-Helal M, Stocks P, Berry NG, et al. HDQ, a potent inhibitor of Plasmodium falciparum proliferation, binds to the quinone reduction site of the cytochrome bc1 complex. Antimicrob Agents Chemother. 2012;56(7):3739-3747.

[104] Li W, Mo W, Shen D, Sun L, Wang J, Lu S, et al. Yeast model uncovers dual roles of mitochondria in action of artemisinin. PLoS Genet. 2005;1(3):e36.

[105] Antoine T, Fisher N, Amewu R, O'Neill PM, Ward SA, Biagini GA. Rapid kill of malaria parasites by artemisinin and semi-synthetic endoperoxides involves ROS-dependent depolarization of the membrane potential. J Antimicrob Chemother. 2014;69(4):1005-1016.

[106] Pidathala C, Amewu R, Pacorel B, Nixon GL, Gibbons P, Hong WD, et al. Identification, design and biological evaluation of bisaryl quinolones targeting *Plasmodium falciparum* type II NADH:quinone oxidoreductase (PfNDH2). J Med Chem. 2012;55(5):1831-1843.

[107] Leung SC, Gibbons P, Amewu R, Nixon GL, Pidathala C, Hong WD, et al. Identification, design and biological evaluation of heterocyclic quinolones targeting *Plasmodium falciparum* type II NADH:quinone oxidoreductase (PfNDH2). J Med Chem. 2012;55(5):1844-1857.

[108] Klingenberg M. Localization of the glycerol-phosphate dehydrogenase in the outer phase of the mitochondrial inner membrane. Eur J Biochem/FEBS. 1970;13(2):247-252.

[109] Yeh JI, Chinte U, Du S. Structure of glycerol-3-phosphate dehydrogenase, an essential monotopic membrane enzyme involved in respiration and metabolism. Proc Natl Acad Sci USA. 2008;105(9):3280-3285.

[110] Fry M, Beesley JE. Mitochondria of mammalian *Plasmodium* spp. Parasitology. 1991;102 Pt 1:17-26.

[111] Uyemura SA, Luo S, Moreno SN, Docampo R. Oxidative phosphorylation, Ca(2+) transport, and fatty acid-induced uncoupling in malaria parasites mitochondria. J Biol Chem. 2000;275(13):9709-9715.

[112] Uyemura SA, Luo S, Vieira M, Moreno SN, Docampo R. Oxidative phosphorylation and rotenone-insensitive malate- and NADH-quinone oxidoreductases in Plasmodium yoelii yoelii mitochondria in situ. J Biol Chem. 2004;279(1):385-393.

[113] Hatefi Y. The mitochondrial electron transport and oxidative phosphorylation system. Annu Rev Biochem. 1985;54:1015-1069.

[114] Kita K, Vibat CR, Meinhardt S, Guest JR, Gennis RB. One-step purification from *Escherichia coli* of complex II (succinate: ubiquinone oxidoreductase) associated with succinate-reducible cytochrome b556. J Biol Chem. 1989;264(5):2672-2677.

[115] Moll R, Schafer G. Purification and characterisation of an archaebacterial succinate dehydrogenase complex from the plasma membrane of the thermoacidophile *Sulfolobus acidocaldarius*. Eur J Biochem/FEBS. 1991;201(3):593-600.

[116] Reddy TL, Weber MM. Solubilization, purification, and characterization of succinate dehydrogenase from membranes of *Mycobacterium phlei*. J Bacteriol. 1986;167(1):1-6.

[117] McNeil MB, Hampton HG, Hards KJ, Watson BN, Cook GM, Fineran PC. The succinate dehydrogenase assembly factor, SdhE, is required for the flavinylation and activation of fumarate reductase in bacteria. FEBS Lett. 2014;588(3):414-421.

[118] Hartman T, Weinrick B, Vilcheze C, Berney M, Tufariello J, Cook GM, et al. Succinate dehydrogenase is the regulator of respiration in *Mycobacterium tuberculosis*. PLoS Pathog. 2014;10(11):e1004510.

[119] Kita K, Oya H, Gennis RB, Ackrell BA, Kasahara M. Human complex II (succinate-ubiquinone oxidoreductase): cDNA cloning of iron sulfur (Ip) subunit of liver mitochondria. Biochem Biophys Res Commun. 1990;166(1):101-108.

[120] Hatefi Y, Stiggall DL. Preparation and properties of succinate: ubiquinone oxidoreductase (complex II). Methods Enzymol. 1978;53:21-27.

[121] Tushurashvili PR, Gavrikova EV, Ledenev AN, Vinogradov AD. Studies on the succinate dehydrogenating system. Isolation and properties of the mitochondrial succinate-ubiquinone reductase. Biochim Biophys Acta. 1985;809(2):145-159.

[122] Suraveratum N, Krungkrai SR, Leangaramgul P, Prapunwattana P, Krungkrai J. Purification and characterization of Plasmodium falciparum succinate dehydrogenase. Mol Biochem Parasitol. 2000;105(2):215-222.

[123] Takeo S, Kokaze A, Ng CS, Mizuchi D, Watanabe JI, Tanabe K, et al. Succinate dehydrogenase in *Plasmodium falciparum* mitochondria: molecular characterization of the SDHA and SDHB genes for the catalytic subunits, the flavoprotein (Fp) and iron-sulfur (Ip) subunits. Mol Biochem Parasitol. 2000;107(2):191-205.

[124] Hagerhall C. Succinate: quinone oxidoreductases. Variations on a conserved theme. Biochim Biophys Acta. 1997;1320(2):107-141.

[125] Kita K, Hirawake H, Miyadera H, Amino H, Takeo S. Role of complex II in anaerobic respiration of the parasite mitochondria from *Ascaris suum* and *Plasmodium falciparum*. Biochim Biophys Acta. 2002;1553(1-2):123-139.

[126] Molenaar D, van der Rest ME, Petrovic S. Biochemical and genetic characterization of the membrane-associated malate dehydrogenase (acceptor) from Corynebacterium glutamicum. Eur J Biochem/FEBS. 1998;254(2):395-403.

[127] Mogi T, Murase Y, Mori M, Shiomi K, Omura S, Paranagama MP, et al. Polymyxin B identified as an inhibitor of alternative NADH dehydrogenase and malate: quinone oxidoreductase from the Gram-positive bacterium *Mycobacterium smegmatis*. J Biochem. 2009;146(4):491-499.

[128] van Dooren GG, Marti M, Tonkin CJ, Stimmler LM, Cowman AF, McFadden GI. Development of the endoplasmic reticulum, mitochondrion and apicoplast during the asexual life cycle of *Plasmodium falciparum*. Mol Microbiol. 2005;57(2):405-419.

[129] Guillemont J, Meyer C, Poncelet A, Bourdrez X, Andries K. Diarylquinolines, synthesis pathways and quantitative structure--activity relationship studies leading to the discovery of TMC207. Future Med Chem. 2011;3(11):1345-1360.

[130] Basco LK, Le Bras J. In vitro activity of mitochondrial ATP synthetase inhibitors against *Plasmodium falciparum*. J Eukaryot Microbiol. 1994;41(3):179-183.

[131] Sturm A, Mollard V, Cozijnsen A, Goodman CD, McFadden GI. Mitochondrial ATP synthase is dispensable in blood-stage Plasmodium berghei rodent malaria but essential in the mosquito phase. Proc Natl Acad Sci USA. 2015;112(33):10216-10223.

[132] Olszewski KL, Mather MW, Morrisey JM, Garcia BA, Vaidya AB, Rabinowitz JD, et al. Branched tricarboxylic acid metabolism in *Plasmodium falciparum*. Nature. 2010;466(7307):774-778.

[133] Olszewski KL, Mather MW, Morrisey JM, Garcia BA, Vaidya AB, Rabinowitz JD, et al. Retraction: Branched tricarboxylic acid metabolism in *Plasmodium falciparum*. Nature. 2013;497(7451):652.

[134] Olszewski KL, Llinas M. Central carbon metabolism of Plasmodium parasites. Mol Biochem Parasitol. 2011;175(2):95-103.

[135] Saunders EC, Ng WW, Chamber JM, Ng M, Naderer T, Kroemer JO, et al. Isoptopomer profiling of *Leishmania mexicana* promastigotes reveals important roles for succinate fermentation and aspartate uptake in TCA cycle anaplerosis, glutamate synthesis and growth. J Biol Chem. 2011;286.

[136] Jäger J, Moser M, Sauder U, Jansonius JN. Crystal structures of *Escherichia coli* aspartate aminotransferase in two conformations. Comparison of an unliganded open and two liganded closed forms. J Mol Biol. 1994;239(2):285-305.

[137] Kamitori S, Okamoto A, Hirotsu K, Higuchi T, Kuramitsu S, Kagamiyama H, et al. Three-dimensional structures of aspartate aminotransferase from *Escherichia coli* and its mutant enzyme at 2.5 A resolution. J Biochem. 1990;108(2):175-184.

[138] Okamoto A, Higuchi T, Hirotsu K, Kuramitsu S, Kagamiyama H. X-ray crystallographic study of pyridoxal 5'-phosphate-type aspartate aminotransferases from *Escherichia coli* in open and closed form. J Biochem. 1994;116(1):95-107.

[139] Smith DL, Almo SC, Toney MD, Ringe D. 2.8-A-resolution crystal structure of an active-site mutant of aspartate aminotransferase from *Escherichia coli*. Biochemistry. 1989;28(20):8161-8167.

[140] Jeffrey PD, Bewley MC, MacGillivray RT, Mason AB, Woodworth RC, Baker EN. Ligand-induced conformational change in transferrins: crystal structure of the open form of the N-terminal half-molecule of human transferrin. Biochemistry. 1998;37(40):13978-13986.

[141] Arnone A, Rogers PH, Hyde CC, Briley PD, Metzler CM, Metzler DE. In Transaminases (eds P. Christen and D. Metzler), pp. 138-155 John Wiley and Sons, NY. 1985.

[142] Ford GC, Eichele G, Jansonius JN. Three-dimensional structure of a pyridoxal-phosphate-dependent enzyme, mitochondrial aspartate aminotransferase. Proc Natl Acad Sci U S A. 1980;77(5):2559-2563.

[143] Malashkevich VN, Toney MD, Jansonius JN. Crystal structures of true enzymatic reaction intermediates: aspartate and glutamate ketimines in aspartate aminotransferase. Biochemistry. 1993;32(49):13451-13462.

[144] McPhalen CA, Vincent MG, Jansonius JN. X-ray structure refinement and comparison of three forms of mitochondrial aspartate aminotransferase. J Mol Biol. 1992;225(2):495-517.

[145] Jain R, Jordanova R, Muller IB, Wrenger C, Groves MR. Purification, crystallization and preliminary X-ray analysis of the aspartate aminotransferase of *Plasmodium falciparum*. Acta Crystallogr Sect F Struct Biol Cryst Commun 2010;66(Pt 4):409-412.

[146] Wrenger C, Muller IB, Schifferdecker AJ, Jain R, Jordanova R, Groves MR. Specific inhibition of the aspartate aminotransferase of Plasmodium falciparum. J Mol Bio wl. 2011;405(4):956-971.

[147] McPhalen CA, Vincent MG, Picot D, Jansonius JN, Lesk AM, Chothia C. Domain closure in mitochondrial aspartate aminotransferase. J Mol Biol. 1992;227(1):197-213.

[148] Battchikova N, Koivulehto M, Denesyuk A, Ptitsyn L, Boretsky Y, Hellman J, et al. Aspartate aminotransferase from an alkalophilic Bacillus contains an additional 20-amino acid extension at its functionally important N-terminus. J Biochem. 1996;120(2): 425-432.

[149] Wrenger C, Müller IB, Butzloff S, Jordanova R, Lunev S, Groves MR. Crystallization and preliminary X-ray diffraction of malate dehydrogenase from *Plasmodium falciparum*. Acta Crystallogr Sect F Struct Biol Cryst Commun. 2012;68(Pt 6):659-662.

[150] Lunev S, Groves MR, Müller IB, Butzloff S, Wrenger C. Oligomeric protein interference demonstrates a measurable phenotype in cultured malarial parasites. Manuscript in preparation.

[151] Woods SA, Schwartzbach SD, Guest JR. Two biochemically distinct classes of fumarase in *Escherichia coli*. Biochim Biophy Acta. 1988;954(1):14-26.

[152] Flint DH, Emptage MH, Guest JR. Fumarase a from *Escherichia coli*: Purification and characterization as an iron-sulfur cluster containing enzyme. Biochemistry. 1992;31(42):10331-10337.

[153] Bulusu V, Jayaraman V, Balaram H. Metabolic fate of fumarate, a side product of the purine salvage pathway in the intraerythrocytic stages of *Plasmodium falciparum*. J Biol Chem. 2011;286(11):9236-9245.

[154] White NJ, Pukrittayakamee S, Hien TT, Faiz MA, Mokuolu OA, Dondorp AM. Malaria. Lancet. 2014;383(9918):723-735.

[155] Hyde JE. Targeting purine and pyrimidine metabolism in human apicomplexan parasites. Curr Drug Targets. 2007;8(1):31-47.

[156] Loffler M, Fairbanks LD, Zameitat E, Marinaki AM, Simmonds HA. Pyrimidine pathways in health and disease. Trends Mol Med. 2005;11(9):430-437.

[157] Reyes P, Rathod PK, Sanchez DJ, Mrema JE, Rieckmann KH, Heidrich HG. Enzymes of purine and pyrimidine metabolism from the human malaria parasite, *Plasmodium falciparum*. Mol Biochem Parasitol. 1982;5(5):275-290.

[158] Gardner MJ, Hall N, Fung E, White O, Berriman M, Hyman RW, et al. Genome sequence of the human malaria parasite *Plasmodium falciparum*. Nature. 2002;419(6906):498-511.

[159] Cassera MB, Zhang Y, Hazleton KZ, Schramm VL. Purine and pyrimidine pathways as targets in *Plasmodium falciparum*. Curr Top Med Chem. 2011;11(16):2103-2115.

[160] Gero AM, Brown GV, O'Sullivan WJ. Pyrimidine de novo synthesis during the life cycle of the intraerythrocytic stage of *Plasmodium falciparum*. J Parasitol. 1984;70(4):536-541.

[161] Flores MV, O'Sullivan WJ, Stewart TS. Characterisation of the carbamoyl phosphate synthetase gene from *Plasmodium falciparum*. Mol Biochem Parasitol. 1994;68(2):315-318.

[162] Flores MV, Atkins D, Wade D, O'Sullivan WJ, Stewart TS. Inhibition of *Plasmodium falciparum* proliferation in vitro by ribozymes. J Biol Chem. 1997;272(27):16940-16945.

[163] Hendry P, McCall MJ, Stewart TS, Lockett TJ. Redesigned and chemically-modified hammerhead ribozymes with improved activity and serum stability. BMC chemical biology. 2004;4(1):1.

[164] Alvarez-Salas LM. Nucleic acids as therapeutic agents. Curr Topics Med Chem. 2008;8(15):1379-1404.

[165] Madani S, Baillon J, Fries J, Belhadj O, Bettaieb A, Ben Hamida M, et al. Pyrimidine pathways enzymes in human tumors of brain and associated tissues: Potentialities for the therapeutic use of N-(phosphonacetyl-L-aspartate and 1-beta-D-arabinofuranosylcytosine. Eur J Cancer Clin Oncol. 1987;23(10):1485-1490.

[166] Banerjee A, Arora N, Murty U. Aspartate carbamoyltransferase of *Plasmodium falciparum* as a potential drug target for designing anti-malarial chemotherapeutic agents. Med Chem Res. 2012;21(9):2480-2493.

[167] Depamede SN, Menz I. Phylogenetic analysis and protein modeling of *Plasmodium falciparum* aspartate transcarbamoylase (ATCase). Res J Microbiol. 2011;6:599-608.

[168] Sun W, Tanaka TQ, Magle CT, Huang W, Southall N, Huang R, et al. Chemical signatures and new drug targets for gametocytocidal drug development. Sci Rep. 2014;4:3743.

[169] Lunev S, Bosch SS, Batista FdeA, Wrenger C, Groves MR. Crystal structure of truncated aspartate transcarbamoylase from *Plasmodium falciparum*. Acta Crystallogr F Struct Biol Commun. 2016;72(Pt 7):523-533.

[170] Simmer JP, Kelly RE, Rinker AG, Jr., Zimmermann BH, Scully JL, Kim H, et al. Mammalian dihydroorotase: nucleotide sequence, peptide sequences, and evolution of the dihydroorotase domain of the multifunctional protein CAD. Proc Natl Acad Sci USA. 1990;87(1):174-178.

[171] Krungkrai J, Krungkrai SR, Phakanont K. Antimalarial activity of orotate analogs that inhibit dihydroorotase and dihydroorotate dehydrogenase. Biochem Pharmacol. 1992;43(6):1295-1301.

[172] Seymour KK, Lyons SD, Phillips L, Rieckmann KH, Christopherson RI. Cytotoxic effects of inhibitors of de novo pyrimidine biosynthesis upon *Plasmodium falciparum*. Biochemistry. 1994;33(17):5268-5274.

[173] Krungkrai SR, Wutipraditkul N, Krungkrai J. Dihydroorotase of human malarial parasite *Plasmodium falciparum* differs from host enzyme. Biochem Biophys Res Commun. 2008;366(3):821-826.

[174] Krungkrai SR, Prapunwattana P, Horii T, Krungkrai J. Orotate phosphoribosyltransferase and orotidine 5'-monophosphate decarboxylase exist as multienzyme complex in human malaria parasite *Plasmodium falciparum*. Biochem Biophys Res Commun. 2004;318(4):1012-1018.

[175] Krungkrai SR, DelFraino BJ, Smiley JA, Prapunwattana P, Mitamura T, Horii T, et al. A novel enzyme complex of orotate phosphoribosyltransferase and orotidine 5'-monophosphate decarboxylase in human malaria parasite *Plasmodium falciparum*: physical association, kinetics, and inhibition characterization. Biochemistry. 2005;44(5):1643-1652.

[176] Queen SA, Jagt DL, Reyes P. In vitro susceptibilities of *Plasmodium falciparum* to compounds which inhibit nucleotide metabolism. Antimicrob Agents Chemother. 1990;34(7):1393-1398.

[177] Rathod PK, Khatri A, Hubbert T, Milhous WK. Selective activity of 5-fluoroorotic acid against Plasmodium falciparum in vitro. Antimicrob Agents Chemother. 1989;33(7):1090-1094.

[178] Scott HV, Gero AM, O'Sullivan WJ. In vitro inhibition of Plasmodium falciparum by pyrazofurin, an inhibitor of pyrimidine biosynthesis de novo. Mol Biochem Parasitol. 1986;18(1):3-15.

[179] Suttle DP, Stark GR. Coordinate overproduction of orotate phosphoribosyltransferase and orotidine-5'-phosphate decarboxylase in hamster cells resistant to pyrazofurin and 6-azauridine. J Biol Chem. 1979;254(11):4602-4607.

[180] Zhang Y, Evans GB, Clinch K, Crump DR, Harris LD, Fröhlich RF, et al. Transition state analogues of Plasmodium falciparum and human orotate phosphoribosyltransferases. J Biol Chem. 2013;288(48):34746-34754.

[181] Zhang Y, Luo M, Schramm VL. Transition states of Plasmodium falciparum and human orotate phosphoribosyltransferases. J Am Chem Soc. 2009;131(13):4685-4694.

[182] Zhang Y, Schramm VL. Pyrophosphate interactions at the transition states of *Plasmodium falciparum* and human orotate phosphoribosyltransferases. J Am Chem Soc. 2010;132(25):8787-8794.

[183] Kumar S, Krishnamoorthy K, Mudeppa DG, Rathod PK. Structure of *Plasmodium falciparum* orotate phosphoribosyltransferase with autologous inhibitory protein-protein interactions. Acta Crystallogr F Struct Biol Commun. 2015;71(Pt 5):600-608.

[184] Miller BG, Wolfenden R. Catalytic proficiency: the unusual case of OMP decarboxylase. Annu Rev Biochem. 2002;71:847-885.

[185] Langley DB, Shojaei M, Chan C, Lok HC, Mackay JP, Traut TW, et al. Structure and inhibition of orotidine 5'-monophosphate decarboxylase from *Plasmodium falciparum*. Biochemistry. 2008;47(12):3842-3854.

[186] Bello AM, Poduch E, Fujihashi M, Amani M, Li Y, Crandall I, et al. A potent, covalent inhibitor of orotidine 5'-monophosphate decarboxylase with antimalarial activity. J Med Chem. 2007;50(5):915-921.

[187] Bello AM, Poduch E, Liu Y, Wei L, Crandall I, Wang X, et al. Structure-activity relationships of C6-uridine derivatives targeting plasmodia orotidine monophosphate decarboxylase. J Med Chem. 2008;51(3):439-448.

[188] Takashima Y, Mizohata E, Krungkrai SR, Fukunishi Y, Kinoshita T, Sakata T, et al. The in silico screening and X-ray structure analysis of the inhibitor complex of *Plasmodium falciparum* orotidine 5'-monophosphate decarboxylase. J Biochem. 2012;152(2):133-138.

[189] Kanchanaphum P, Krungkrai J. Kinetic benefits and thermal stability of orotate phosphoribosyltransferase and orotidine 5'-monophosphate decarboxylase enzyme complex in human malaria parasite *Plasmodium falciparum*. Biochem Biophys Res Commun. 2009;390(2):337-341.

[190] Ali MH, Imperiali B. Protein oligomerization: how and why. Bioorg Med Chem. 2005;13(17):5013-5020.

[191] Levy ED, Boeri Erba E, Robinson CV, Teichmann SA. Assembly reflects evolution of protein complexes. Nature. 2008;453(7199):1262-1265.

[192] Hashimoto K, Nishi H, Bryant S, Panchenko AR. Caught in self-interaction: evolutionary and functional mechanisms of protein homooligomerization. Phys Biol. 2011;8(3):035007.

[193] Perica T, Chothia C, Teichmann SA. Evolution of oligomeric state through geometric coupling of protein interfaces. Proc Natl Acad Sci U S A. 2012;109(21):8127-8132.

[194] Nishi H, Hashimoto K, Madej T, Panchenko AR. Evolutionary, physicochemical, and functional mechanisms of protein homooligomerization. Prog Mol Biol Transl Sci. 2013;117:3-24.

[195] Caffrey DR, Somaroo S, Hughes JD, Mintseris J, Huang ES. Are protein-protein interfaces more conserved in sequence than the rest of the protein surface? Protein Sci. 2004;13(1):190-202.

[196] Valdar WS, Thornton JM. Protein-protein interfaces: analysis of amino acid conservation in homodimers. Proteins. 2001;42(1):108-124.

[197] Agrawal N, Dasaradhi PV, Mohmmed A, Malhotra P, Bhatnagar RK, Mukherjee SK. RNA interference: biology, mechanism, and applications. Microbiol Mol Biol Rev. 2003;67(4):657-685.

[198] Hammond SM. Dicing and slicing: the core machinery of the RNA interference pathway. FEBS Lett. 2005;579(26):5822-5829.

[199] Barnes RL, Shi H, Kolev NG, Tschudi C, Ullu E. Comparative genomics reveals two novel RNAi factors in *Trypanosoma brucei* and provides insight into the core machinery. PLoS Pathog. 2012;8(5):e1002678.

[200] Mueller AK, Hammerschmidt-Kamper C, Kaiser A. RNAi in Plasmodium. Curr Pharm Des. 2014;20(2):278-283.

[201] Kolev NG, Tschudi C, Ullu E. RNA interference in protozoan parasites: achievements and challenges. Eukaryot Cell. 2011;10(9):1156-1163.

[202] Baum J, Papenfuss AT, Mair GR, Janse CJ, Vlachou D, Waters AP, et al. Molecular genetics and comparative genomics reveal RNAi is not functional in malaria parasites. Nucleic Acids Res. 2009;37(11):3788-3798.

5

Tackling the Problems Associated with Antimalarial Medicines of Poor Quality

Kamal Hamed and Kirstin Stricker

Abstract

The use of poor-quality antimalarials has devastating consequences, including increased morbidity, mortality, and drug resistance. Unfortunately, this issue appears to be widespread, especially in parts of Africa and Asia, jeopardizing the progress and investments already made in global malaria control in these regions. In developing countries, inadequate laws and regulatory oversight, along with the lack of human, technical, and financial resources, do not encourage the manufacture and distribution of high-quality medicines. The problem of poor-quality medicines can only be addressed by a multipronged approach that includes tackling poor regulation and ineffective/poorly implemented laws at national and international levels. In addition, pharmaceutical companies must be responsible for ensuring that the quality of antimalarials meets the stringent guidelines established by regulatory authorities, for testing their medicines accordingly and for releasing to market only medicines that pass these requirements. The chapter also discusses how the implementation of strategies such as the WHO Prequalification Program, the African Medicine Registration Harmonization initiative, and the ethical production of medicines by pharmaceutical companies help to ensure that antimalarial therapies marketed in low-income, malaria-endemic countries are quality assured.

Keywords: antimalarial medicines, malaria, quality, Africa, Asia

1. Introduction

Safe, effective, high-quality, and affordable medicines are essential for the achievement of positive, equitable health outcomes [1]. They are necessary for the prevention and treatment of serious public health threats, and for the achievement of the global health goals [2]. However, there is growing concern regarding the increasing availability and use of poor-quality medicines, particularly in developing countries in Africa, Asia, and South America [3–7].

Poor-quality medicines include those that have been falsified (i.e., deliberately and fraudulently mislabeled with respect to identity and/or source) and substandard medicines (i.e., products resulting from poor manufacturing with no intent to deceive and usually with inadequate or too much active pharmaceutical ingredient) [2].

Falsified medicines have resulted in billions of dollars in illegal annual revenues going to criminals and have caused prolonged, severe illness and deaths. Falsified drugs particularly affect the most disadvantaged people in poor countries [5].

In particular, the use of substandard antimalarial agents has been reported [3, 4, 7–18]. A World Health Organization (WHO) survey of antimalarial medicine quality in six countries from sub-Saharan Africa discovered that nearly 30% of the fully tested samples of medications failed to comply with internationally recognized quality specifications [8]. Similarly, a review reported that approximately one third of antimalarial medication samples from sub-Saharan Africa, as well as from Southeast Asia, failed chemical assay analysis [3].

Factors contributing to poor-quality medicines are numerous [3]. In many developing countries, for example, first-line artemisinin-based combination therapy (ACT) cannot be afforded by many patients [4, 5]. Consequently, patients tend to procure cheaper alternatives that may be falsified or substandard and that may contain subtherapeutic amounts of the active pharmaceutical ingredients (APIs) or only one of the two active ingredients of the ACT [2, 12]. Thus, the use of such poor-quality antimalarial agents leads to increases in morbidity and mortality [19]. In addition, subtherapeutic concentrations of drugs in vivo may be contributing to the selection of resistant parasites [3, 20, 21]. In the face of seemingly ineffective agents, societies are at risk of losing confidence in antimalarial medicines, their doctors and the healthcare system, and thus jeopardizing years of global public health success and investment [2].

In many countries, inadequate laws and regulatory oversight, along with the lack of human, technical, and financial resources, do not encourage the manufacture and distribution of high-quality medicines [2, 22]. The WHO has estimated that nearly a third of countries lack the ability to oversee medicine manufacture, importation, or distribution [23]. With this in mind, the WHO is playing an important role in establishing quality standards for registration and quality control of antimalarials by a prequalification program [24]. Initiatives such as the African Medicine Registration Harmonization (AMRH), in which partners collaborate with the WHO, have also been started in an attempt to improve quality standards of medicines at local and regional levels [25]. In addition, pharmaceutical companies must be responsible for ensuring that the quality of antimalarials meets the stringent guidelines established by regulatory authorities, for testing their medicines accordingly and for releasing to market only medicines that pass these requirements [2, 22].

This chapter will discuss the extent and consequences of poor-quality antimalarial medicines. In addition, the ways in which this issue might be tackled are also discussed, with a focus on the role of pharmaceutical companies, the WHO, and local and regional initiatives.

2. Defining poor-quality antimalarials

A variety of definitions have been used to classify the different types of poor-quality medicines [3, 26, 27]. The WHO has attempted to develop a consensus on definitions of poor-quality medicines, and has outlined two classes of drugs, namely those that are falsified, and those that are substandard [26].

Falsified medicines have been fraudulently manufactured with fake packaging, and contain little or no active ingredient (and often other potentially harmful substances) [3, 26]. Falsified antimalarial tablets and ampoules containing little or no API are a major problem in some areas [25]. They may be impossible to distinguish from the genuine product and may lead to under-dosing and high levels of treatment failure. In some extreme cases, the falsified antimalarials may contain toxic ingredients [26].

Substandard medicines have been poorly manufactured by a legitimate producer with no intent to deceive, but they usually have inadequate or excessive amounts of active ingredient(s) and/or excipients [3, 26]. The WHO also includes degraded drugs within this class [26]. The degraded drugs were originally of good quality, but become poor quality as a result of unsuitable or extended storage after manufacturing, or through interaction with inadequate excipients [3, 26].

3. The growing problem of poor-quality antimalarials

The problem of poor-quality antimalarial agents, particularly those containing artemisinins, is widespread and varies among countries. There are numerous reports of falsified and substandard antimalarial agents in particular in Africa and Asia [8–18].

One WHO survey evaluated the quality of selected antimalarials in six countries in sub-Saharan Africa (Cameroon, Ethiopia, Ghana, Kenya, Nigeria, and United Republic of Tanzania) [8]. Samples were collected and tested for quality by reliable quality control laboratories according to specifications set up in recognized pharmacopeias. The researchers found that 28.7% of the 267 fully tested samples collected between April and June 2008 failed to comply with prespecified internationally acceptable quality criteria. A similar proportion of ACTs and sulfadoxine-pyrimethamine (SP) were subject to quality defects (29% for ACTs and 28% for SP; **Figure 1**). Prevailing problems associated with ACTs were related to the content of the APIs and the presence of impurities. For SP, it was mainly problems related to dissolution. Interestingly, only 4% of the drugs with the WHO prequalification status failed quality analysis, compared with 60% of drugs not prequalified by the WHO. Therefore, control of the quality of antimalarial medicines throughout the distribution system, according to proper specifications, is an important prerequisite for ensuring optimal treatment outcomes [8].

In Southeast Asia, a similar problem with poor-quality medicines has been reported in a review of published and unpublished data from studies evaluating samples of antimalarials [3]. In seven Southeast Asian countries, 497 (35%) of 1437 samples failed chemical analysis, 423 (46%)

of 919 samples failed packaging analysis, and 450 (36%) of 1260 samples were falsified [3]. The same review also found that, in sub-Saharan Africa (21 countries), 796 (35%) of 2297 samples failed chemical analysis, 28 (36%) of 77 samples failed packaging analysis, and 79 (20%) of 389 samples were falsified [3].

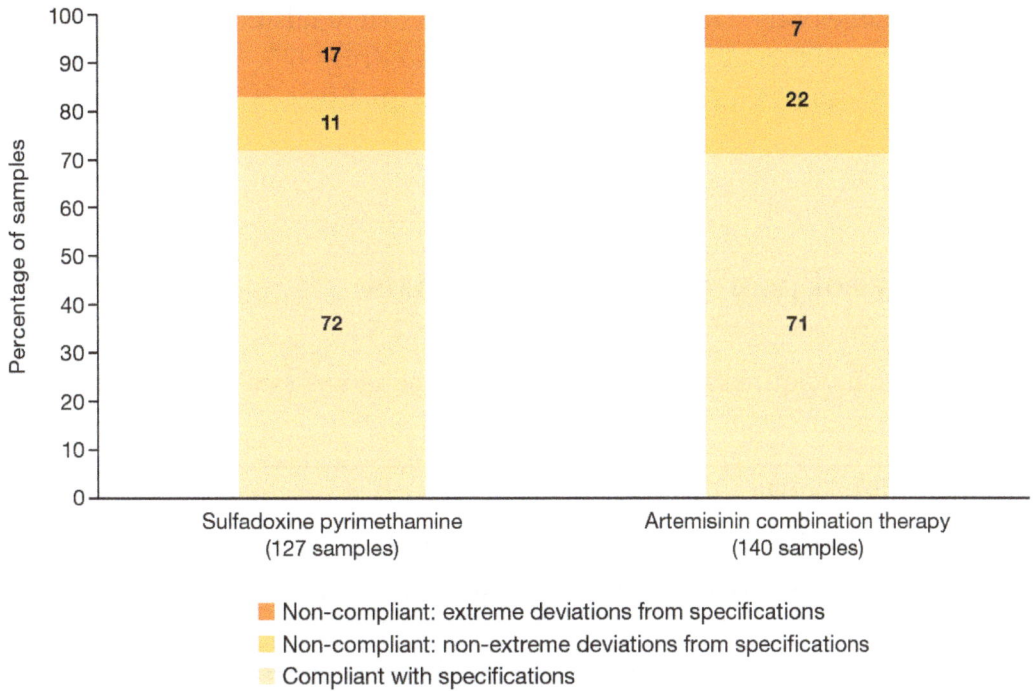

Figure 1. Proportions of compliant, moderately noncompliant and extremely noncompliant samples of artemisinin-based combination therapies (ACTs) and sulfadoxine-pyrimethamine (SP) in sub-Saharan Africa [8]. Extreme deviations were defined as a deviation by at least 20% from the declared content to one or more active ingredients, and/or dissolved percentage of one or more active ingredients less than the pharmacopoeial limit (Q) minus 25%.

The World-Wide Antimalarial Resistance Network (WWARN) has developed a comprehensive, open-access, global database, with a linked Antimalarial Quality Surveyor (an online visualization tool) in order to more fully understand the evidence relating to poor-quality antimalarials [15]. A systematic literature search from 1946 to March 2013 identified 251 published antimalarial reports, of which 130 had sufficient information to estimate the frequency of poor-quality antimalarials [15]. Out of 9348 antimalarials sampled, 30.1% (2813) failed chemical or packaging quality tests. Of the 2813 failed samples, 39.3% were classified as falsified, 2.3% as substandard, and 58.3% as poor quality without evidence available to categorize them as either falsified or substandard. Oral artesunate was the medicine most commonly reported as falsified (with 61.9% failing). The survey found that 60.6% (63) of the 104 malaria-endemic countries had no publicly available reports on antimalarial drug quality. Further investigation of the quality of antimalarials is required in the Americas, and in central and southern African regions, as there have been very few studies conducted in these malarious areas [15].

Studies from individual countries have also reported the existence of poor-quality antimalarials. One recent study used mystery shoppers and overt surveys to identify the quality of antimalarials in Cambodia [12]. Of 291 samples tested, 31.3% did not contain an appropriate amount of the API, i.e., the API content was not within the 85–115% range when measured by high performance liquid chromatography, and the samples were therefore considered to be of poor quality.

A recent study of the quality of artemisinin-based antimalarials from Tanzania's private sector found that, while none of the 1737 antimalarial samples were falsified, 4.1% were outside the 85–115% artemisinin API range [17]. WHO prequalified drugs (25.7% of the total) were more likely to be of higher quality, with only 0.5% WHO prequalified drugs being of poor quality, compared with 5.4% of those not WHO prequalified.

4. Consequences of poor-quality antimalarials

The use of poor-quality antimalarials has serious consequences (see **Table 1**) [3, 19, 28–36].

Increases in morbidity and mortality
Financial loss for patients, healthcare system, pharmaceutical companies
Loss of public confidence in pharmaceutical brand, medicines, pharmacies, and healthcare providers
Increased drug resistance

Table 1. Consequences of poor-quality antimalarials.

4.1. Morbidity and mortality

Exposure to low-quality antimalarials results in poor treatment outcomes, with increased morbidity and mortality. The literature contains several case reports of patients placed at risk or dying as a result of poor-quality antimalarials [28–30]. A study in 39 sub-Saharan African countries estimated that approximately 122,350 (4%) of the deaths in children aged <5 years that occurred in 2013 were associated with poor-quality antimalarial agents [19].

The impact of falsified and substandard medicines is likely to extend beyond such increases in morbidity and mortality. The continued use of poor-quality antimalarials that carry subtherapeutic levels of active ingredient will most likely lead to drug resistance [26, 31–36]. Partial artemisinin-resistant *Plasmodium falciparum* malaria has been reported in several Asian countries in the Greater Mekong Subregion [31–35]. The change in parasite sensitivity is manifest in the form of delayed parasite clearance, and has been associated with mutations in the Kelch 13 (K13) propeller region [37]. Indeed, the Greater Mekong Subregion is a major source from which drug-resistant malaria, including artemisinin-resistant *P. falciparum*, is known to emanate [38]. This occurs for multiple reasons, among which the local prevalence of falsified or substandard artemisinins is an important exacerbatory factor [38]. Based on the new WHO Global Technical Strategy for malaria 2016–2030, countries in the Greater Mekong Subregion have established a Strategy for Malaria Elimination in the Greater Mekong (2015–

2030) in response to the threat of multidrug resistance in this region [36, 39]. The goals of the strategy are to eliminate *P. falciparum* malaria by 2025, and all malaria by 2030, in all countries in the Greater Mekong.

4.2. Resistance

Resistance can be prevented or its outset slowed by the use of combination antimalarials, with different mechanisms of action [26]. Consequently, the standard of care for uncomplicated *P.falciparum* (i.e. move P. from previous page to page 6, line 1 so as not to break *P. falciparum (P. [space] falciparum)* malaria is treatment with ACTs [26]. The use of artemisinin monotherapies in subtherapeutic doses for over 30 years and the availability of substandard artemisinins are thought to be a major driving force in the selection of the resistant phenotype in these regions [9, 10, 33]. Moreover, some therapies declared as combinations in effect have been proven to be artemisinin monotherapies [9]. Resistance to artemisinin compromises the efficacy of the ACT and adds pressure on the partner drug [26].

Resistance to chloroquine has also been confirmed in *Plasmodium vivax* in 10 countries [36]. ACTs are now recommended for the treatment of chloroquine-resistant *P. vivax*, with the exception of treatment with artesunate and SP, where resistance to the partner drug may compromise the efficacy of the combination therapy.

4.3. Economic burden

The use of poor-quality antimalarials can have a negative financial impact on patients and their families [3, 16, 40]. Replacement or additional drugs, repeated courses of poor-quality antimalarials, repeated consultations at health facilities, and lost work days can all impose an unwanted economic burden [3, 16, 40], Indeed, recent modeling assuming current incidence rates of malaria indicates that widespread artemisinin resistance can be expected to lead to 116,000 excess deaths annually [41]. This burden may be particularly severe in some developing countries, where the majority of the population has to pay for their medicines and the cost of the medication represents a substantial proportion of the household income [40].

Poor-quality antimalarials also have negative financial consequences for healthcare systems, pharmaceutical companies, governments and societies, and their use may potentially jeopardize the investments made in the past decades to control and eliminate malaria [3, 16, 40]. The lost productivity and increased healthcare costs associated with the use of poor-quality antimalarials generally occur in resource-constrained countries that are already disproportionately bearing the global cost of malaria [36, 40]. These countries generally lack the increased financial resources needed to inspect, analyze and police the antimalarial supply chain [7].

In particular, the development and spread of resistance to antimalarial medicines has increased the cost of controlling malaria [36, 40, 41]. A decision-tree model estimated the direct medical costs for the effective treatment of malaria using ACT in nonresistant areas to be $US114 million (2013 costs). In comparison, it was estimated that these costs would increase by 28% if ACT was failing at a rate of 30%, and treatment of severe malaria reverted to quinine [41]. Productivity losses were estimated to be $US385 million for each year during which failing ACT was used as first-line therapy [41]. Most of this cost was associated with the lost productivity associated with excess morbidity after treatment had failed.

The development of resistance to all current antimalarials would necessitate the development of new, and potentially more expensive, alternatives by pharmaceutical companies, further adding to the economic burden they incur when a poor-quality alternative is used instead of their legitimate high-quality product [40].

If clinical trials use poor-quality medicines, not only are resources wasted, but patients may be harmed [42]. In addition, the erroneous conclusions reached in these trials may inappropriately inform public health policy [42].

5. Tackling the problem of poor-quality antimalarials

A wide variety of issues have contributed to the proliferation of poor-quality medicines in developing countries (**Table 2**) [2, 3]. In order for the quality of antimalarials to be assured, these issues need to be addressed.

Inadequate testing of quality

- Lack of inexpensive surveillance testing systems
- Lack of prequalified laboratories

Poor consumer and healthcare worker knowledge about product authenticity

Inadequate standardization of procedures within quality surveys

Self-prescription of drugs

Availability of products via the Internet

Expensive drugs with large profit margins

Trading in free-trade zones or free ports with minimum regulation

Poor or inadequate national, regional and global legislation, with few legal penalties

Absence of drug regulatory authorities

Unethical practices by manufacturers of antimalarials

Lack of political will and cooperation from stakeholders

Stockouts, thefts, and the erratic supply of antimalarials

Table 2. Factors contributing to the manufacture and distribution of poor-quality antimalarials [2, 3, 16].

It is essential that antimalarial medications be produced according to good manufacturing practice, contain the correct drug(s) and excipients in appropriate doses, and have bioavailability that is similar to the reference product; in addition, the drugs must be stored under appropriate conditions, and be dispensed before their expiry date [26].

Some of the factors that contribute to the availability of poor-quality medicines can only be addressed by collaborative action between law enforcement bodies, regulatory authorities, and customs and excise agencies [26]. Encouragingly, some initiatives and mechanisms are already in place to help ensure that quality assured antimalarials are available for use in malaria-endemic countries.

5.1. Detection methods and technology

Tests capable of accurately detecting and classifying poor-quality medicines at the point of entry into countries and at public and private pharmacies are essential for understanding the types, names, extent, and amount of poor-quality medicines being dispensed both nationally and globally [2, 7].

Such tests can be conducted using quick, inexpensive methods in the field with the aim of examining packaging and detecting drug contents [7]. These tools would also empower those inspecting the medicines throughout the supply chain [7]. Rather than having to wait for the samples to be sent to national or international laboratories, results would be available more or less immediately [7]. Current methods for testing the quality of drugs in the field include visual packaging inspection, lot number reporting via mobile phones, thin-layer chromatography, colorimetric tests, and simplified spectroscopic methods [2, 7]. Portable instruments used to screen for the quality of antimalarial agents include Raman spectrometers and the Global Pharma Health Fund GPHF-Minilab® [40]. Other simple, technologies for testing the quality of antimalarials in the field are in development [43, 44].

More accurate methods of testing the quality of medicines involve laboratories that are equipped for exhaustive chemical analysis [2]. Such investigations can be difficult in developing countries, given the sophisticated and expensive equipment, the type of reagents, and the level of technical expertise that are required. For example, Kenya, Tanzania, South Africa, and Uganda are currently the only countries in Africa with WHO prequalified laboratories for drug quality testing [19, 45].

5.2. Field reports

Quality surveys can serve as an important source of information about the quality of medicines available. Data on the quality of antimalarials, if properly collected, interpreted and used, are essential for the planning of effective interventions [46]. However, reports that have not employed rigorous scientific techniques will potentially bias results [47]. To ensure consistency and accuracy, the WHO has recently produced draft guidelines for the conduct of surveys of quality medicines [46].

5.3. Legislation and regulation

Existing laws in many countries are insufficiently strict to deter the manufacturing and distribution of poor-quality medicines; where this legislation exists, it may not be implemented [22]. Such absence of legislation prohibiting the manufacture and distribution of poor-quality medicines encourages their continued manufacturer, since there is no fear of being apprehended and prosecuted [2, 22].

Appropriate national medicine regulatory authorities would help to ensure that all pharmaceutical products on the market were safe, effective and meet approved quality standards [48]. Such regulation would control registration and postmarketing surveillance (quality monitoring and pharmacovigilance) of medicines, as well as the licensing and inspection of manufacturers, importers, exporters, wholesalers, distributors, pharmacies and retail outlets, control of clinical trials, and control of the promotion (**Figure 2**) [48]. It has also been suggested that an international legal convention against poor-quality medicines would address both regulatory and criminal international governance challenges [7].

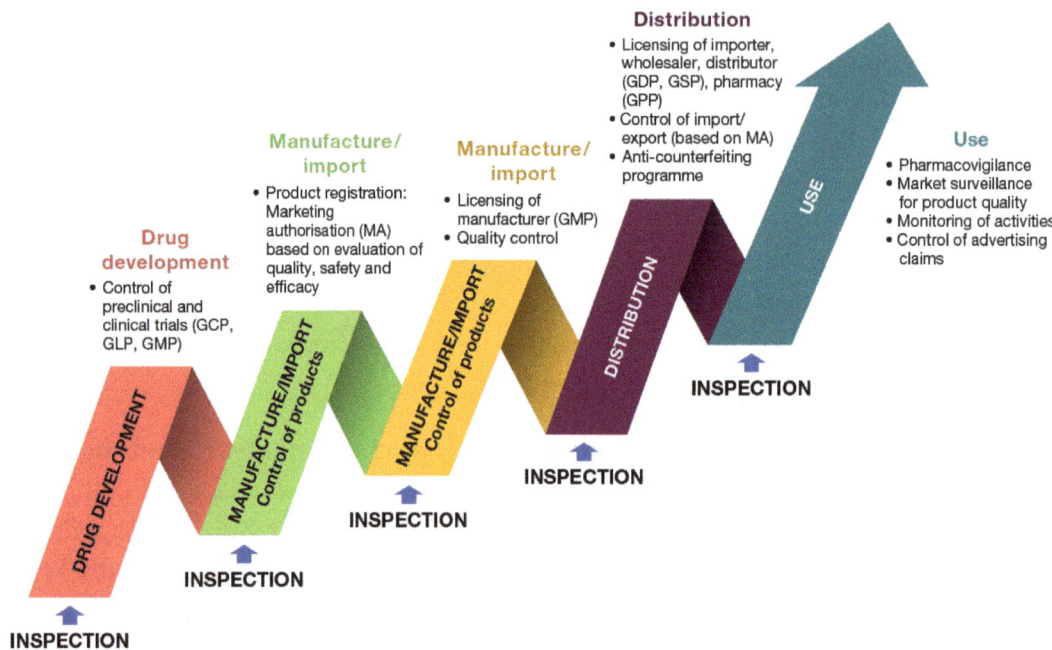

Figure 2. Regulatory system for medicines [48]. GCP, good clinical practices; GDP, good distribution practices; GLP, good laboratory practices; GMP, good manufacturing practices; GPP, good pharmaceutical practices; GSP, good storage practices.

However, the WHO has estimated that 30% of member countries lack any capacity to oversee medicine manufacture, importation, or distribution [23]. At present, only about 20% of member countries have well-developed medicine regulation at varying levels of development and operational capacity.

In particular, the lack of global harmonization of drug registration processes is contributing to the increased availability of poor-quality antimalarials. Regulatory authorities such as the European Medicines Agency (EMA) and the United States Food and Drug Administration (FDA) provide guidelines for the registration of new drugs for the pharmaceutical industry. Such guidelines include steps for assuring drug quality [49, 50]. For example, the FDA regulates and controls new drugs according to the new drug application process and the review and ultimate approval of generic drugs is controlled by regulations for abbreviated new drug applications.

However, similar rigorous standards are not applied universally, and particularly in sub-Saharan Africa. Africa currently has more than 50 independent local regulatory health authority agencies, with different administrative and technical requirements, processes and timelines for medicine registration and regulatory review, and with variable transparency of the registration process. A recent WHO assessment in 26 sub-Saharan African countries found that drug approval regulation was not carried out to the extent required to ensure the quality, efficacy, and safety of medicines [48]. Few countries in sub-Saharan Africa relied on the decisions made by other regulators, such as those stringently applied by the EMA or FDA, or by the WHO through its Prequalification of Medicines Program [48].

5.4. The role of the WHO

Many look to the WHO for leadership in regulating the quality of medicines, especially in light of its successful implementation of the public health treaty on tobacco control [7].

Due to the association of oral artemisinin monotherapies with the development of resistance, the WHO urges regulatory authorities in malaria-endemic countries *"to take measures to halt the production and marketing of these oral monotherapies, and promote access to quality-assured artemisinin-based combination therapies"* [51]. The number of countries that allow the marketing of oral artemisinin monotherapies has dropped markedly since the World Health Assembly adopted a resolution supporting the ban in 2007. As of November 2015, marketing of artemisinin monotherapies was still allowed by seven countries: Angola, Cape Verde, Colombia, Gambia, Sao Tome and Principe, Somalia, and Swaziland [51]. However, a continued strengthening of pharmaceutical regulation and the enforcement of existing regulations will be required for the complete withdrawal of oral artemisinin monotherapies from all countries.

In an attempt to standardize the quality of medicines that reach the market, in terms of their efficacy, safety, and method of manufacture, the WHO are managing the Prequalification of Medicines Program [24]. This program's quality evaluation criteria are based on international pharmaceutical standards and a mix of the best practices applied by the world's leading regulatory authorities [52]. Products that meet all of the criteria of the WHO Prequalification of Medicines Program are considered to be quality assured and are added to a WHO list of prequalified medicinal products [53]. This list is used by international procurement agencies and by countries to guide bulk purchasing of medicines. Currently, over 40 of the prequalified medicinal products on this list are antimalarial agents [53]. This program has validated the entry of a number of generic products into markets and procurement pools [52]. Such validation has provided an incentive for other manufacturers of generic products to raise their quality standards and increase the availability of affordable medicines.

In addition to prequalifying medicines, this program also prequalifies pharmaceutical quality control laboratories and active pharmaceutical ingredients, as well as advocating for medicines of guaranteed quality [24].

5.5. The AMRH initiative

One of the means of improving quality standards is to engage regional networks in developing countries with larger, more powerful and better resourced organizations such as the WHO. One example of such a network is the African Medicine Registration Harmonization Initiative (AMRH) [25, 54]. This program aims to harmonize the registration of medicinal products in Africa across regional economic communities (RECs) [25, 54]. In Africa, the RECs range in size from five to more than twenty-five member states—and all have been invited to participate in the AMRH program.

Partners involved in the AMRH program include the WHO, the New Partnership for Africa's Development, the African Union Commission, the Pan-African Parliament, the World Bank, the Bill and Melinda Gates Foundation, the UK Department for International Development, and the Clinton Health Access Initiative [25]. The WHO is to provide leadership for the development of common technical standards, documents, tools, and processes in line with international standards. The WHO also provides technical assistance for capacity-building and organizes joint assessment and inspection activities [25].

The first REC to secure funding from the AMRH initiative trust fund was the East African Community (EAC). The EAC Medicines Registration Harmonization (MRH) project was formally launched in 2012 in Tanzania and aims to achieve a harmonized medicines registration process in its member countries (Uganda, Kenya, the United Republic of Tanzania, Rwanda, and Burundi) based on common documents, processes, and shared information [25]. Given the progress made in the EAC MRH project, the AMRH initiative plans to expand to other RECs in Africa. It is hoped that five or six groupings will eventually cover the entire African continent. Continued support by concerned governments and international partners will be crucial for its success [25].

5.6. The role of pharmaceutical companies

Poor manufacturing and quality-control practices in the production of genuine drugs (either branded or generic) have considerable impact on the quality of medicines [40]. Pharmaceutical companies are responsible for ensuring that quality meets the guidelines of stringent health authorities, for testing their medicines accordingly and for releasing only medicines that pass these requirements [55]. Chinese and Indian manufacturers are commonly cited as sources of poor-quality antimalarials, but manufacturers in other countries may also be involved [7, 40]. It is essential that pharmaceutical companies behave ethically at all times and follow relevant guidelines and codes of conduct provided by regulatory authorities if the quality of medicines is to be assured.

Reputable pharmaceutical companies must ensure that medicines are under strict surveillance, and with quality control measures in place at all stages of the drug supply chain. Novartis, for example, ensures the quality control of medicines in a three-step process that involves verification, authentication, and pharmaceutical forensic investigations. Verification occurs at the local level to attest to the genuineness of the packaging materials and the plausibility of the manufacturing data (batch number, manufacturing, and expiry date). Authentication, done in the field, involves analyzing the product (tablets, liquids) with vibrational spectrometers. In the case of substantiation of falsification of medicines, a pharmaceutical forensic investigation then occurs, and any substantiated falsification incidents are escalated to the key stakeholders and national health authorities and the WHO are notified.

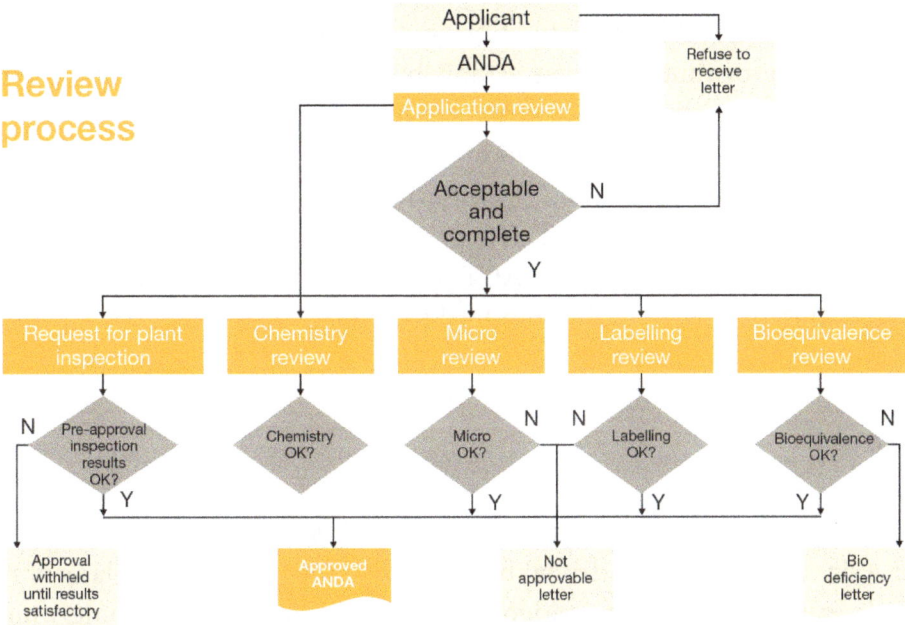

Figure 3. Process for review and approval of generic drugs (ANDA) [58]. Source: US Food and Drug Administration (public domain).

In countries where stringent regulatory authorities exist, pharmaceutical companies developing new drugs must follow a new drug application process that requires both preclinical and clinical studies [50]. In contrast, the approval of generic drugs or new formulations of existing drugs occurs via an abbreviated process that does not require clinical efficacy and safety studies (**Figure 3**) [56]. One of the dangers with some generic products is that they may contain the correct amounts of the drug, but, because of their formulation, they are not adequately absorbed, resulting in lower efficacy. Consequently, this abbreviated process requires proof that the generic product (or new formulation of a reference product) and the reference product have comparable bioavailability. If this is established, the products are said to be bioequivalent [56, 57].

Different types of evidence may be used to establish bioequivalence for pharmaceutically equivalent drug products, including in vivo or in vitro testing, or both [56]. If a generic product or new formulation shows equivalent exposure to the original marketed compound, it is assumed that its efficacy and safety will also be equivalent [56]. To this end, the WHO recommended that not only must all antimalarial medicines be manufactured according to good manufacturing practice and have the correct drug and excipient content, but they must also be proven to have bioavailability that is comparable to that of the reference listed product [26].

An example of a study that was conducted in line with these bioequivalence guidelines involves the antimalarial artemether-lumefantrine [58]. Because development of this compound adhered to these guidelines, this formulation received the WHO prequalification status in June 2014 [53]. The novel fixed-dose tablet formulation of the antimalarial artemether-lumefantrine 80/480 mg was developed in order to reduce the pill burden at each dose and potentially enhance adherence. It was then tested in a bioequivalence study in healthy volunteers against four standard tablets of artemether-lumefantrine 20/120 [59]. Bioequivalence between the two formulations was established, with the prespecified criteria for bioequivalence being met. These prespecified criteria were that the 90% confidence intervals for the geometric mean ratio (novel formulation versus four standard tablets) of the primary pharmacokinetic endpoints (AUC and C_{max}) for artemether and lumefantrine were contained within the acceptance interval of 0.80–1.25. These outcomes established that the rate and extent of absorption of both components of the ACT in the novel formulation of artemether-lumefantrine are comparable to those in the standard tablets.

6. Conclusion

There is a pressing need to reduce the use of poor-quality antimalarial medicines, especially in Africa and Asia. The problem is driven by several factors, including a lack of national and international drug legislation, and inadequate quality assurance by some pharmaceutical companies. This chapter has reviewed the steps and studies needed to ensure development of high-quality medicines based on health authority regulations (including WHO prequalification). The problem of poor-quality medicines can only be addressed by a multipronged approach that includes tackling poor regulation and ineffective/poorly implemented laws at national and international levels. Sustained national and international financing must underpin any such future approach. A legal framework or treaty that protects all countries against poor-quality medicines is also urgently required. Such a framework would facilitate the production of high-quality antimalarials and protect all countries against those who produce, distribute, and sell poor-quality products. In addition, pharmaceutical companies must be responsible for ensuring that the quality of antimalarials meets the stringent guidelines established by regulatory authorities, for testing their medicines accordingly and for releasing only medicines that pass these requirements into the market. The harmonization of the registration process across all nations would help ensure that patients throughout the world obtain access to high-quality antimalarials.

Surveillance of the quality of antimalarials is an essential component of the global fight against malaria. The establishment of a highly qualified, well-resourced international organization that works in collaboration with national medical regulatory bodies, pharmaceutical companies, and international agencies may help to ensure access to high-quality antimalarials on a global level. The implementation of strategies such as the WHO Prequalification Program, the AMRH initiative, and the ethical production of medicines by pharmaceutical companies will help to ensure that antimalarial therapies marketed in low-income, malaria-endemic countries are quality assured. Future research must focus on innovative technologies that accurately and affordably support the detection of poor-quality medicines at all levels of the supply chain, including prequalified reference laboratories. It is to be hoped that the implementation of such a multipronged approach by policy makers and leaders at the international and national levels will ensure the continued global availability of affordable, high-quality drugs to patients with malaria.

Acknowledgements

KH is an employee of Novartis Pharmaceuticals Corporation and KS is an employee of Novartis Pharma AG.

Author details

Kamal Hamed[1*] and Kirstin Stricker[2]

*Address all correspondence to: kamal.hamed@novartis.com

1 Novartis Pharmaceuticals Corporation, East Hanover, NJ, USA

2 Novartis Pharma AG, Basel, Switzerland

References

[1] Hamburg M. Foreword to the global pandemic of falsified medicines: laboratory and field innovations and policy implications. Am J Trop Med Hyg. 2015;92(6 Suppl.):1.

[2] Nayyar GM, Breman JG, Herrington JE. The global pandemic of falsified medicines: laboratory and field innovations and policy perspectives. Am J Trop Med Hyg. 2015;92(6 Suppl.):2–7.

[3] Nayyar GM, Breman JG, Newton PN, Herrington JE. Poor-quality antimalarial drugs in southeast Asia and sub-Saharan Africa. Lancet Infect Dis. 2012;12(6):488–496.

[4] Newton PN, Green MD, Mildenhall DC, Plancon A, Nettey H, Nyadong L, et al. Poor quality vital anti-malarials in Africa—an urgent neglected public health priority. Malar J. 2011;10:352.

[5] Newton PN, Green MD, Fernandez FM, Day NP, White NJ. Counterfeit anti-infective drugs. Lancet Infect Dis. 2006;6(9):602–613.

[6]   Hajjou M, Krech L, Lane-Barlow C, Roth L, Pribluda VS, Phanouvong S. Monitoring the quality of medicines: results from Africa, Asia, and South America. Am J Trop Med Hyg. 2015;92 (6 Suppl.):68–74.

[7]   Nayyar GM, Attaran A, Clark JP, Culzoni MJ, Fernandez FM, Herrington JE, et al. Responding to the pandemic of falsified medicines. Am J Trop Med Hyg. 2015;92(6 Suppl.):113–118.

[8]   Sabartova J, Toumi A. WHO report: survey of the quality of selected antimalarial medicines circulating in six countries of sub-Saharan Africa. 2015. Available from: http://www.who.int/medicines/publications/qamsareport/en/ [Accessed: July 7, 2016].

[9]   El-Duah M, Ofori-Kwakye K. Substandard artemisinin-based antimalarial medicines in licensed retail pharmaceutical outlets in Ghana. J Vector Borne Dis. 2012;49(3):131–139.

[10] Bate R, Coticelli P, Tren R, Attaran A. Antimalarial drug quality in the most severely malarious parts of Africa—a six country study. PLoS One. 2008;3(5):e2132.

[11] Dondorp AM, Newton PN, Mayxay M, Van Damme W, Smithuis FM, Yeung S, et al. Fake antimalarials in Southeast Asia are a major impediment to malaria control: multinational cross-sectional survey on the prevalence of fake antimalarials. Trop Med Int Health. 2004;9(12):1241.

[12] Yeung S, Lawford HL, Tabernero P, Nguon C, van Wyk A, Malik N, et al. Quality of antimalarials at the epicenter of antimalarial drug resistance: results from an overt and mystery client survey in Cambodia. Am J Trop Med Hyg. 2015;92(6 Suppl.):39–50.

[13] Chikowe I, Osei-Safo D, Harrison JJ, Konadu DY, Addae-Mensah I. Post-marketing surveillance of anti-malarial medicines used in Malawi. Malar J. 2015;14:127.

[14] Osei-Safo D, Agbonon A, Konadu DY, Harrison JJ, Edoh M, Gordon A, et al. Evaluation of the quality of artemisinin-based antimalarial medicines distributed in Ghana and Togo. Malar Res Treat. 2014;2014:806416.

[15] Tabernero P, Fernandez FM, Green M, Guerin PJ, Newton PN. Mind the gaps—the epidemiology of poor-quality anti-malarials in the malarious world—analysis of the WorldWide Antimalarial Resistance Network database. Malar J. 2014;13:139.

[16] Karunamoorthi K. The counterfeit anti-malarial is a crime against humanity: a systematic review of the scientific evidence. Malar J. 2014;13:209.

[17] ACT Consortium Drug Quality Project Team and the IMPACT2 Study Team. Quality of artemisinin-containing antimalarials in Tanzania's private sector-results from a nationally representative outlet survey. Am J Trop Med Hyg. 2015;92(6 Suppl.):75.

[18] Ravinetto R, Ngeleka Mutolo D, de Spiegeleere B, Marini R, Hasker E, Schiavetti B. The quality of paediatric medicines supplied by private wholesalers in Kinshasa, DRC. Trop Med Int Health. 2015;20(1 Suppl.):136.

[19] Renschler JP, Walters KM, Newton PN, Laxminarayan R. Estimated under-five deaths associated with poor-quality antimalarials in sub-Saharan Africa. Am J Trop Med Hyg. 2015;92(6 Suppl.):119–126.

[20] Dondorp AM, Nosten F, Yi P, Das D, Phyo AP, Tarning J, et al. Artemisinin resistance in Plasmodium falciparum malaria. N Engl J Med. 2009;361(5):455.

[21] White NJ, Pongtavornpinyo W, Maude RJ, Saralamba S, Aguas R, Stepniewska K, et al. Hyperparasitaemia and low dosing are an important source of anti-malarial drug resistance. Malar J. 2009;8:253.

[22] Attaran A. Stopping murder by medicine: introducing the Model Law on Medicine Crime. Am J Trop Med Hyg. 2015;92(6 Suppl.):127.

[23] World Health Organization. What encourages counterfeiting of medicines? 2013. Available from: https://www.wiltonpark.org.uk/wp-content/uploads/WP1185-WHO-What-encourages-counterfeiting-of-medicines.pdf. [Accessed: July 7, 2016].

[24] World Health Organization. Prequalification of medicines by WHO. Factsheet No. 278. 2013. Available from: http://www.who.int/mediacentre/factsheets/fs278/en. [Accessed: July 7, 2016].

[25] African Medicine Registration Harmonization Programme. AMRH Programme. 2014. Available from: http://amrh.org/. [Accessed: July 7, 2016].

[26] World Health Organization. Guidelines for the treatment of malaria. 2015. Available from: www.who.int/malaria/publications/atoz/9789241549127/en/. [Accessed: July 7, 2016].

[27] Attaran A, Barry D, Basheer S, Bate R, Benton D, Chauvin J, et al. How to achieve international action on falsified and substandard medicines. BMJ. 2012;345:e7381.

[28] Newton PN, McGready R, Fernandez F, Green MD, Sunjio M, Bruneton C, et al. Manslaughter by fake artesunate in Asia-will Africa be next? PLoS Med. 2006;3(6):e197.

[29] Keoluangkhot V, Green MD, Nyadong L, Fernandez FM, Mayxay M, Newton PN. Impaired clinical response in a patient with uncomplicated falciparum malaria who received poor-quality and underdosed intramuscular artemether. Am J Trop Med Hyg. 2008;78(4):552–555.

[30] Chaccour CJ, Kaur H, Mabey D, Del Pozo JL. Travel and fake artesunate: a risky business. Lancet. 2012;380(9847):1120.

[31] Ye R, Hu D, Zhang Y, Huang Y, Sun X, Wang J, et al. Distinctive origin of artemisinin-resistant Plasmodium falciparum on the China-Myanmar border. Sci Rep. 2016;6:20100.

[32] Tun KM, Imwong M, Lwin KM, Win AA, Hlaing TM, Hlaing T, et al. Spread of artemisinin-resistant Plasmodium falciparum in Myanmar: a cross-sectional survey of the K13 molecular marker. Lancet Infect Dis. 2015;15(4):415.

[33] Dondorp AM, Yeung S, White L, Nguon C, Day NP, Socheat D, et al. Artemisinin resistance: current status and scenarios for containment. Nat Rev Microbiol. 2010;8(4): 272.

[34] Noedl H, Se Y, Schaecher K, Smith BL, Socheat D, Fukuda MM. Evidence of artemisinin-resistant malaria in western Cambodia. N Engl J Med. 2008;359(24):2619.

[35] Phyo AP, Nkhoma S, Stepniewska K, Ashley EA, Nair S, McGready R, et al. Emergence of artemisinin-resistant malaria on the western border of Thailand: a longitudinal study. Lancet. 2012;379(9830):1960.

[36] World Health Organization. World Malaria Report. 2015. Available from: http://www.who.int/malaria/publications/world-malaria-report-2015/report/en/ [Accessed: July 7, 2016].

[37] Mita T, Tachibana S, Hashimoto M, Hirai M. Plasmodium falciparum kelch 13: a potential molecular marker for tackling artemisinin-resistant malaria parasites. Expert Rev Anti Infect Ther. 2016;14(1):125–135.

[38] Cui L, Yan G, Sattabongkot J, Chen B, Cao Y, Fan Q, Parker D, Sirichaisinthop J, Su XZ, Yang H, Yang Z, Wang B, Zhou G. Challenges and prospects for malaria elimination in the Greater Mekong Subregion. Acta Trop. 2012;121(3):240–245.

[39] World Health Organization. Strategy for malaria elimination in the Greater Mekong Subregion: 2015–2030. 2015. Available from: http://www.wpro.who.int/mvp/documents/strat_mal_elim_gms/en/. [Accessed: July 7, 2016].

[40] Johnston A, Holt DW. Substandard drugs: a potential crisis for public health. Br J Clin Pharmacol. 2014;78(2):218.

[41] Lubell Y, Dondorp A, Guérin PJ, Drake T, Meek S, Ashley E, Day NPJ, White NJ, White LJ. Artemisinin resistance—modelling the potential human and economic costs. Malar J. 2014;13:452.

[42] Newton PN, Schellenberg D, Ashley EA, Ravinetto R, Green MD, ter Kuile FO, et al. Quality assurance of drugs used in clinical trials: proposal for adapting guidelines. BMJ. 2015;350:h602.

[43] Weaver AA, Lieberman M. Paper test cards for presumptive testing of very low quality antimalarial medications. Am J Trop Med Hyg. 2015;92(6 Suppl.):17.

[44] Ho NT, Desai D, Zaman MH. Rapid and specific drug quality testing assay for artemisinin and its derivatives using a luminescent reaction and novel microfluidic technology. Am J Trop Med Hyg. 2015;92(6 Suppl.):24.

[45] World Health Organization. WHO list of prequalified quality control laboratories. 38th edition, 2016. Available from: www.who.int/prequal/lists/PQ_QCLabsList.pdf [Accessed: February 22, 2016].

[46] World Health Organization. Guidelines on the conduct of surveys of the quality of medicines: draft for comment. 2016. Available from: http://www.who.int/medicines/

areas/quality_safety/quality_assurance/Guidelines-on-medicines-quality-surveys-QAS15-630_30062015.pdf. [Accessed: July 7, 2016].

[47] Newton PN, Lee SJ, Goodman C, Fernandez FM, Yeung S, Phanouvong S, et al. Guidelines for field surveys of the quality of medicines: a proposal. PLoS Med. 2009;6(3):e52.

[48] World Health Organization. Assessment of medicines regulatory systems in sub-Saharan African countries. 2010. Available from: www.who.int/healthsystems/Assessment26African_countries.pdf?ua=1. [Accessed: July 7, 2016].

[49] European Medicines Agency. EMA Scientific Guidelines. 2015. Available from: http://www.ema.europa.eu/ema/index.jsp?curl=pages/regulation/general/general_content_000043.jsp&mid=WC0b01ac05800240cb [Accessed: July 7, 2016].

[50] United States Food and Drug Administration. FDA drug development guidelines. 2015. Available from: http://www.fda.gov/Drugs/DevelopmentApprovalProcess/HowDrugsareDevelopedandApproved/ApprovalApplications/InvestigationalNewDrugINDApplication/ucm176522.htm. [Accessed: July 7, 2016].

[51] World Health Organization. Withdrawal of oral artemisin-based monotherapies. 2016. Available from: http://www.who.int/malaria/areas/treatment/withdrawal_of_oral_artemisinin_based_monotherapies/en/. [Accessed: July 7, 2016].

[52] World Health Organization. Improving quality for better treatment and greater access: prequalifications of medicine programme. 2012. Available from: http://apps.who.int/prequal/info_general/documents/advocacy/Advocacy_booklet_2012.pdf. [Accessed: July 7, 2016].

[53] World Health Organization. WHO list of prequalified medicinal products. 2016. Available from: http://apps.who.int/prequal/. [Accessed: July 7, 2016].

[54] World Health Organization. WHO support for medicines regulatory harmonization in Africa: focus on East African Community. 2014. Available from: http://www.who.int/medicines/publications/druginformation/DI_28-1_Africa.pdf. [Accessed: July 7, 2016].

[55] World Medical Association. WMA Declaration of Helsinki—Ethical Principles for Medical Research Involving Human Subjects. 2016. Available from: http://www.wma.net/en/30publications/10policies/b3/. [Accessed: July 7, 2016].

[56] United States Food and Drug Administration. Product-specific recommendations for generic drug development. 2016. Available from: http://www.fda.gov/Drugs/GuidanceComplianceRegulatoryInformation/Guidances/ucm075207.htm. [Accessed: July 7, 2016].

[57] European Medicines Agency. Guideline on the investigation of bioequivalence. 2015. Available from: www.ema.europa.eu/docs/en_GB/document_library/Scientific_guideline/2010/01/WC500070039.pdf. [Accessed: July 7, 2016].

[58] United States Food and Drug Administration. The FDA Process for Approving Generic Drugs. 2007. Available from: http://www.fda.gov/Training/ForHealthProfessionals/ucm090320.htm. [Accessed: July 7, 2016].

[59] Lefevre G, Bhad P, Jain JP, Kalluri S, Cheng Y, Dave H, et al. Evaluation of two novel tablet formulations of artemether-lumefantrine (Coartem) for bioequivalence in a randomized, open-label, two-period study. Malar J. 2013;12:312.

6

Transyears Competing with the Seasons in Tropical Malaria Incidence

Lyazzat Gumarova, Germaine Cornelissen,
Borislav D Dimitrov and Franz Halberg

Abstract

Communicable and non-communicable diseases show coperiodisms (shared cycles) with the sun's and earth's magnetism. About 11-year cycles and components with periods a few weeks or a few months longer than one year (near- and far-transyears, respectively) are the cases in point. Published data on the incidence of malaria in Burundi, Papua New Guinea, and Thailand are analysed by the linear-nonlinear cosinor to assess the relative prominence of transyears versus the calendar year. An about 2.3-year component characterizes malaria incidence in Burundi and Papua New Guinea (Thailand data were only sampled yearly). Long-term trends cannot be distinguished from the presence of an about 11-year cycle found in a 100-year long record from Chizhevsky on mortality from cholera in Russia, albeit its second harmonic is statistically significant in Burundi's data. Whereas far- and near-transyears characterize malaria incidence in Burundi more prominently than the calendar year, only a candidate near-transyear of small amplitude is barely detected in Papua New Guinea, where the calendar year is most prominently expressed. Both regions are located near the equator. Selectively-assorted geographic differences such as these, observed herein for a communicable disease, have been previously observed for non-communicable conditions, such as sudden cardiac death.

Keywords: Chronoepidemiology, Malaria, time series analysis, public health, infectious diseases

1. Introduction

Signatures of cycles in the sun's and the earth's magnetism, found in the aetiology of both communicable and non-communicable diseases, are selectively assorted geographically [1]. Far-transyears and near-transyears (components with periods a few months or a few weeks longer than the calendar year, respectively) are both known to characterize interplanetary and terrestrial magnetism and their biospheric signatures [1–3]. A geographic study of the incidence of sudden cardiac death reveals the prominence of the transyear over the calendar year in Minnesota and Tokyo, whereas the opposite holds in Hong Kong, North Carolina (USA), and the Republic of Georgia [2, 4].

About 11-year (Horrebow-Schwabe) cycles of relative sunspot numbers [5–7] have also been reported to characterize communicable diseases such as malaria, as suggested earlier by Dimitrov et al. [8]. In their analysis of cerebral malaria in Papua New Guinea (latitude between 0° and 12°S, longitude 140°–160°E), these authors also reported the presence of a strong calendar-yearly component, in the absence of a marked transyear. By contrast, a transyear over calendar year prominence at -3° from the equator characterized a time series of natality in Mindanao, Philippines (8°N, 125°E) [2,3]. In a study of malaria in Thailand, a period of about 4 years was prominent, while geographic differences prevailed; "seasonal" cycles were only synchronous in small clusters [9].

Gomez-Elipe et al. [10] forecast malaria incidence based on monthly case reports and environmental factors in Karuzi, a province of the Burundi highlands (at 3°6′5″ S, 30°9′53″ E), recorded from 1997 to 2003. The analysis is complicated by the occurrence of a large outbreak, resulting in outlying values. The authors developed a satisfactory model to predict malaria incidence (notifications of malaria cases from local health facilities) in an area of unstable transmission by studying the association between environmental variables (rain, temperature, and a vegetation index, NDVI) and disease dynamics. Their autoregressive integrated moving average model predicted malaria incidence during a given month based on the incidence during the previous month together with NDVI, mean maximum temperature, and rainfall during the previous month with a 93% forecasting accuracy (R^2adj = 82%, $P < 0.0001$). While their model was useful for forecasting the malaria incidence rate in the study area, we ask whether cycles in malaria incidence found in Karuzi are similar to those found in other geographic sites located near the equator, where populations are exposed to factors that strongly influence the origin and magnitude of malaria epidemics, such as a weakened immunity of the population associated with famine and massive displacements, failures of control measures and epidemiologic disease surveillance, and unstable environmental factors such as rainfall, temperature, and vegetation [11].

Herein, we revisit published data on the incidence of malaria in different geographic locations near the equator. For this purpose, we turn to data in Papua New Guinea [8], Thailand, and Karuzi, Burundi [10], to explore any differences in terms of the relative prominence of transyears versus the calendar year. Our meta-analysis raises the question whether space weather may also contribute to communicable diseases like malaria in certain geographic regions at certain but not at other longitudes and/or as a function of prevailing climatologic factors.

2. Materials and methods

Data from Papua New Guinea consist of the total monthly admissions for cerebral malaria and of those from selected facilities, recorded between 1987 and 1996 [8]. Data from Thailand are those reported by WHO (www.sears.who.int/EN/), available yearly between 1971 and 2010 for the percentage of microscopically diagnosed malaria positive slides found in blood smears examined, the number of cases of *Plasmodium falciparum* infections (including mixed infections), the number of *P. falciparum* infections per 100 slides examined, the percentage of *P. falciparum* infections per 100 malaria positives, and the number and percentage of malaria-related deaths, among others. Data from Karuzi, Burundi, are those published by Gomez-Elipe et al. [10], available from 1997 to 2003.

Data were analysed by the extended cosinor [12–15]. Least squares spectra examined the entire time structure (globally) to identify candidate cycles as spectral peaks. Nonlinear least squares based on Marquardt's algorithm [16] provided estimates of the periods involved with a measure of uncertainty as "conservative" 95% confidence intervals (CIs).

3. Results

After square root transformation, the monthly incidence of malaria in Burundi was characterized by a near- and far-transyear, and by components with periods of about 5.2 and 2.3 years. Results from the nonlinear analyses are summarized in **Table 1**. The corresponding model fitted to the data is illustrated in **Figure 1**. As illustrated in **Figure 2** (left and middle), the near- and far-transyears with periods of about 1.15 and 1.5 years, respectively, are more prominently expressed than the 1.0-year synchronized (calendar) component, as gauged by amplitude ratios.

The about 5.2-year component found in Burundi (**Figure 1**) may correspond to the second harmonic of the decadal cycle reported by Dimitrov et al. [8] for cases of cerebral malaria in Papua New Guinea. A component with a period slightly longer than 2 years was also reported by Dimitrov et al. [8] for the data in Papua New Guinea, together with a prominent yearly rhythm, as seen from least squares spectra of the original data and of the detrended data, obtained by removing either a linear or a quadratic trend (**Figure 3(A)–(C)**). The large-amplitude low-frequency component reflects a trend, a low-frequency cycle, or both, which may be difficult to separate in view of the brevity of the series. There is also a smaller spectral peak (below the noise level) that may correspond to a near-transyear, perhaps the second harmonic of the slightly longer-than-2-year component.

All components fitted concomitantly					
Period	[95% CI]		Amplitude	[95% CI]	
Original data					
4.78	3.89	5.68	7.04	3.68	10.40
2.26	1.95	2.58	4.80	1.38	8.21
1.50	1.34	1.66	4.82	1.44	8.19
1.13	1.02	1.24	3.90	0.63	7.17
After square-root transformation					
5.18	4.21	6.15	1.05	0.65	1.45
2.34	1.93	2.74	0.55	0.14	0.96
1.54	1.35	1.73	0.59	0.17	1.00
1.15	1.04	1.27	0.50	0.11	0.90

Table 1. Nonlinear results of monthly incidence of malaria in Burundi.

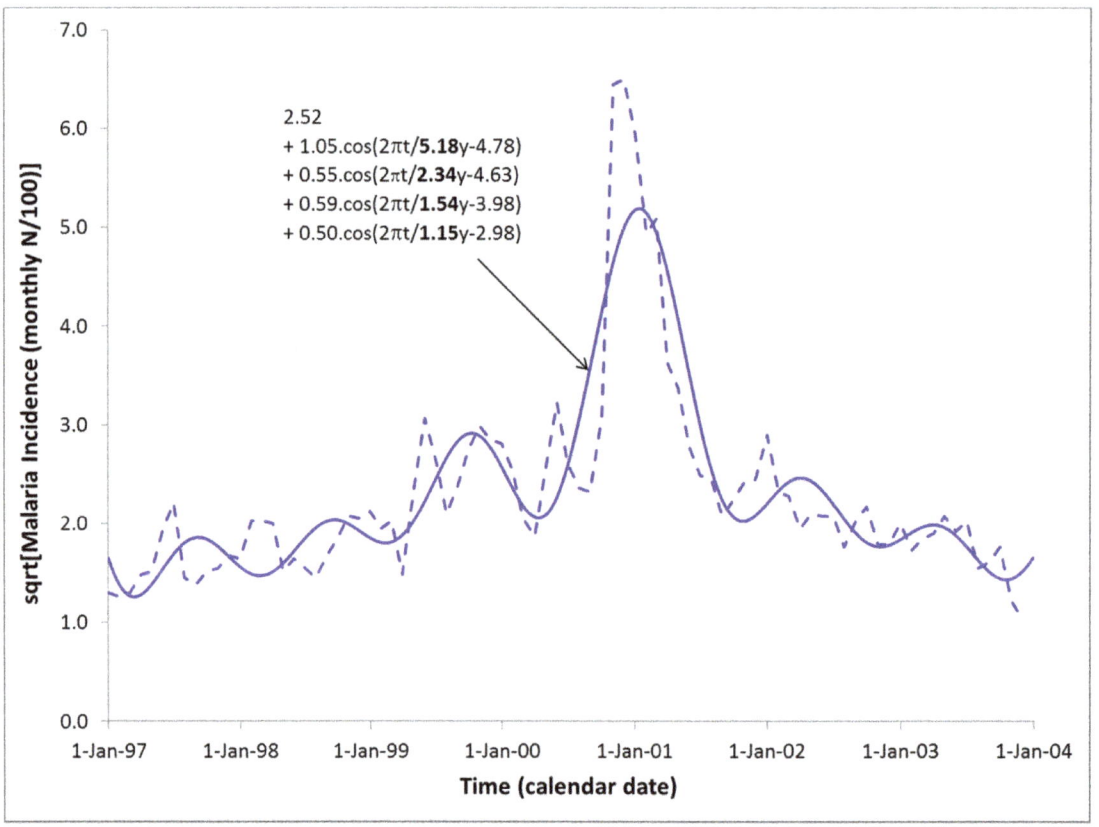

$$2.52$$
$$+ 1.05 \cdot \cos(2\pi t / 5.18y - 4.78)$$
$$+ 0.55 \cdot \cos(2\pi t / 2.34y - 4.63)$$
$$+ 0.59 \cdot \cos(2\pi t / 1.54y - 3.98)$$
$$+ 0.50 \cdot \cos(2\pi t / 1.15y - 2.98)$$

Figure 1. In view of a large outbreak resulting in influential (outlying) values, the monthly data on malaria incidence in Burundi recorded between 1997 and 2004 are transformed by taking their square root prior to analysis by the extended (linear-nonlinear) cosinor. Components with periods of about 5.2, 2.3, 1.5, and 1.15 years identified by least squares spectra and validated nonlinearly are included in a model plotted with the data. © Halberg Chronobiology Center.

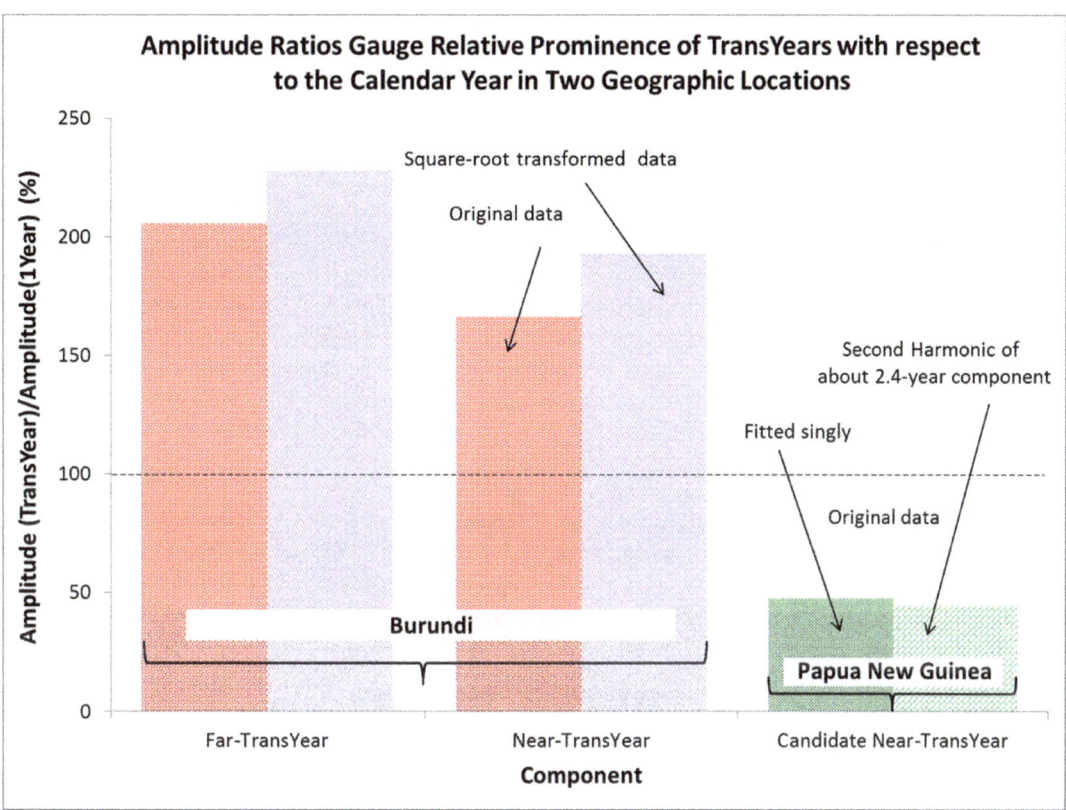

Figure 2. Amplitude ratios compare the relative prominence of the far- and near-transyear versus the calendar year in malaria incidence in Burundi (left and middle) and in Papua New Guinea (right). Despite the fact that both geographic sites are located near the equator, transyears are more prominent in Burundi but are only barely detected in Papua New Guinea. © Halberg Chronobiology Center.

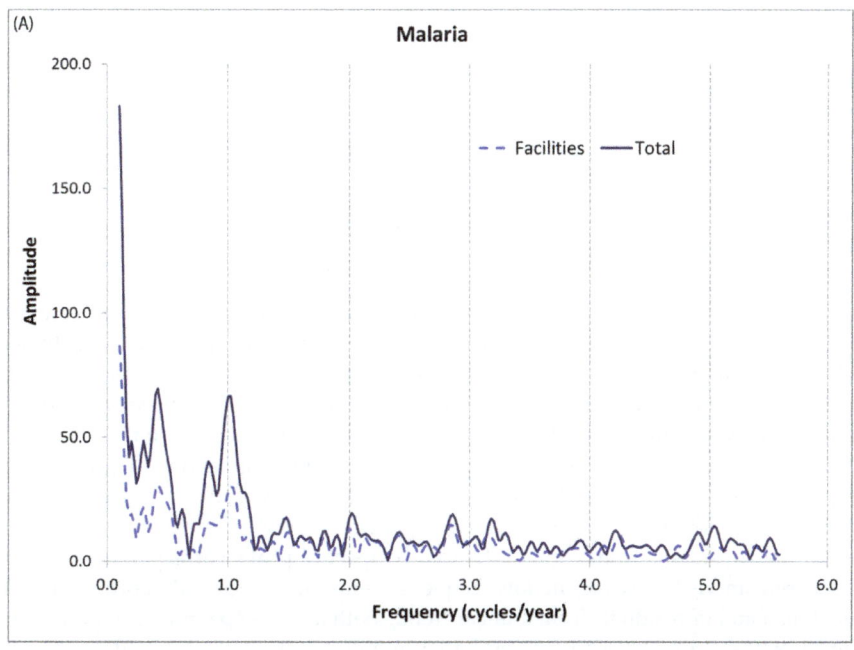

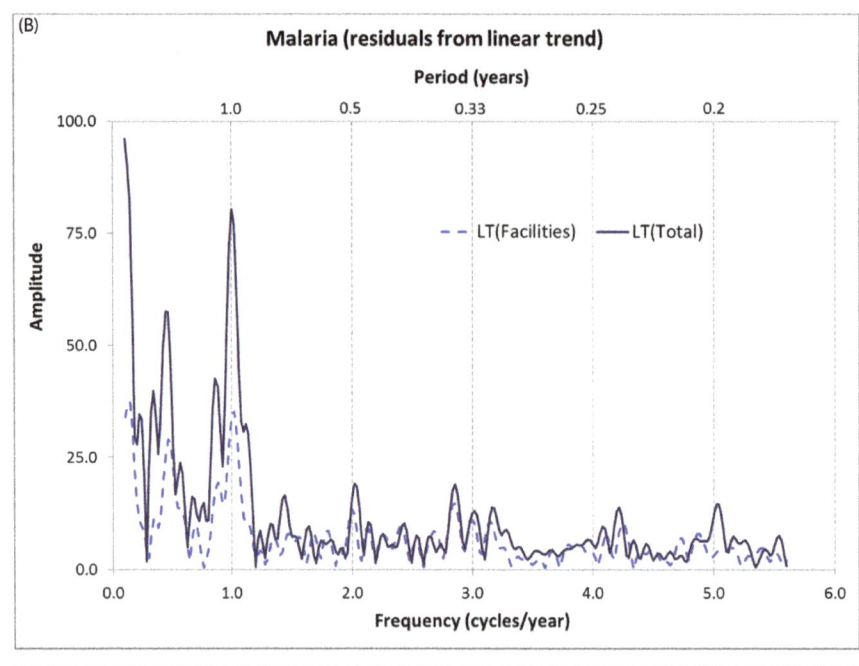

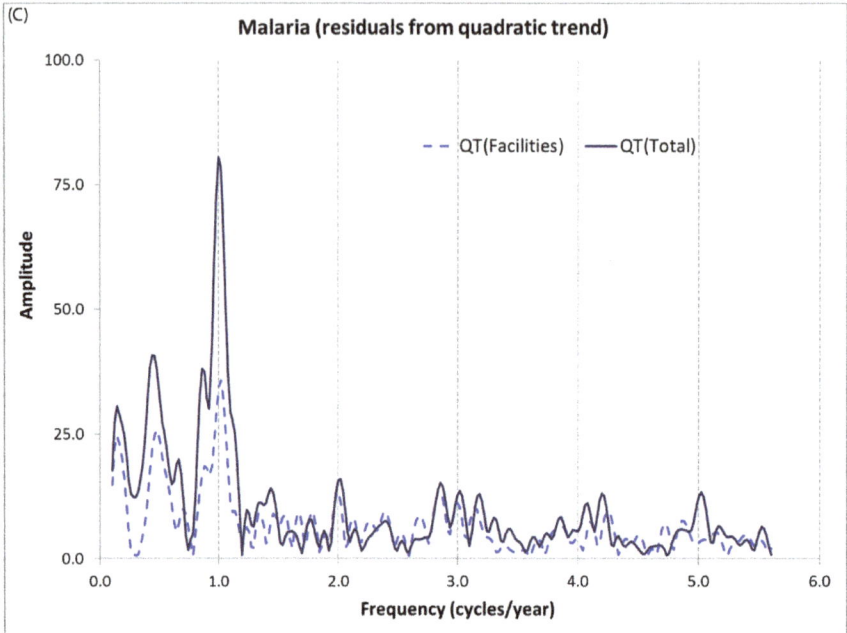

Figure 3. (A) Least squares spectrum of the monthly incidence of cerebral malaria in Papua New Guinea (original data). Spectral peaks correspond to a prominent 1-year component and a cycle with a period slightly longer than 2 years. The large amplitude of the low-frequency component may reflect the increasing trend seen in a plot of the data as a function of time (not shown). © Halberg Chronobiology Center. **(B)** Least squares spectrum of the monthly incidence of cerebral malaria in Papua New Guinea (residuals from a linear trend). In addition to the spectral peaks corresponding to the year and about 2.3-year components seen in the spectrum of the original data (**Figure 3(A)**), there is a smaller peak corresponding to a cycle with a period of about 1.15 years, which may also be the second harmonic of the about 2.3-year cycle. © Halberg Chronobiology Center. (C) Least squares spectrum of the monthly incidence of cerebral malaria in Papua New Guinea (residuals from a quadratic trend). Spectral peaks corresponding to the yearly and about 2.3-yearly components remain visible, while the low-frequency amplitude is considerably reduced by comparison to spectra of the original data and of residuals from a linear trend. With a series spanning no more than 10 years, it is not possible to distinguish between a quadratic trend and a cycle with a period of about 10 years or longer. © Halberg Chronobiology Center.

	Facilities						Total					
	Period	[95% CI]		Amplitude	[95% CI]		Period	[95% CI]		Amplitude	[95% CI]	
Trial period = 2 years												
Original	2.392	2.084	2.700	30.93	-1.07	62.94	2.420	2.127	2.714	70.05	4.10	135.99
+LinTrend	2.147	1.961	2.332	29.30	7.67	50.93	2.229	2.019	2.440	58.76	14.02	103.50
+QuadTrend	2.104	1.900	2.308	26.24	4.56	47.91	2.228	1.977	2.478	42.14	3.87	80.40
Trial periods = 10, 2 and 1 year(s)												
Original	15.346	8.607	22.085	93.50	63.98	123.02	17.629	8.924	26.333	247.54	118.83	376.26
	2.055	1.840	2.270	22.88	2.11	43.65	2.448	2.190	2.707	41.14	8.30	73.98
	0.985	0.952	1.017	33.80	13.14	54.46	0.992	0.970	1.013	77.53	45.86	109.19
+LinTrend	7.895	4.377	11.414	35.44	13.66	57.21	11.879	1.871	21.887	116.30	-12.49	245.09
	2.147	1.925	2.370	24.73	3.24	46.23	2.338	2.079	2.596	41.20	7.44	74.96
	0.986	0.953	1.019	33.43	12.55	54.32	0.993	0.971	1.016	77.20	44.40	110.00
+QuadTrend	6.160	2.488	9.831	24.81	0.15	49.47	5.161	3.597	6.725	35.28	0.88	69.69
	2.126	1.892	2.360	25.36	3.22	47.50	2.190	1.970	2.409	41.46	8.50	74.42
	0.987	0.954	1.021	34.12	12.43	55.82	0.996	0.975	1.018	80.29	47.96	112.63
Trial periods = 10, 2 and 1(fixed) year(s)												
Original	15.614	8.684	22.544	94.12	63.97	124.28	21.895	5.081	38.708	309.80	0.33	619.26
	2.056	1.852	2.260	23.46	3.29	43.62	2.200	1.980	2.419	38.13	7.06	69.21
	1.000			32.42	12.40	52.44	1.000			77.49	46.83	108.16
+LinTrend	7.822	4.518	11.127	35.02	14.10	55.94	11.405	2.988	19.821	106.28	15.08	197.47
	2.137	1.926	2.347	25.13	4.27	45.99	2.265	2.036	2.493	41.27	8.52	74.01
	1.000			32.37	12.13	52.62	1.000			77.00	45.43	108.56
+QuadTrend	6.036	2.846	9.226	24.63	1.54	47.72	5.149	3.666	6.632	35.45	2.27	68.64
	2.117	1.898	2.337	25.81	4.30	47.33	2.185	1.977	2.393	41.61	9.82	73.40
	1.000			33.27	12.16	54.37	1.000			80.06	48.92	111.20
Trial period = 1.2 years												
Original	1.189	1.031	1.346	15.84	-6.75	48.44	1.187	1.058	1.316	40.22	-27.36	107.81
+LinTrend	1.136	1.052	1.220	19.40	-3.05	41.84	1.154	1.074	1.235	43.06	-3.13	89.24
+QuadTrend	1.130	1.044	1.215	18.64	-3.52	40.80	1.152	1.078	1.226	38.61	0.84	76.37
Trial period = 2.4(&2ndH) years												
Original	2.397	2.162	2.631	30.72	-6.26	67.70	2.405	2.197	2.612	69.37	-6.57	145.31
	1.198			15.39	-21.34	52.12	1.202			38.49	-37.30	114.28
+LinTrend	2.220	2.077	2.363	26.78	2.68	50.87	2.287	2.147	2.428	54.38	5.26	103.51
	1.110			15.93	-8.10	39.97	1.144			38.98	-10.19	88.16
+QuadTrend	1.982	1.925	2.040	23.21	3.03	43.40	2.300	2.164	2.436	39.01	-1.81	79.84
	0.991			35.91	15.58	56.24	1.150			36.29	-3.61	76.20
Trial period = 10,2.4(&2ndH) years on residuals from 1-year fit												
Original	14.160	8.695	19.625	88.98	65.46	112.51	17.656	9.159	26.153	245.83	121.36	370.30
	2.357	2.110	2.603	19.79	-1.41	40.98	2.408	2.240	2.577	40.60	9.60	71.60
	1.178			7.90	-12.43	28.22	1.204			18.59	-11.26	48.45
+LinTrend	8.008	4.596	11.421	35.59	15.31	55.87	12.612	0.755	24.470	118.08	-28.72	364.87
	2.165	2.048	2.283	23.80	3.95	43.66	2.204	2.095	2.314	38.99	8.10	69.87
	1.083			16.21	-2.85	35.27	1.102			28.80	-0.59	58.18
+QuadTrend	6.042	3.160	8.923	24.49	3.33	45.65	5.133	3.829	6.437	35.08	4.44	65.71
	2.160	2.042	2.278	24.38	4.03	44.73	2.195	2.097	2.293	39.90	10.60	69.21
	1.080			16.94	-2.79	36.67	1.097			30.62	2.22	59.03

Table 2. Nonlinear results from several models fitted to monthly incidence of malaria in Papua New Guinea.

Nonlinear results from several models fitted to the data in Papua New Guinea are summarized in **Table 2**. A 1.0-year synchronized component is most prominent, whereas transyears are not detected with statistical significance (**Figure 2**, right). As seen from **Table 2**, the period of the circannual component has a CI overlapping the exact 1.0 (calendar) year. Accordingly, its period can be fixed in composite models. The period of the about 2.3-year component assumes consistent estimates irrespective of the model considered. As expected from the brevity of the series spanning only 10 years, this is not the case for the decadal component. Indeed, the low-frequency (about 10-year?) component is somewhat problematic: analyses of the original data tend to estimate its period between 17 and 22 years, shortened to about 11 years in some models including a linear trend, or toward 5 years when considering a quadratic trend. Nevertheless, for the total number of cases, the period estimate converges toward 11.4 years when a linear trend is included in the model, albeit with a very wide CI. A near-transyear with a period of about 1.15 years is also detected when fitted as a single component or as the second harmonic of the about 2.3-year cycle, but its amplitude is much smaller than that of the yearly rhythm and it cannot be detected with statistical significance as part of a composite model including the yearly and decadal cycles. Only in the case of facilities when a linear trend is included in the model and analyses are carried out on residuals from the yearly component is the near-transyear detected with borderline statistical significance, the decadal cycle having an estimated period of 8.0 [CI: 4.6, 11.4] years.

As a compromise, a model consisting of a linear trend, a fixed 1-year component and about 10-year and 2.3-year components was used to approximate the data. For all cases (total), the period estimates were 11.4 [CI: 3.0, 19.8] and 2.26 [CI: 2.04, 2.49] years. Using these estimates, a composite model was fitted by the linear cosinor, including the candidate 1.1-year component. The model as a whole and all its components are detected with statistical significance for both facilities and all cases (*P*<0.001). Results from this multiple-component fit were used to approximate the data, as illustrated in **Figure 4**.

Whatever model is considered, malaria in Papua New Guinea is characterized by a prominent yearly component, a cycle with a period slightly longer than 2 years and a trend that may correspond to a longer cycle, possibly with a period of about 10 years. No far-transyear is detected and a near-transyear may be the second harmonic of the about 2.3-year cycle, much less prominent than the calendar year, in sharp contrast with results in Burundi, also located near the equator. Thus the incidence of malaria differed not only by the absence in Burundi of a calendar-year component found in Papua New Guinea, but also by the presence of prominent far- and a near-transyears in Burundi, but only a candidate near-transyear in cerebral malaria incidence in Papua New Guinea. Accordingly, the near-transyear-to-calendar year amplitude

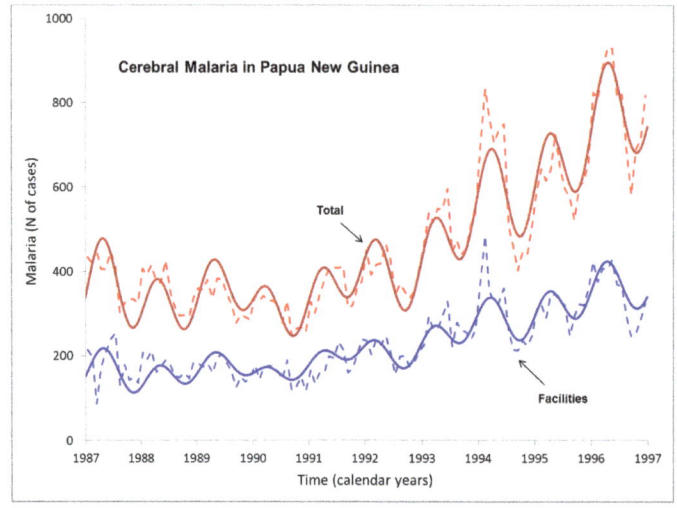

Figure 4. Monthly data on the incidence of cerebral malaria in Papua New Guinea are fitted with a model consisting of a linear trend, a 1.0-year synchronized rhythm, about 11.4-year and about 2.3-year components, and a candidate 1.1-year near-transyear. Whereas the contribution of each component to the composite model can be seen by the naked eye, this is not the case for the near-transyear that only has a very small amplitude. © Halberg Chronobiology Center.

ratio, if the presence of a near-transyear in Papua New Guinea is accepted, was smaller than 100% (**Figure 2** (right)).

Variable	Period	[95% CI]		Amplitude	[95% CI]		[1-parameter limits]
API	17.21	12.97	21.45	0.98	0.00	1.95	0.51	1.45
	9.60	7.64	11.56	0.66	-0.24	1.56	0.23	1.09
SPR%	18.42	13.70	23.13	1.02	-0.07	2.12	0.50	1.55
	10.07	8.02	12.12	0.73	-0.28	1.73	0.24	1.21
SfR	16.62	11.36	21.88	0.13	-0.03	0.30	0.05	0.21
	8.27	7.24	9.30	0.15	-0.01	0.32	0.07	0.23
Pf%	25.71	18.97	32.44	4.84	2.11	7.57	3.53	6.15
	9.15	8.14	10.16	3.18	0.49	5.87	1.89	4.48
Pf%	22.70	13.29	32.11	5.50	0.40	10.60	3.35	7.66
	15.94	11.04	20.84	3.71	-1.57	8.99	1.48	5.94
	8.81	8.02	9.60	2.80	0.91	4.69	2.00	3.60

All models fitted with a linear trend.

API: Annual parasite incidence (malaria positives in 1000 population).

SPR%: Slide positivity rate (positives per 100 slides examined).

SfR: Slide falciparum rate (Pf infection per 100 slides examined).

Pf%: Pf infections per 100 malaria positives.

Table 3. Nonlinear results of yearly incidence of malaria in Thailand.

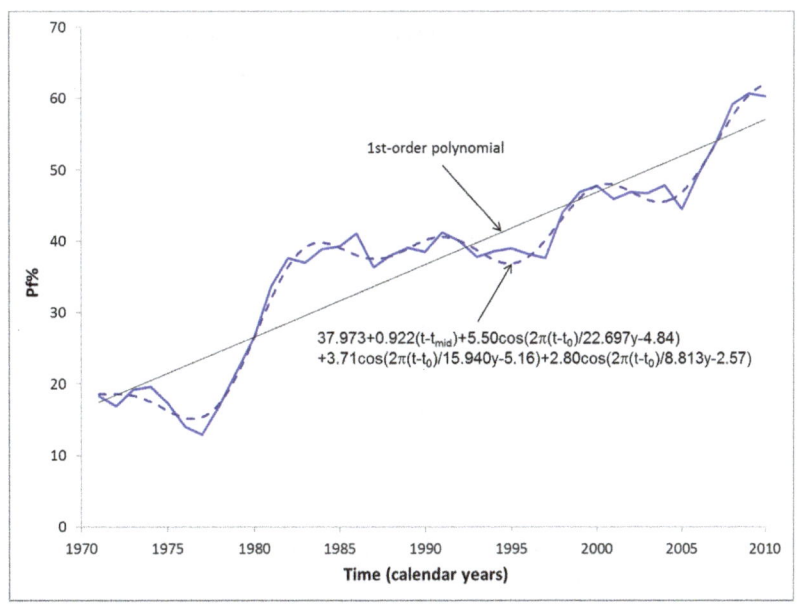

Figure 5. The yearly data on the percentage of *Plasmodium falciparum* infections (expressed per 100 malaria positives) in Thailand are fitted with a model consisting of a linear trend and cycles with periods of about 22.7, 15.9, and 8.8 years. © Halberg Chronobiology Center.

Tentative decadal components were also found by linear-nonlinear cosinor in the yearly data from Thailand (**Table 3**). Results for the percentage of *P. falciparum* infections per 100 malaria positives are illustrated in **Figure 5**.

4. Discussion

Malaria is transmitted in tropical and subtropical areas where Anopheles mosquitoes can survive and multiply. Malaria parasites can complete their growth cycle in the mosquitoes. Temperature is particularly critical. Generally, in warmer regions closer to the equator, transmission is more intense, and malaria can be transmitted year-round. It is not surprising then that components with periods other than 1 year may also be detected, reflecting the influence of solar and other factors not directly related to temperature.

Our interest in the relative contributions of the seasons vs. helio-, interplanetary and terrestrial magnetism was stimulated by the report by Dimitrov et al. [8] of a sharp calendar-yearly peak in the spectrum of monthly admissions of cerebral malaria in Papua New Guinea (latitude -6°; 1987–1996) with no comparable transyears (components longer than a year with a CI of their period not overlapping the calendar year). Decadal and longer cycles cannot be examined in the short series of malaria incidence in Burundi analysed herein, although, as noted, an about 5-year cycle can be the second harmonic of the Horrebow-Schwabe cycle. An about 2-year component is also found in interplanetary and geomagnetism as well as in the El Niño Southern Oscillation (ENSO) and may show cross-wavelet coherence with malaria in certain regions of Thailand [9].

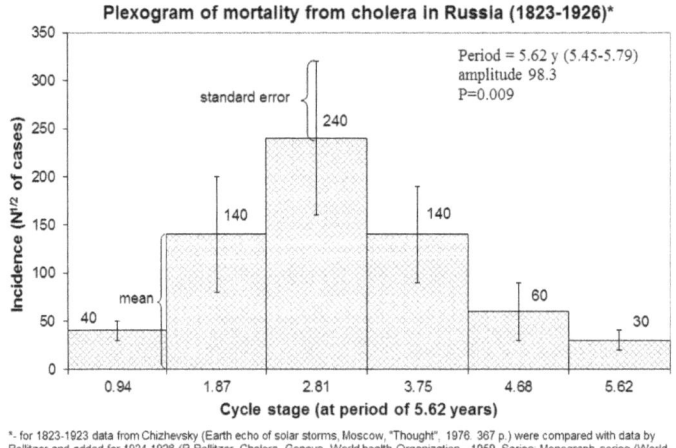

Figure 6. An about 5.6-year component was also detected in yearly data from Chizhevsky on mortality from cholera in Russia [19, 20]. © Halberg Chronobiology Center.

An about 5-year component in his time series on cholera incidence was communicated to Alexander Leonidovich Chizhevsky [17] by Vladimir Boleslavovich Shostakovich (**Figure 6**) [18]. Decadal and multidecadal signatures are found in diphtheria, croup, relapsing fever, and cholera at a time when these diseases were rampant in meta-analyses [18] of statistics assembled descriptively by Chizhevsky [17]. Chizhevsky also reports on data from Dr. SI Ivanchenko regarding the incidence of malaria in the North Caucasus from 1916 to 1930. He noted an inverse relationship between the incidence of malaria and air ionization. Albeit short, the record can be characterized by a decadal component, as illustrated in **Figure 7**.

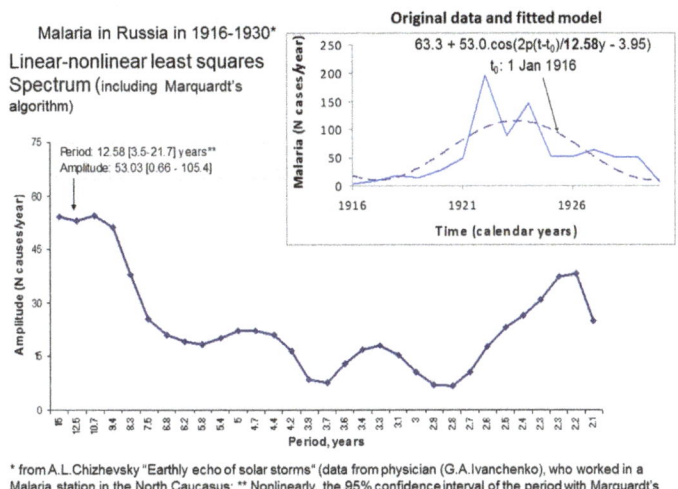

* from A.L.Chizhevsky "Earthly echo of solar storms" (data from physician (G.A.Ivanchenko), who worked in a Malaria station in the North Caucasus; ** Nonlinearly, the 95% confidence interval of the period with Marquardt's conservative approach was ridiculously wide); the 1-parameter CI of the period extends from 7.1 – 18.1

Figure 7. A decadal component characterizes the incidence of malaria in Russia between 1916 and 1930, as seen from the low-frequency spectral peak, resolved nonlinearly as an about 12.6-year component, which is fitted to the data (top right). Note a secondary smaller spectral peak corresponding to a period of about 2.3 years, as observed also in the data from Burundi (**Figure 1**) and Papua New Guinea (**Figure 3**). © Halberg Chronobiology Center.

In the case of malaria, it is surprising to see the presence of a calendar yearly component in the tropical region of Papua New Guinea, which is absent in Karuzi, Burundi (at 3° from the equator at a latitude, but not a longitude similar to that of Papua New Guinea). The original publication on malaria in Burundi [10] used data on rain and temperature and a vegetation index to predict malaria incidence. The terrestrial environmental variables could also be related to solar activity, as reviewed by Clayton [19] and Abbot [20].

Both the near- and far-transyears are features of the solar wind's speed and of geomagnetics. Space weather and geomagnetism may act via rainfall and its consequences. Just as helio-, interplanetary, or geomagnetism can influence sudden cardiac death [2], they may also influence communicable diseases, probably via the host, whose steroidal defence shows a decadal cycle [21] and/or by the invading microorganism. Bacterial mutations can also undergo a cycle mirroring that of sunspots [22–24].

Funding support:

Funding for this study is from Halberg Chronobiology Fund (GC), University of Minnesota Supercomputing Institute (GC). Processing charges are funded by the Academic Unit of Primary Care and Populations Sciences, University of Southampton, UK.

Author details

Lyazzat Gumarova[1,2], Germaine Cornelissen[1], Borislav D Dimitrov[3*] and Franz Halberg[1,4]

*Address all correspondence to: b.dimitrov@soton.ac.uk

1 Halberg Chronobiology Center, University of Minnesota, Minneapolis, MN, USA

2 Al-Farabi Kazakh National University, Almaty, Kazakhstan

3 Primary Care and Population Sciences, University of Southampton, Southampton, UK

4 Deceased

References

[1] Halberg F, Cornelissen G, Katinas GS, Hillman D, Otsuka K, Watanabe Y, Wu J, Halberg Francine, Halberg J, Sampson M, Schwartzkopff O, Halberg E. Many rhythms are control information for whatever we do: an autobiography. *Folia Anthr* 2012; 12: 5–134.

[2] Halberg F, Cornelissen G, Katinas G, Tvildiani L, Gigolashvili M, Janashia K, Toba T, Revilla M, Regal P, Sothern RB, Wendt HW, Wang ZR, Zeman M, Jozsa R, Singh RB, Mitsutake G, Chibisov SM, Lee J, Holley D, Holte JE, Sonkowsky RP, Schwartzkopff O, Delmore P, Otsuka K, Bakken EE, Czaplicki J, International BIOCOS Group. Chrono-biology's progress: season's appreciations 2004-2005. Time-, frequency-, phase-, variable-, individual-, age- and site-specific chronomics. *J Appl Biomed* 2006; 4: 1–38.

[3] Cornelissen G, Halberg F, Mikulecky M, Florida P, Faraone P, Yamanaka T, Murakami S, Otsuka K, Bakken EE. Yearly and perhaps transyearly human natality patterns near the equator and at higher latitudes. *Biomed Pharmacother* 2005; 59 (Suppl 1): S117–S122.

[4] Halberg F, Otsuka K, Watanabe Y, Katinas G, Wang ZR, Cornelissen G. The cosmos with Aeolian cycles, tipping the scale between death and survival: an indispensable control. *World Heart J* 2013; 5 (4): 231–240.

[5] Schwabe H. Sonnen-Beobachtungen im Jahre Solar observations in 1843. *Astron Nachr* 1844; 21: 254–256 (no. 495).

[6] Thiele ThN. De Macularum Solis antiquioribus quibusdam observationibus Hafniae institutis (Early sunspot observations of Copenhagen's institutions). *Astron Nachr* 1859; 50: 259–261.

[7] Cornelissen G, Halberg F, Sonkowsky R, Siegelova J, Homolka P, Dusek J, Fiser B. Meta-analysis of Horrebow's and Schwabe's scholarship with a view of sampling require-

ments. In: Halberg F, Kenner T, Fiser B, Siegelova J (Eds.). Proceedings, *Noninvasive Methods in Cardiology*, Masaryk University, Brno, Czech Republic 2009; 141–158.

[8] Dimitrov B, Valev D, Werner R, Atanassova PA. Cyclic patterns of cerebral malaria admissions in Papua New Guinea for the years 1987–1996. *Epidemiol Infect* 2013; 141 (11): 2317–2327.

[9] Childs DZ, Cattadori IM, Suwonkerd W, Prajakwong S, Boots M. Spatiotemporal patterns of malaria incidence in northern Thailand. *Trans R Soc Trop Med Hyg* 2006; 100: 623–631.

[10] Gomez-Elipe A, Otero A, Van Herp M, Aguirre-Jaime A. Forecasting malaria incidence based on monthly case reports and environmental factors in Karuzi, Burundi, 1997–2003. *Malar J* 2007; 6: 129.

[11] Nájera JA, Kouznetsov RL, Delacollette C. Malaria epidemics, detection and control, forecasting and prevention. In: *WHO/MAL/98.1084*. Geneva: World Health Organization; 1998.

[12] Halberg F. Chronobiology: methodological problems. *Acta Med Rom* 1980; 18: 399–440.

[13] Cornelissen G, Halberg F. Chronomedicine. In: Armitage P, Colton T (Eds.) *Encyclopedia of Biostatistics*, 2nd ed. Chichester, UK: John Wiley & Sons Ltd 2005; 796–812.

[14] Refinetti R, Cornelissen G, Halberg F. Procedures for numerical analysis of circadian rhythms. *Biol Rhythm Res* 2007; 38 (4): 275–325.

[15] Cornelissen G. Cosinor-based rhythmometry. *Theor Biol Med Model* 2014; 11: 16. 24 pp.

[16] Marquardt DW. An algorithm for least-squares estimation of nonlinear parameters. *J Soc Ind Appl Math* 1963; 11: 431–441.

[17] Chizhevsky AL. *The Terrestrial Echo of Solar Storms*. Moscow: "Mysl"; 1976. 349 pp.

[18] Gumarova L, Cornelissen G, Hillman D, Halberg F. Geographically selective assortment of cycles in pandemics: meta-analysis of data collected by Chizhevsky. *Epidemiol Infect* 2013; 141: 2173–2184.

[19] Clayton HH. *Variation in Solar Radiation and The Weather*. Washington, DC: Smithsonian Miscellaneous Collections 1920; 71: No. 3. 53 pp.

[20] Abbot CG. *Solar Variation and Weather, A Summary of the Evidence, Completely Illustrated and Documented*. Washington, DC: Smithsonian Miscellaneous Collections 146, No. 3 (Publ. 4545); 1963. 67 pp. + 4 plates.

[21] Cornelissen G, Halberg F, Breus T, Syutkina EV, Baevsky R, Weydahl A, Watanabe Y, Otsuka K, Siegelova J, Fiser B, Bakken EE. Non-photic solar associations of heart rate variability and myocardial infarction. *J Atmos Solar-Terr Phys* 2002; 64: 707–720.

[22] Faraone P, Cornelissen G, Katinas GS, Halberg F, Siegelova J. Astrophysical influences on sectoring in colonies of microorganisms. *Scr Med (Brno)* 2001; 74: 107–114.

[23] Faraone P, Halberg F, Cornelissen G, Schwartzkopff O, Katinas GS. Anticipations on the deepenings of astrophysical influence on appearing of sectors in microbial colonies named CSD (some statistical correlations and reminiscences about lost CSD-data). *CIFA News* 2002; 31 (Suppl): 1–15.

[24] Faraone P, Cornelissen G, Konradov A, Vladimirskii B, Chibisov S, Katinas G, Halberg F. A transyear in air bacteria and staphylococci. Science without borders. Trans Int Acad Sci H&E, 2003/2004; 1: 437 -439.

7

Inactivation of Malaria Parasites in Blood: PDT vs Inhibition of Hemozoin Formation

Régis Vanderesse, Ludovic Colombeau,
Céline Frochot and Samir Acherar

Abstract

Malaria causes hundreds of thousands of human deaths every year, and the World Health Assembly has made it a priority. To help eliminate this disease, there is a pressing need for the development and implementation of new strategies to improve the prevention and treatment, due in part to antimalarial drug resistances. This chapter focuses on two strategies to inactivate the malaria parasite in blood, which are photodynamic therapy (PDT) and inhibition of hemozoin formation. The PDT strategy permits either a control of the proliferation of mosquito larvae to develop some photolarvicides for the prevention or a photoinactivation of the malaria parasite in red blood cells (RBCs) to minimize infection transmission by transfusion. The inhibition of hemozoin formation strategy is used for the development of new antimalarial drug by understanding its formation mechanism.

Keywords: hemozoin, photodynamic therapy, blood decontamination, heme-drug interaction, preventive treatment, curative treatment

1. Introduction

Malaria in humans is an infectious disease caused by parasites of the genus *Plasmodium*, and it is spread to humans by the bite of the female anopheles mosquito. Among the species of *Plasmodium*, five are capable of inducing human disease. These are the species: *falciparum*, *vivax*, *malariae*, *ovale*, and *knowlesi*. The first is the most widespread and the most virulent, which is responsible of 80% of infections and about 90% of deaths, especially in Africa.

In 2000, malaria was seen as one of the most critical constraints on global development and considered as a priority challenge of the "Millennium Development Goals" (MDGs). The main objective was to halt and begin to reverse the incidence of malaria by 2015 (Target 6C). The *World Malaria Report 2015* written by the World Health Organization (WHO) summarizes advances that have taken place in each WHO region over the 2000–2015 period [1]. Malaria is endemic in 95 countries mainly in Africa (88%). This report shows that this goal was achieved with an almost 37% and 60% drop in malaria incidence and in death rates, respectively, over this period. In 2015, 214 million cases of malaria were recorded including 438 000 that have led to the death of the patients, reflecting a decline of 18% and 48% in cases and deaths, respectively, over the 2000–2015 period. In May 2015, the *Global Technical Strategy for Malaria 2016–2030* was endorsed by the World Health Assembly. This strategy has its goal to reach a 90% reduction in global malaria incidence and mortality by 2030.

With regard to preventing malaria in countries at risk, the WHO recommends sleeping under an insecticide-treated mosquito net (ITN) and protecting by indoor residual spraying (IRS). Furthermore, the recommended treatment is an artemisinin-based combination therapy (ACT).

Despite a slight decrease, this disease remains a leading cause of death of children in Africa due in part to antimalarial drug resistances. Declines in cases and deaths caused by malaria are due to the development of new strategies such as the use of photodynamic therapy (PDT) for the control of the infection vector or to induce inactivation of *Plasmodium falciparum* and targeting the hemozoin inhibition, with the aim of preventing and treating malaria.

2. Inhibition of hemozoin formation

2.1. Generalities on the hemozoin production by *P. falciparum*

Hemoglobin, the main component of red blood cells (RBCs), represents almost 95% of the protein part of the cytosol (liquid fraction of the cell cytoplasm) up to reach 5 mM concentration in the cytoplasm (>300 mg/mL) [2]. Hemoglobin essential for cellular respiration is composed of a protein portion (globin) and a complex molecular structure centered on an iron atom (heme, ferriprotoporphyrin IX, Fe(II)PPIX which carries oxygen, and carbon dioxide from breathing).

During its life cycle in the red blood cell (RBC), the human malaria parasite (**Figure 1**), *P. falciparum*, gobbles up between 60 and 80% of hemoglobin from the host cell cytoplasm [3] by using a cytostome (cell mouth) for the purpose of transporting it to its acidic digestive food vacuole (pH ≈ 5.0–5.4 [4, 5]). At this acidic pH maintained by means of an ATPase pump enabling activation of a proton gradient, the hemoglobin is degraded into amino acids that are used for the production of parasite proteins, thereby allowing the release of free heme which is toxic to the parasite [6–9]. The hemoglobin degradation mechanism was studied in detail, and it was shown that it implies enzymes (proteases) present in the food vacuole of the parasite such as two aspartic (plasmepsins I and II) and cysteine (falcipain) proteases [10–14].

The heme detoxification is a crucial step for the survival and growth of the parasite [15]. Heme is assumed to generate the formation of reactive oxygen species (ROS), *via* the Fenton reaction catalyzed by its iron atom [16–18], and hydroxyl radicals that may lead to peroxidation of lipid membranes [19–21]. It was postulated also that specific heme-H_2O_2 reaction might produce free radicals [21] which may result in oxidation of lipids, proteins, and DNA [22, 23].

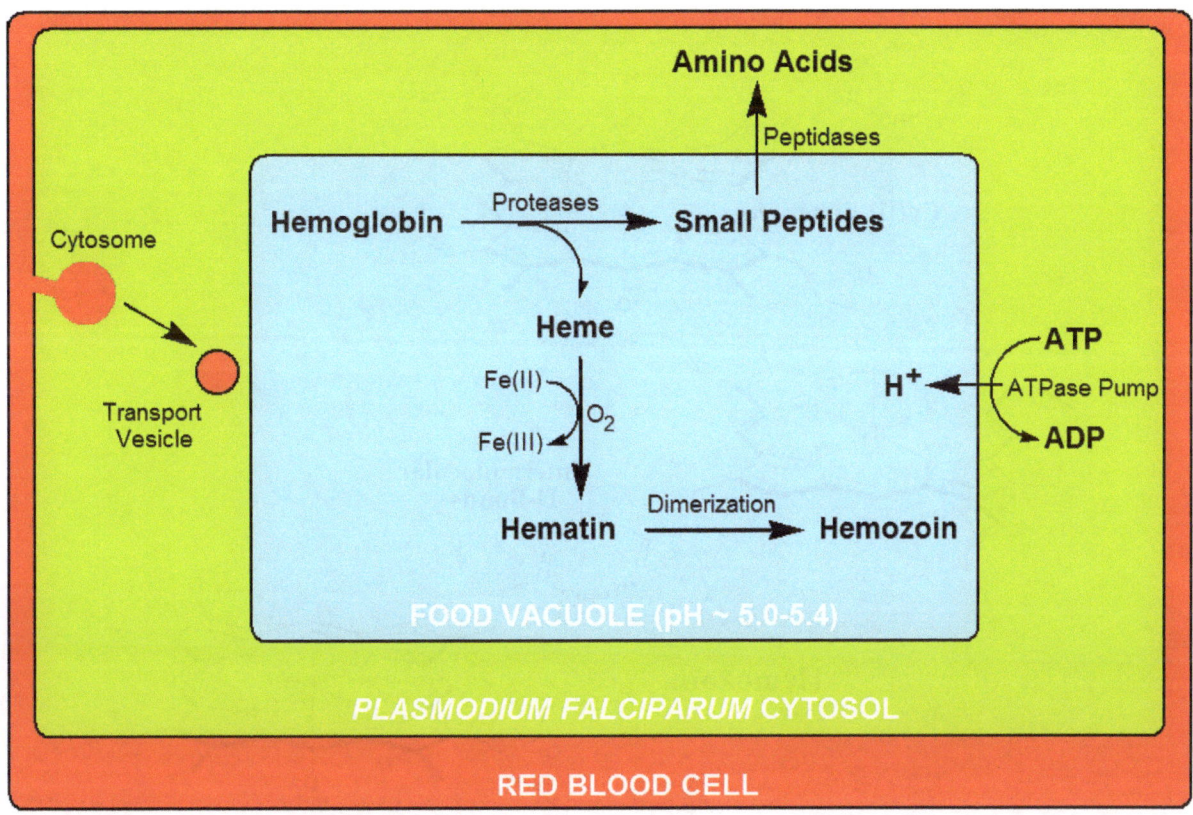

Figure 1. Hemoglobin degradation by *Plasmodium falciparum* in RBC.

The detoxification of heme begins with the self-oxidation of the Fe(II) in heme group into Fe(III) to form potentially toxic hydroxyferriprotoporphyrin IX (hematin, HO-Fe(III)PPIX; **Figure 2**) [8, 24, 25]. This detoxification ends with the formation of highly insoluble brown crystals known as hemozoin (malaria pigment; **Figure 2**) [26, 27] according to biomineralization or biocrystallization processes [28, 29] and not *via* a polymerization as previously believed; the x-ray structure is identical to a synthetic Fe(III)PPIX compound called β-hematin [30]. In 2000, the crystalline structure of β-hematin was determined to be a cyclic dimer of Fe(III)PPIX, involving two coordination bonds between the propionate side chain of one and the Fe(III) atom of the other [28]. These cyclic dimers are self-assembled in the crystal lattice *via* inter-molecular hydrogen bonds which link the propionic acid side chains of each Fe(III)PPIX, thereby losing their toxic potential (heme detoxification), and then eliminated from the food vacuole. In 2010, the crystal structure of *P. falciparum* hemozoin has been solved by Klonis et al. after a reanalysis of x-ray crystallographic data for β-hematin [31].

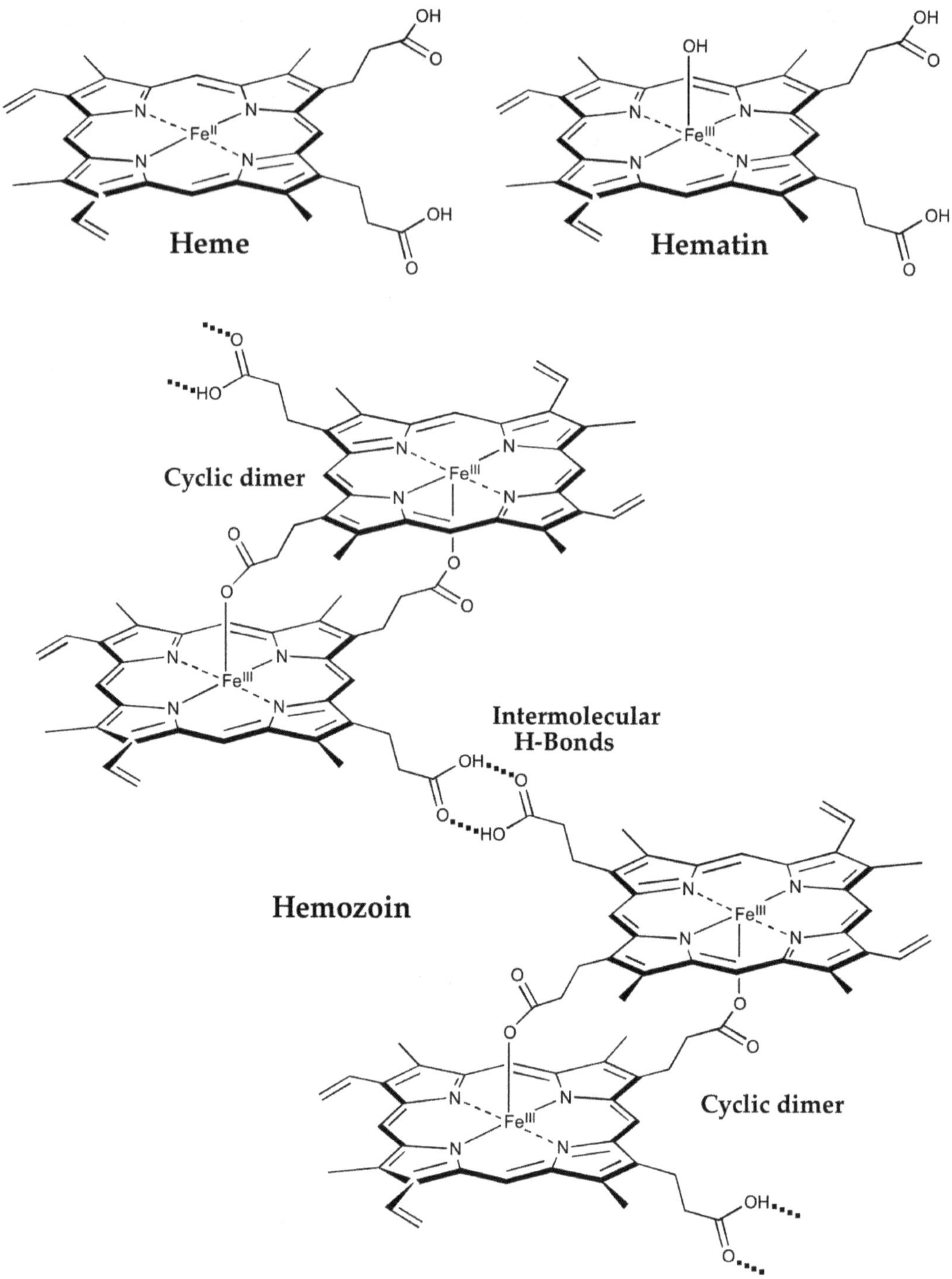

Figure 2. Chemical structure of heme, hematin, and hemozoin.

The mechanism concerning formation of β-hematin (hemozoin) in vivo and in vitro is still ambiguous and will be discussed in the following section.

2.2. Mechanistic assumptions about the hemozoin formation

The heme detoxification by *P. falciparum* results in the formation of hemozoin by template-mediated crystallization ("biocrystallization"), and a number of studies have been conducted in order to understand the hemozoin formation. Hemozoin or β-hematin (synthetic hemozoin) was used for these studies, and various mechanisms about the β-hematin formation have been postulated for the in vivo process.

Before beginning the discussion about mechanistic assumptions of the hemozoin formation, it is worth noting that when comparing the natural hemozoin and its synthetic version (β-hematin), we see a considerable difference in their size and shape. The natural hemozoin consists of small crystals ranging in size from 50 to 500 nm, whereas for the synthetic β-hematin, these crystals are bigger (50 nm to 20 μm) and depend on solvent used for the recrystallization. This difference in size can lead to diverse immunomodulatory responses [32].

The various studies of this mechanism gave rise to a number of assumptions [11, 33, 34] such as spontaneous [35, 36], autocatalyzed [37, 38], enzyme-catalyzed [39], lipid-catalyzed [40–43], and initiated or catalyzed by histidine-rich proteins (HRPs) [44–48], which can be divided into two main types: non-biological and biological conditions (**Figure 3**).

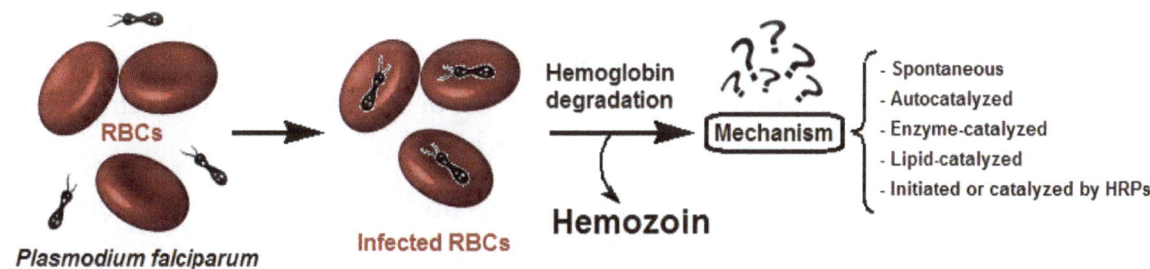

Figure 3. Postulated mechanisms about the hemozoin formation by *Plasmodium falciparum*.

The first category (non-biological conditions) is based on the assumption that β-hematin formation can happen spontaneously without any external help [35]. This observation comes from studies conducted in acetate solution, which shows that the β-hematin can be formed at a moderate low pH compared to the acidic digestive food vacuole [36].

The second category includes of all other mechanisms and provides a presumption that the β-hematin formation can catalyze itself or requires the presence of biological material (bio-crystallization). The first idea about an autocatalytic process is, among other things, due to a recent observation of the continued growth of a preexisting hemozoin crystal [37].

As regards the second idea, it began in 1992 with the work of Slater and Cerami [39] which have shown that heme can react with trophozoite lysate extracts at pH 5–6 to generate hemozoin and that chloroquine, an antimalarial drug, can inhibit this formation. The authors concluded that the creation of the two propionate-Fe(III) linkages during the heme detoxification is catalyzed by an enzyme named heme polymerase. The use of extracts from *Plasmodium berghei* (rodent malaria) by Chou and Fitch gave equivalent results [49].

Despite being challenged, this heme polymerase theory attempted to explain hemozoin propagation without clarifying its initiation. This breach paved the way for other hypotheses about the formation of hemozoin involving a protein or enzyme [38]. Firstly, Hempelman in 2007 introduced the concept of "biocrystallization" instead of "polymerization" to describe the hemozoin formation process [29]. One of the hypotheses suggested that biocrystallization is caused by enzymes, which postulate the presence of proteins such as histidine-rich proteins (HRPs). Sullivan and coworkers [48] showed that HRPs I, II, and III, present in the parasite's digestive vacuole, may be able to promote the formation of hemozoin in vitro. In 2008, Jani et al. [46] identified a novel heme detoxification protein (HDP) from *P. falciparum*, which is considered as one of the most powerful of the hemozoin-producing enzymes. As an example, we could cite the work of Choi and coworkers in 2002 and Nakatani et al. in 2014 concerning the elucidated reaction mechanisms of HRP II and HDP [44, 47]. These authors have shown that some histidine residues are active sites in these proteins and can bind with heme to promote the heme dimerization by bringing two molecules. This dimer would be used as a crystal growth initiator of hemozoin. Recently, Chugh and coworkers have established that HDP and falcipain-2 can work in tandem within the digestive food vacuole of the parasite to transform hemoglobin efficiently into hemozoin [45].

Finally, the last proposed mechanism is the biocrystallization catalyzed by lipids [40–43, 50]. These lipids, produced by the parasite after digesting the transport vesicles and trapped in its food vacuole, have been characterized with spectroscopic studies [7, 41] and known as a neutral lipid blend (NLB) and monopalmitoylglycerol (MPG). In 2007, Pisciotta et al. proved that Fe(III)PPIX can be processed into β-hematin through the action of these lipids with the yield of 80% or more [51] as assumed by Sullivan two years before [27].

The design and development of new antimalarial drugs first begin with the understanding of the mechanism of action of *P. falciparum* after invading RBCs and giving rise to hemozoin formation *via* the heme detoxification. Although this mechanism is not completely elucidated and still requires much work, these assumptions allow researchers to develop new strategies with a view to solving the problem of antimalarial drug resistance concerning chloroquine and artemisinin, the two most antimalarial drugs used to treat malaria.

By way of example, new strategies envisaged include the use of PDT (Section 3) in order to kill mosquito larvae (prevention Section 3.2) or to inactivate malaria parasites in the RBCs (treatment Section 3.3) but also the design of new antimalarial drugs that are able to inhibit the β-hematin formation by heme-drug interaction (treatment Section 4).

3. Photodynamic therapy for preventive and curative treatments

3.1. Generalities

The therapeutic effects of light are known since ancient times and were widely used in combination with natural substances for centuries in Chinese, Egyptian, or Indian civilizations for the treatment of numerous diseases such psoriasis, vitiligo, and rickets [52]. The integration of the concepts of "phototherapy" and then "photosensitivity" in modern medicine is much more recent, since it originated in the work of Niels Finsen, a Danish doctor who demonstrated in the 1890s the positive influence of light on the healing process (Nobel Prize for Medicine in 1903) [53]. However, the concept of exogenous photosensitizer (PS), that is to say, therapeutic molecule introduced for the specific purpose of interacting with light to generate the desired therapeutic effect, was introduced only a few years later, at the turn of the twentieth century by Raab and von Tappeiner as related by Spikes in a very good historical review [54]. In 1900, Oscar Raab, a student at the Department of Pharmacology of the University of Munich in the group of Hermann von Tappeiner, tried to characterize the influence of acridine on the development of *Paramecium caudatum* and *Plasmodium malariae*, a paramecium responsible for malaria. Very quickly, Raab noted that, according to the hour of the treatment and the weather conditions, the impact of administered acridine on the survival of microorganisms seemed extremely variable. He quickly demonstrated that the mechanism of cell death induced by acridine requires activation by light irradiation. Later, von Tappeiner identified oxygen as the third component (with the PS and light source) involved in photo-induced mechanism. He proposed the term "photodynamic therapy" (photodynamische Wirkung in the original) to define all therapeutic protocols involving these three elements [55]. von Tappeiner's team experimented eosin as PS to treat tumors in six patients, and some promising results were obtained [56]. Unfortunately, in this period, the concept did not arouse reactions on behalf of the scientific world in Western medicine [57].

In summary, PDT is an innovative medical treatment involving the concomitant action of three components that are photoactivatable molecule called PS, light of a suitable wavelength, and oxygen present in the biological medium. After light excitation of the PS and energy transfer from the excited PS to oxygen, reactive oxygen species are produced especially singlet oxygen ($^1O_2$) that can destroy cancer cells in proximity. It is interesting to notice that the PS itself is nontoxic and turns out to be toxic only with light. Light is also nontoxic by itself. The selectivity of action of PDT allows through a localized light radiation to eradicate tumor cells while preserving healthy cells. PS fluorescence properties are also an asset that is utilized to visualize the diseased tissue. The mechanisms are summarized in **Figure 4**.

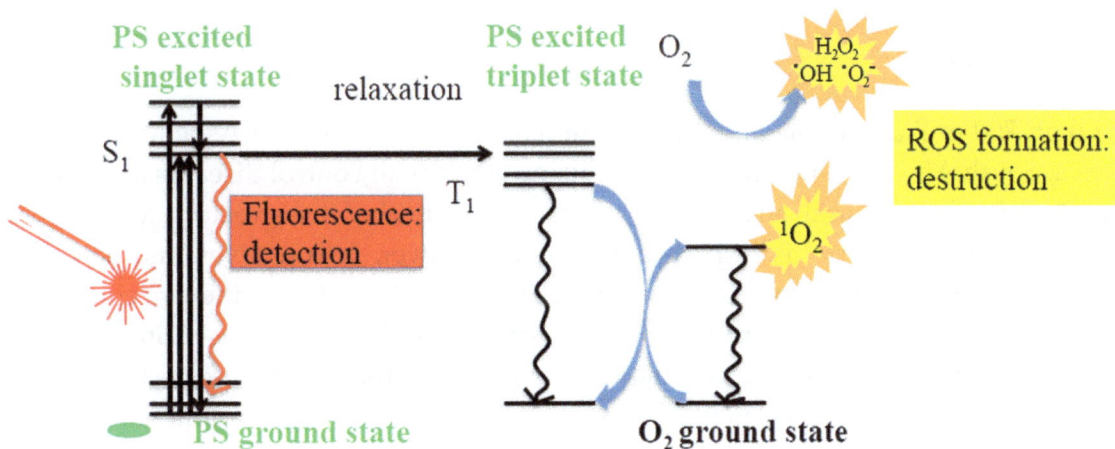

Figure 4. Mechanism of PDT (simplified Perrin-Jablonski diagram).

This technique was used clinically for many years, and in 1993, bladder cancer Photofrin PDT receives government approval in Canada. Since then, PDT has been developed in many countries of the world. PDT is an obvious treatment for dermatology applications, and it is used daily for skin diseases such as actinic keratoses, acne, and wine stain [57]. PDT has been also widely employed as a treatment for age-related macular degeneration (ARMD). However, since 2006, intravitreal injections of Avastin, humanized monoclonal antibody having anti-angiogenic activity, significantly reduced the use of PDT to treat ARMD. In urology, the French company Steba Biotech has invested heavily to develop a new PS, the TOOKAD® (currently in phase 3) for the treatment of prostate cancer. The first clinical applications demonstrate the technical feasibility [58]. In gastroenterology, PDT demonstrated its effectiveness for the treatment of superficial cancers of the esophagus in patients ineligible for further treatment, with a postradiation recurrence, severe dysplasia in Barrett, and unresectable cholangiocarci-noma [59]. In gynecology, the interest of PDT has been shown in the treatment of cervical dysplasia of low- and high-grade cervical lesions [60]. Our team developed folic acid-targeted photosensitizers that could be very efficient to treat peritoneal carcinosis, and a preclinical evaluation is under progress [61, 62]. In pulmonology, the number of studies on the treatment of lung cancer is still limited, and the role of PDT in the therapeutic arsenal of the practitioner remains to be demonstrated. PDT appears to be a promising treatment for malignant pleural mesothelioma (MPM). Thus, PDT has been tested in phase I and phase II clinical trials to MPM patients in combination with extrapleural pneumonectomy or pleurectomy/decortication and an intravenous chemotherapy. The first work of the team of Professor Friedberg (University of Pennsylvania, Philadelphia, USA) has shown promising results with a median overall survival of 31 months [63]. PDT is not only a powerful technique to destroy human cells but also for viruses [64], yeasts [65], molds [66], bacteria [67], protozoa [68], parasites [69], and insects (Section 3.2). PDT is used in the development of new strategies to treat malaria and more generally to treat tropical diseases, either by controlling the propagation vector of the disease (Section 3.2), by inactivation of microorganisms responsible for these diseases, or by inactivating parasites (Section 3.3).

3.2. Prevention: destruction of mosquito larvae

3.2.1. Generalities

More than 700 million people are affected annually by mosquitoes in Asia, Mexico, Central America, South America, and Africa. A promising strategy to control diseases transmitted by mosquitoes (malaria, filarial, and dengue fever) is the control of these vectors. Mosquitoes are vectors of pathogens: *Aedes* is responsible for dengue fever, yellow fever, and encephalitis; *Anopheles* for malaria and encephalitis; and *Culex* for yellow fever and encephalitis [70]. Pesticides such as DDT (dichlorodiphenyltrichloroethane) have been used in affected area leading to decline of the mosquito population. Nevertheless, the use of these pesticides induces risks for safety reasons, development of resistance in major vectors, environmental and human health problems, etc. There is a need for developing improved insecticide, and the use of light with a PS is a possibility. In this case, the PS is called a photopesticide. One of the first re-searchers who described the potential of photosensitive molecules as insecticides was probably A. Barbieri in 1928 [71]. In 1979, rose bengal was used to treat Culex larvae [72]. In 1983, a review was written by J. Robinson about the photosensitizing dyes used as insect control agent [73]. The concept is to make a gulp down a small amount of PS to a mosquito larva, and then, after PS excitation by sunlight, the larva dies. Reviews have been published recently on this topic [70, 74]. The use of porphyrins has been described from the late 1980s [75, 76]. Different porphyrin derivatives have been then tested such as chlorophyllin, pheophorbide, and hematoporphyrin in laboratory conditions but also in semi-field conditions. A synthetic *meso*-substitute developed by Lucantoni et al. in 2012 had a potent photosensitizing activity on *Aedes aegypti* larvae that are responsible for the dengue in laboratory conditions [77].

3.2.2. Anopheles mosquitoes: the primary vector for malaria

Malaria is spread to humans by the bite of the female anopheles mosquito. In 2012, Fabris et al. described the photolarvicidal activity of a new PS called C12-porphyrin (5-(4-*N*-dodecyl-pyridyl)-10,15,20-tri(4-*N*-methylpyridyl)-21*H*,23*H*-porphyrin tetraiodide) [78]. This molecule was first supplied by Frontier Scientific Inc. (US Patent no. 6 573 258), and our team improved the synthesis and performed the photophysical properties study [79]. The structure of molecule is presented in **Figure 5**.

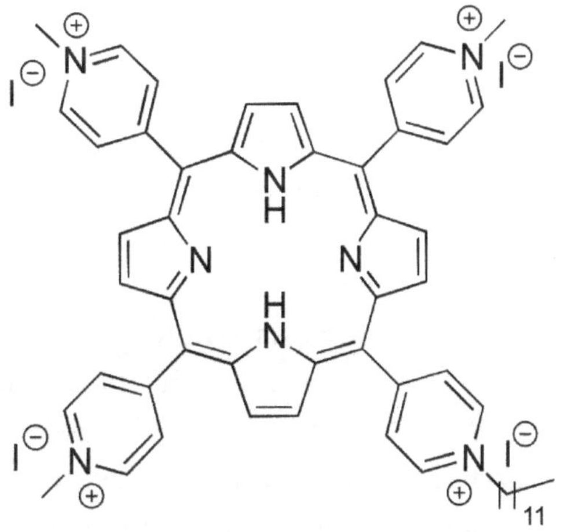

Figure 5. Chemical structure of C12-porphyrin.

In collaboration with the Institut de Recherche en Sciences de la Santé (IRSS) located in Burkina Faso, Fabris et al. studied the potential of C12-porphyrin as a photolarvicide for the control of *Anopheles*. Two different formulations with C12 were prepared: one is composed of Eudragit S100, an anionic methacrylic acid/methyl methacrylate copolymer, and the other is a fraction of cat food pellets. Both of them proved to be very efficient in laboratory conditions. The porphyrin-mediated photoinactivation of anopheles larvae could represent an interesting approach in the achievement of reduction of malaria morbidity and mortality.

3.3. Prevention: photoinactivation of parasites in blood

3.3.1. Generalities

With the emergence of many antibiotics, PDT declined for the treatment of parasite-related diseases, and it is only in recent decades that it knew a regain of interest with the increasing problem of antibiotic resistance [80]. Antibiotic resistance is a global problem that reduces the power of conventional treatments of many diseases (both nosocomial and community-acquired infections). It concerns all pathogens including bacteria, fungi, and viruses.

To circumvent this bio-resistance, an attractive approach is PDT as non-antibiotic strategy to inactivate microorganisms (bacteria, viruses, parasites, etc.). This process is called antimicrobial photodynamic therapy (aPDT) [81, 82] or antibacterial PDT [83, 84] but is also known as photodynamic inactivation (PDI) [85–87] or photodynamic antimicrobial chemotherapy (PACT) [88–91]. This treatment can be effective in the case of chronic ulcers, infected burns, acne vulgaris, and a variety of local bacterial infections but also in the case of periodontitis [92], dengue [93], tuberculosis [94], viral infection [95], and malaria [96–99]. A very large variety of microorganisms have been studied and are listed by Alves et al. in a recent review [70] in which the insect pest elimination, water disinfection, and elimination of food-borne pathogens are described. A state of the art of PDT (potential) applications in animal models and clinical infectious diseases has been submitted by Dai et al. in 2009 [95], and numerous PSs are described [99, 100].

3.3.2. Inactivation of P. falciparum in human RBCs

Malaria is no more considered as poverty-related disease in Western countries, and attention has been paid to developing blood decontamination methods, vaccines, or new therapies. The spread of malaria disease, particularly with *P. falciparum*, in high-risk countries by blood transfusion is very worrying, especially as global traveling is continuously increasing. Inhabitants of tropical and subtropical regions where malaria is endemic can develop an immune response. However, they can carry a significant amount of parasites that can be transmitted by transfusion even if the blood is frozen (3 weeks' survival) [101, 102]. Decontamination of blood can be carried out according to several protocols including solvent-detergent methods, filtration, deleucocytation, photochemical techniques, etc. PSs such as psoralens, porphyrins, acridines, phenothiazines, porphyrins, and others can be used as additive for blood sterilization, and numerous protocols have been described, some of them could be found in [103, 104].

The life cycle of *Plasmodium* can be characterized by two phases: (a) the asexual proliferative phase in humans (intermediate host), called schizogony. This phase takes place in two different locations in humans and chronologically first within hepatocytes in the liver (exoerythrocytic cycle) and in circulating erythrocytes (RBC cycle). It also stands in the mosquito as a result of the sexual phase, (b) a sexual differentiation phase followed by asexual reproduction, called sporogony, which begins in humans and continues in the mosquito by the maturation of these in male and female gametes. As already mentioned, in erythrocytes, *P. falciparum* ingests 30–80% of hemoglobin, which is then digested in the food vacuole (an acidic organelle) and detoxified into hemozoin. This hemozoin itself could be a PS for killing *P. falciparum*, and Leblanc et al. [105] demonstrated that a simple irradiation of infected cultured RBCs by a near IR laser (800 nm) could induce a ~0.5 log reduction in parasitemia, but this is not enough for decontamination of blood.

Historically, Ehrlich's group was the first to use methylene blue (**Figure 6**) as a PS [106] and Rounds et al. conducted a pioneering work on the photokilling potency of a ruby laser and methylene blue on cells infected by *P. lophurae* [107]. Since then, a wide variety of dyes have been explored. Merocyanine 540 was one of the first PSs used for the decontamination of blood [108] which reduced the concentration of parasites by 3 log when exposed to light. However, the overlapping between hemoglobin and the PS absorption made it not suitable for deparasitization.

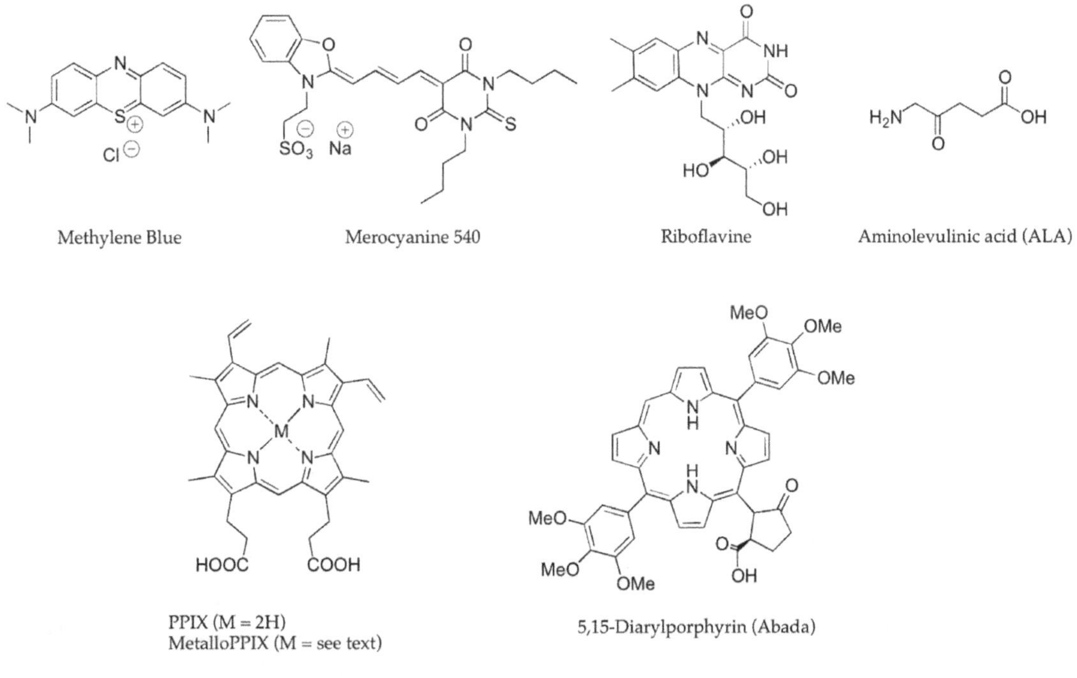

Figure 6. PS used for blood decontamination.

Riboflavin or vitamin B2 (**Figure 6**) deficiency is closely related to malaria [109, 110], and its administration can prevent hemozoin formation in the asexual cycle in the food vacuole of erythrocytes. Akompong et al. observed that addition of riboflavin can induce a 65% decrease of the food vacuole volume and subsequently damage to light-exposed contaminated blood [111]. In 2013, Goodrich's group tested the "Mirasol® pathogen reduction technology" (PRT) system against *P. falciparum* and *P. yoelii* [112]. This PRT system uses riboflavin and UV light for the destruction of a broad range of blood-borne pathogens and receives the European Community mark for both platelet and plasma applications. For *P. falciparum*, the percentage of parasitemia was 0.97 and <0.0005% before and after treatment, respectively. Similar results were obtained in vivo with blood of mice infected by *P. yoelii*. Recently, the "International Society for Medical Laser Applications" ordered a clinical trial named "Antimicrobial photodynamic therapy as a new treatment option for Malaria" in India on a group of 50 patients receiving an antimicrobial photodynamic treatment (riboflavin + 447 nm blue laser) over a period of 5 days plus conventional treatments [113].

In a recent research, Sigala et al. [114] demonstrated that sequencing of *P. falciparum* genome and some gene deletions did not affect the heme formation indicating that the host enzymes are involved and can be a parallel pathway for the life cycle of *P. falciparum*. They showed the involvement of protoporphyrin IX (PPIX; **Figure 6**) in this parallel pathway and proposed a new treatment based on the chemoluminescence of luminol and aminolevulinic acid (ALA; **Figure 6**), which is the initial building block of PPIX [115] to produce ROS. The combination of ALA, luminol, and stimulating factor (4-iodophenol or dihydroartemisinin) decreased the parasitemia in the range of 75–80% [114]. ALA has also been described by Smith and Kain as a potentiate PS for killing *P. falciparum* in the presence of white light. The culture incubated by 0.2 mM ALA for 8 hours and exposed to light for 30 min exhibited a parasitemia less than 0.002% after 2 days [116].

PS	Conditions	Effects	Reference
Hemozoin	800 nm; 485 mW/cm²; 60 min	~0.5 log reduction in parasitemia	[105]
Methylene blue	694 nm; 70 J/cm²	Preferential uptake by infected erythrocytes by imaging	[107]
Merocyanine 540	485 nm; 26 W/m²; 30 min	1000-fold reduction in parasitemia	[108]
Riboflavin	No irradiation /48h	65% decrease in food vacuole volume	[111]
Riboflavin	UV ; 6.24 J/mL ; 72 h	<0.002% survival	[112]
ALA	White light; 0.57 W/cm²; 30 min	<0.0005% survival	[116]
ALA	Chemoluminescence by luminol	75–80% death	[114]
SnPPIX	No irradiation	IC_{50} = 6.5 µM (85 µM for chloroquine) on trophozoite lysate	[118]
Zn-PPIX	No irradiation	IC_{50} = 330 nM on RBC	[119]
Diarylporphyrin	No irradiation	IC_{50} = 20 nM on erythrocytes	[120]
Pheophorbide Ph4-OH	660 nm; 7 W/cm²; 20 min	Total eradication with 2 µM/L	[121]
PC4 phthalocyanine	>600 nm; 60 J/cm²; 10 min	<0.025% survival with 2 µM/L	[122]

Table 1. Bibliographic data.

In 1996, Martiney et al. [117] described a slight inhibition of hemozoin formation by using Zn-PPIX without light. Using trophozoite lysate of *P. falciparum*, Begum et al. obtained similar results with SnPPIX with an IC_{50} = 6.5 µM (to be compared to 85 µM for chloroquine) [118]. Recently, Garcia's group [119] encapsulated metal-PPIX (2H, Fe, Co, Cu, Mn, Ni, and Zn) in marine atelocollagen using the coacervation technique. They obtained an IC_{50} = 330 nM (for Zn-PPIX) on RBC and found that encapsulated Zn-PPIX was 80-fold more effective than the nonencapsulated Zn-PPIX and similar to chloroquine. In 2013, Abada et al. evaluated a series of 11 diversely substituted porphyrins against *P. falciparum* [120]. Only the 5,15-di-(3,4,5-trimethoxyphenyl)-10-(5-oxopyrrolidine-2(*S*)-carboxylate) (**Figure 6**) porphyrin has an efficiency comparable to chloroquine with an IC_{50} value of 20 nM with a slight delay of infected mice survival.

The photosensitized inactivation of *P. falciparum* has been investigated by Grellier et al. [121] by using *N*-(4-butanol) pheophorbide derivative (Ph4-OH) as PS. Illumination at 660 nm (7 mW cm^{-2}) of parasitized whole blood induced a total eradication using 2 μM Ph4-OH and 20 min illumination, 4 μM Ph4-OH and 10 min illumination, or 8 μM Ph4-OH and 5 min illumination. The blood remained uncontaminated for at least 2 weeks. These results are better than those obtained with merocyanine 540 [108] and comparable to that obtained with phthalocyanines. In fact, Lustigman and BenHur [122] described the phthalocyanine HOSiP-cOSi(CH$_3$)$_2$(CH$_2$)$_3$N(CH$_3$)$_2$ (Pc 4) as PS for blood decontamination and obtained an inactivation (≥99.8%) of *P. falciparum* clones 7G8 and HB3 by 10 and 40 min irradiation with a xenon short-arc lamp (>600 nm). The same team evaluated an IC_{50} of 24 nM in the dark [123]. The main results are summarized in **Table 1** (when available).

Besides the decontamination of blood or dialysis, numerous studies have been conducted to understand the physiology of the human malaria parasite *Plasmodium*, and some PSs have been used. For example, 4,4-difluoro-5,7-dimethyl-4-bora-3a,4a-diaza-s-indacene-3-hexadecanoic acid (BODIPY FL C$_{16}$) has been used as a marker for chloroquine resistance [124] or spatial distribution of oxidative stress in infected erythrocytes [125]. Other examples are 5,6-chloromethyl-2,7-dichlorodihydrofluorescein diacetate (CM-H2DCFDA), 5',6'-carboxy-10-dimethylamino-3-hydroxy-spiro[7*H*-benzo[c]xanthene-7,1'(3*H*)-isobenzofuran]-3'-one (SNARF), and 2,7-bis-(2-carboxyethyl)-5,6-carboxyfluorescein acetoxymethyl ester (BCECF) for the measurement of the parasite's food vacuolar pH [126].

4. Curative treatment: drugs inhibiting β-hematin formation

Among various strategies, we will focus in the following part only on antimalarial drugs that inhibit the β-hematin formation by heme-drug interaction (purely π-π interactions). This strategy of drug development uses the heme scaffold itself as a hematin crystallization inhibitor (**Figure 2**). We can quote quinine, chloroquine, rufigallol and exifone and artemisinin, which are currently used as antimalarial drugs *via* this strategy (**Figure 7**).

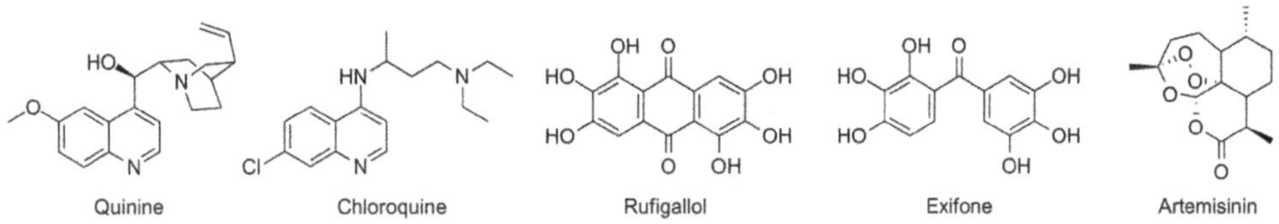

Figure 7. Structures of current antimalarial drugs.

Several studies and reviews [97] reported that porphyrins can inhibit the process of heme crystallization in the acidic food vacuole of the malaria parasite. As current antimalarial drugs, porphyrins are able to inhibit the β-hematin formation by strong π-π stacking interactions. Several porphyrins have been studied for their use in heme aggregation inhibition.

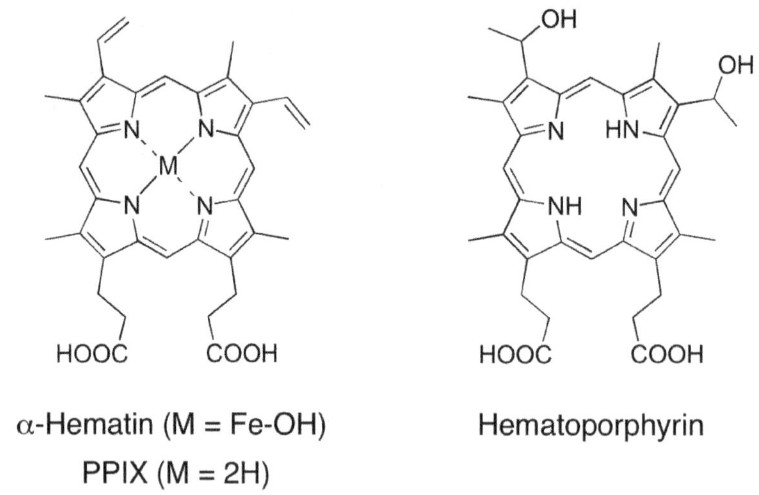

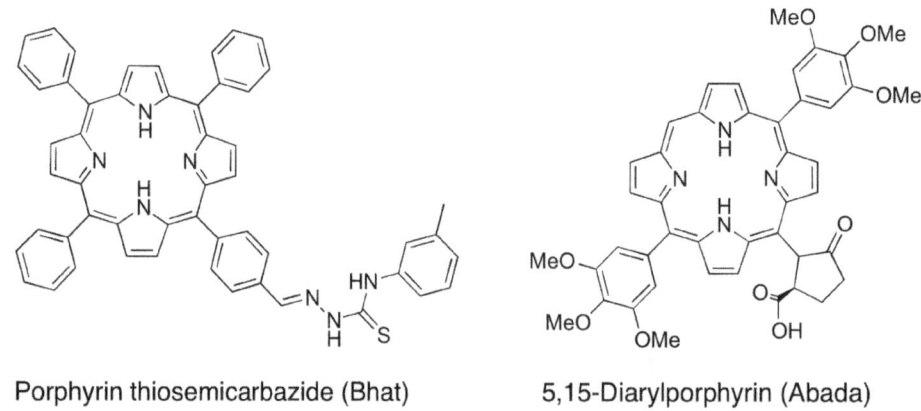

α-Hematin (M = Fe-OH)
PPIX (M = 2H)

Hematoporphyrin

Figure 8. Structures of hematin, PPIX, and hematoporphyrin.

In 1997, Basilico et al. [127] evaluated the effect of two non-iron metalloporphyrins (PPIX and hematoporphyrin) on the crystallization of α-hematin (**Figure 8**) to β-hematin also called synthetic hemozoin (**Figure 2**). Crystallization of hematin may be achieved in 4.5 M sodium acetate buffer at 60°C [35]. Heme and β-hematin may be differentiated by their IR spectroscopic characteristics [128]. IR spectra of β-hematin show two bands at 1662 and 1209 cm^{-1}, which disappear in IR spectra of heme. From this property, Basilico et al. demonstrated that free-base porphyrins inhibit heme crystallization with hematoporphyrin more actively than PPIX. The presence of hydroxyl groups can explain the better inhibitory ability of hematoporphyrin.

In 1999, Tamarelli's team also showed that Fe(III)PPIX is reduced to Fe(II)PPIX as a novel endogenous antimalarial because Fe(II)PPIX molecules inhibit the crystallization process causing the death of the parasite [129].

Porphyrin thiosemicarbazide (Bhat)

5,15-Diarylporphyrin (Abada)

Figure 9. Structure of antimalarial drugs designed by Bhat (left) and Abada (right).

Some researchers are interested in the synthesis of free-base porphyrins. In 2008, Bhat et al. [130] synthesized and evaluated the antimalarial activity of a series of porphyrin thiosemicarbazides. Only one compound (**Figure 9 left**) possesses an ability to inhibit β-hematin formation similar to chloroquine and quinine, the control drugs that are usually used in the malaria treatment. More recently, Abada et al. [120] synthesized a new 5,15-diarylporphyrin (**Figure 9 right**) with a good activity against *Plasmodium* with 20 nM IC_{50} value. The in vivo evaluation on *P. berghei* in mice model showed that this compound allowed delaying the death of the animal on about two days.

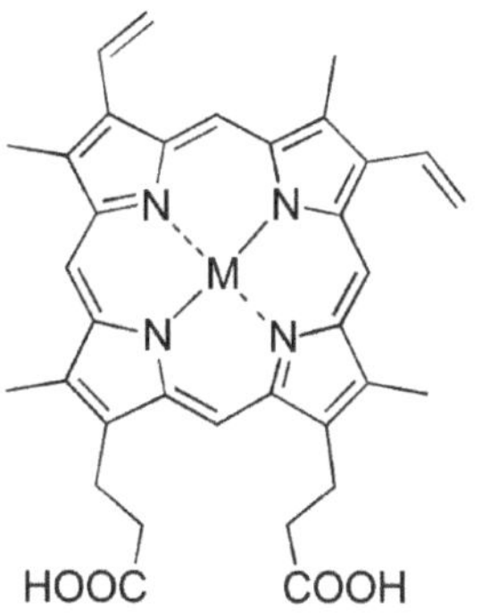

PPIX (M = 2H)
MetalloPPIX (M = see text)

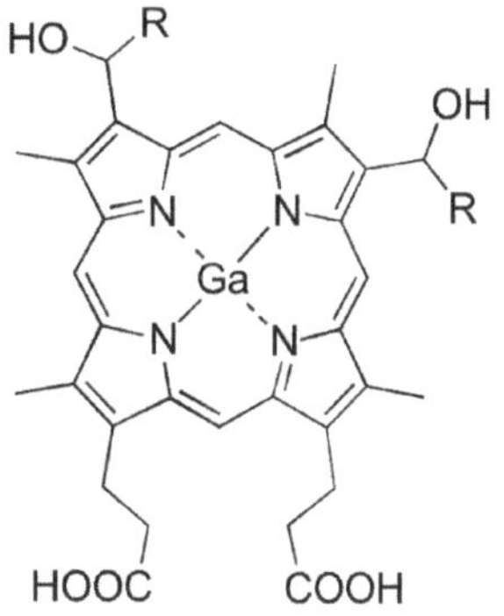

GaHPIX (R = CH_3)
GaDPIX (R = CH_2OH)

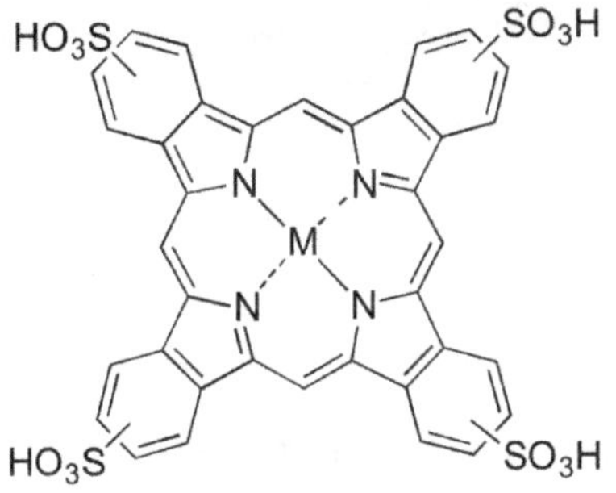

PcS (M = 2H)
Ni(II)PcS (M = Ni(II))

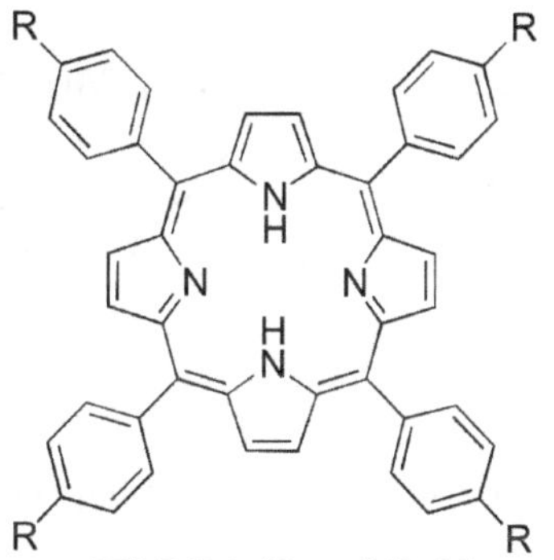

TPPC4 (R = CO_2H)
TPPS4 (R = SO_3H)

Figure 10. Structure of porphyrins and phthalocyanines developed by Wright and Begum.

In 2000, Wright's team highlighted the presence of other metal ions than Fe(III) can influence the conversion of heme to β-hematin. A number of metallo-PPIX, including Fe(III), Cr(III), Co(III), Cu(II), Mn(III), Mg(II), Zn(II), and Sn(IV) showed in vitro an ability to inhibit the β-hematin formation (**Figure 10**) [131]. In 2003 [132], phthalocyanines, phthalocyanine tetrasulfonate (PcS) and Ni(II)PcS, and anionic porphyrins, *meso*-tetra(4-sulfonatophenyl) porphyrin (TPPS4) and *meso*-tetra(4-carboxyphenyl) porphyrin (TPPC4), came to complete the previous study (**Figure 10**). All of them are inhibitors of heme crystallization. Among them, Mg(II), Zn(II), and Sn(IV) acted six times more efficiently than the free ligand PPIX and were more efficient than the chloroquine standard as well. These results showed that metalloporphyrins with high oxidation state could form complexes with heme through the Fe-propionate linkages while being efficient crystallization inhibitors.

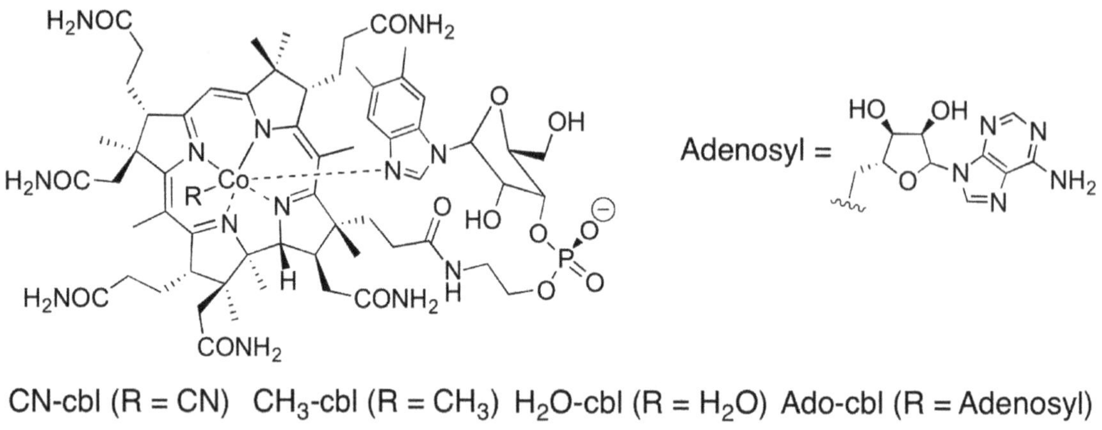

CN-cbl (R = CN) CH$_3$-cbl (R = CH$_3$) H$_2$O-cbl (R = H$_2$O) Ado-cbl (R = Adenosyl)

Figure 11. Structure of cobalamin derivatives.

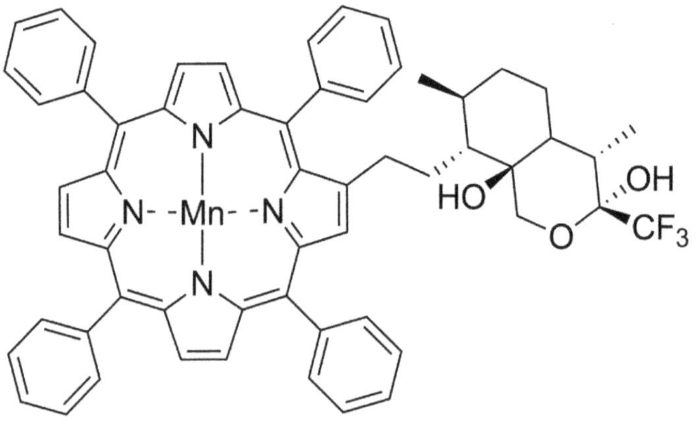

Figure 12. Mn(II) complexes of alkylated tetraphenylporphyrin with a fluorinated artemisinin.

The same behavior was observed by Begum et al. [118] who evaluated the antimalarial activity of free-base PPIX, deuteroporphyrin IX (DPIX), and hematoporphyrin IX (HPIX) and their corresponding complexes with Ga(III), Ag(III), Pd(II), Co(III), Mn(III), Sn(IV), Cr(III), and Fe(III) ions (**Figure 10**). Once again, SnPPIX at 15.5 µM had a better activity than the chloroquine control. Both GaPPIX and GaDPIX showed an antimalarial activity also.

In the same way, Chemaly et al. [133] observed that cobalamins (cbls) also called vitamin B12 (corrin ring with a chemical structure close to the heme but the central iron atom is replaced by an atom of cobalt) possess antimalarial activity. Methylcobalamin (CH$_3$-cbl), adenosylcobalamin (Ado-cbl), and aquacobalamin (H$_2$O-cbl) (**Figure 11**) showed increased efficacy over the chloroquine; cyanocobalamin (CN-cbl) was a little more efficient than chloroquine. The in vivo evaluation of vitamin B12 derivatives on the growth of *P. falciparum* (Ado-cbl > CH$_3$-cbl > H$_2$O-cbl > CN-cbl) was slightly lower than chloroquine or quinine.

Rodriguez et al. [134] showed that Mn(II) complexes of alkylated tetraphenylporphyrin with a fluorinated artemisinin derivative (**Figure 12**) were effective inhibitors of β-hematin formation with an IC_{50} of 2.6 nM.

Benoit-Vical et al. [135, 136] showed a similar behavior with anionic metalloporphyrins. Alone the *meso*-tetrakis(4-sulfonatophenyl)porphyrin (TPPS) and *meso*-tetrakis(3,5-disulfonatomesityl)porphyrin (TMPS) complexed to manganese (**Figure 13**) inhibited slightly the β-hematin formation. However, the fact of combining them with β-artemether enhanced strongly the in vitro and in vivo antimalarial activity of β-artemether.

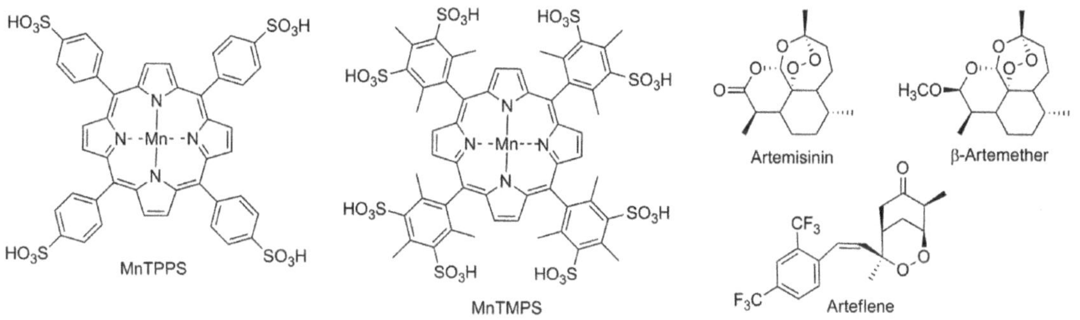

Figure 13. Structure of MnTPPS, MnTMPS, and other antimalarial derivatives.

5. Conclusion and perspectives

Malaria eradication is one of the great issues for humankind in the decades ahead. Based on figures from the *World Malaria Report 2015*, today more than ever, we are on the right track to reach this objective. The decline in cases and deaths caused by malaria stems from the relentless efforts of researchers to understand how the *P. falciparum* affects the RBCs. These different studies generated a wide range of strategies to prevent and treat malaria. Transfusion-transmitted malaria (TTM) must be understood as a high-risk situation, not only in African countries at risk but also around the world due to the increased immigration and travel from malaria-endemic areas. As mentioned in Section 3.3.2, malaria parasites can be transmitted by transfusion even if the blood is frozen (3 weeks' survival). In Europe, for example, all donated bloods are subjected to a large number of safety procedures including nucleic acid testing, blood filtration, or bacterial culture, but these are not done in many developing countries because of limited funds. All blood products are currently available in sterilized forms, except red blood cell (RBC) and platelet concentrates (PCs). The treatment of whole blood with a photosensitizer and light is a promising strategy. Very recent studies showed that this treatment can be achieved by riboflavin plus irradiation [137] and does not alter the quality of the blood [138]. As we already mentioned in Section 3.3.2, a first clinical study worldwide employing antimicrobial PDT is under progress in India using riboflavin as a photosensitizer and 447 nm blue laser. This chapter report focuses on innovative approaches using PDT or the design of new antimalarial drugs that is able to inhibit the β-hematin formation *via* heme-drug interaction.

Author details

Régis Vanderesse[1], Ludovic Colombeau[2], Céline Frochot[2] and Samir Acherar[1*]

*Address all correspondence to: samir.acherar@univ-lorraine.fr

1 Macromolecular Physical Chemistry Laboratory, University of Lorraine, Nancy Cedex, France

2 Reactions and Process Engineering Laboratory, University of Lorraine, Nancy Cedex, France

References

[1] WHO. World Malaria Report. 2015. Available from: http://www.who.int/malaria/publications/world-malaria-report-2015/report/en/

[2] Francis SE, Sullivan DJ, Goldberg DE. Hemoglobin metabolism in the malaria parasite *Plasmodium falciparum*. Annu Rev Microbiol, 1997;51:97–123. DOI: 10.1146/annurev.micro.51.1.97

[3] Krugliak M, Zhang JM, Ginsburg H. Intraerythrocytic *Plasmodium falciparum* utilizes only a fraction of the amino acids derived from the digestion of host cell cytosol for the biosynthesis of its proteins. Mol Biochem Parasitol, 2002;119:249–256. DOI: 10.1016/s0166-6851(01)00427-3

[4] Klonis N, Tan O, Jackson K, Goldberg D, Klemba M, Tilley L. Evaluation of pH during cytostomal endocytosis and vacuolar catabolism of haemoglobin in *Plasmodium falciparum*. Biochem J, 2007;407:343–354. DOI: 10.1042/BJ20070934

[5] Krogstad DJ, Schlesinger PH, Gluzman IY. Antimalarials increase vesicle pH in *Plasmodium falciparum*. J Cell Biol, 1985;101:2302–2309. DOI: 10.1083/jcb.101.6.2302

[6] Chou AC, Fitch CD. Mechanism of hemolysis induced by ferriprotoporphyrin IX. J Clin Invest, 1981;68:672–677. DOI: 10.1172/JCI110302

[7] Fitch CD, Chevli R, Banyal HS, Phillips G, Pfaller MA, Krogstad DJ. Lysis of *Plasmodium falciparum* by ferriprotoporphyrin-IX and a chloroquine-ferriprotoporphyrin-IX complex. Antimicrob Agents Chemother, 1982;21:819–822. DOI: 10.1128/AAC.21.5.819

[8] Har-el R, Marva E, Chevion M, Golenser J. Is hemin responsible for the susceptibility of Plasmodia to oxidant stress? Free Radic Res Commun, 1993;18:279–290. DOI: 10.3109/10715769309147495

[9] Orjih AU, Banyal HS, Chevli R, Fitch CD. Hemin lyses malaria parasites. Science, 1981;214:667–669. DOI: 10.1126/science.7027441

[10] Banerjee R, Liu J, Beatty W, Pelosof L, Klemba M, Goldberg DE. Four plasmepsins are active in the *Plasmodium falciparum* food vacuole, including a protease with an active-site histidine. Proc Natl Acad Sci USA, 2002;99:990–995. DOI: 10.1073/pnas.022630099

[11] Coronado LM, Nadovich CT, Spadafora C. Malarial hemozoin: from target to tool. Biochim Biophys Acta, 2014;1840:2032–2041. DOI: 10.1016/j.bbagen.2014.02.009

[12] Eggleson KK, Duffin KL, Goldberg DE. Identification and characterization of falcilysin, a metallopeptidase involved in hemoglobin catabolism within the malaria parasite *Plasmodium falciparum*. J Biol Chem, 1999;274:32411–32417. DOI: 10.1074/jbc. 274.45.32411

[13] Goldberg DE. Hemoglobin degradation. Curr Top Microbiol Immunol, 2005;295:275–291. DOI: 10.1007/3-540-29088-5_11

[14] Goldberg DE, Slater AF, Beavis R, Chait B, Cerami A, Henderson GB. Hemoglobin degradation in the human malaria pathogen *Plasmodium falciparum*: a catabolic pathway initiated by a specific aspartic protease. J Exp Med, 1991;173:961–969. DOI: 10.1084/jem.173.4.961

[15] Meshnick SR. Artemisinin: Mechanisms of action, resistance and toxicity. Int J Parasitol, 2002;32:1655–1660. DOI: 10.1016/S0020-7519(02)00194-7

[16] Kirschner-Zilber I, Rabizadeh E, Shaklai N. The interaction of hemin and bilirubin with the human red-cell membrane. Biochim Biophys Acta, 1982;690:20–30. DOI: 10.1016/0005-2736(82)90234-6

[17] Shinar E, Rachmilewitz EA. Oxidative denaturation of red blood cells in thalassemia. Semin Hematol, 1990;27:70–82. PMID: 2405497

[18] Vincent SH. Oxidative effects of heme and porphyrins on proteins and lipids. Semin Hematol, 1989;26:105–113. PMID: 2658086

[19] Klouche K, Morena M, Canaud B, Descomps B, Beraud JJ, Cristol JP. Mechanism of *in vitro* heme-induced LDL oxidation: effects of antioxidants. Eur J Clin Invest, 2004;34:619–625. DOI: 10.1111/j.1365-2362.2004.01395.x

[20] Sadrzadeh SMH, Anderson DK, Panter SS, Hallaway PE, Eaton JW. Hemoglobin potentiates central-nervous-system damage. J Clin Invest, 1987;79:662–664. DOI: 10.1007/s12029-013-9496-4

[21] Tappel AL. Unsaturated lipide oxidation catalyzed by hematin compounds. J Biol Chem, 1955;217:721–733. DOI: 10.1007/BF02633109

[22] Aft RL, Mueller GC. Hemin-mediated DNA strand scission. J Biol Chem, 1983;258:12069–12072. DOI: 10.1016/j.ejps.2012.04.014

[23] Aft RL, Mueller GC. Hemin-mediated oxidative-degradation of proteins. J Biol Chem, 1984;259:301–305. PMID: 6323403

[24] Atamna H, Ginsburg H. Origin of reactive oxygen species in erythrocytes infected with *Plasmodium falciparum*. Mol Biochem Parasitol, 1993;61:231–241. DOI: 10.1016/0166-6851(93)90069-A

[25] Foley M, Tilley L. Quinoline antimalarials: mechanisms of action and resistance and prospects for new agents. Pharmacol Ther, 1998;79:55–87. DOI: 10.1016/s0163-7258(98)00012-6

[26] Scheibel LW, Sherman IW. Metabolism and organellar function during various stages of the life cycle: proteins, lipids, nucleic acids, and vitamins, in: Malaria: Principles and Practice of Malariology. Churchill-Livingstone, Edinburgh, 1988. p. 219–252.

[27] Sullivan DJ. Hemozoin: a biocrystal synthesized during the degradation of hemoglobin, in: Biopolymers Online, Wiley-VCH Verlag GmbH & Co. KGaA, 2005. p. 129–163. DOI: 10.1002/3527600035.bpol9007

[28] Egan TJ, Mavuso WW, Ncokazi KK. The mechanism of beta-hematin formation in acetate solution, parallels between hemozoin formation and biomineralization processes. Biochemistry (Mosc), 2001;40:204–213. DOI: 10.1021/bi0013501

[29] Hempelmann E. Hemozoin biocrystallization in *Plasmodium falciparum* and the antimalarial activity of crystallization inhibitors. Parasitol Res, 2007;100:671–676. DOI: 10.1007/s00436-006-0313-x

[30] Bohle DS, Dinnebier RE, Madsen SK, Stephens PW. Characterization of the products of the heme detoxification pathway in malarial late trophozoites by X-ray diffraction. J Biol Chem, 1997;272:713–716. DOI: 10.1074/jbc.272.2.713

[31] Klonis N, Dilanian R, Hanssen E, Darmanin C, Streltsov V, Deed S, et al. Hematin-hematin self-association states involved in the formation and reactivity of the malaria parasite pigment, hemozoin. Biochemistry (Mosc), 2010;49:6804–6811. DOI: 10.1021/bi100567j

[32] Coban C, Yagi M, Ohata K, Igari Y, Tsukui T, Horii T, et al. The malarial metabolite hemozoin and its potential use as a vaccine adjuvant. Allergol Int, 2010;59:115–124. DOI: 10.2332/allergolint.10-RAI-0194

[33] Egan TJ. Recent advances in understanding the mechanism of hemozoin (malaria pigment) formation. J Inorg Biochem, 2008;102:1288–1299. DOI: 10.1016/j.jinorgbio.2007.12.004

[34] Egan TJ. Haemozoin formation. Mol Biochem Parasitol, 2008;157:127–136. DOI: 10.1016/j.molbiopara.2007.11.005

[35] Egan TJ, Ross DC, Adams PA. Quinoline antimalarial-drugs inhibit spontaneous formation of beta-hematin (malaria pigment). FEBS Lett, 1994;352:54–57. PMID: 7925942

[36] Orjih AU, Mathew TC, Cherian PT. Erythrocyte membranes convert monomeric ferriprotoporphyrin IX to beta-hematin in acidic environment at malarial fever temperature. Exp Biol Med, 2012;237:884–893. DOI: 10.1258/ebm.2012.012013

[37] Chen MM, Shi L, Sullivan Jr DJ. Haemoproteus and Schistosoma synthesize heme polymers similar to Plasmodium hemozoin and β-hematin. Mol Biochem Parasitol, 2001;113:1–8. DOI: 10.1016/S0166-6851(00)00365-0

[38] Dorn A, Stoffel R, Matile H, Bubendorf A, Ridley RG. Malarial haemozoin/beta-haematin supports haem polymerization in the absence of protein. Nature, 1995;374:269–271. DOI: 10.1038/374269a0

[39] Slater AFG, Cerami A. Inhibition by chloroquine of a novel heme polymerase enzyme-activity in malaria trophozoites. Nature, 1992;355:167–169. DOI: 10.1038/355167a0

[40] Ambele MA, Egan TJ. Neutral lipids associated with haemozoin mediate efficient and rapid beta-haematin formation at physiological pH, temperature and ionic composition. Malar J, 2012;11:Article Number 337. DOI: 10.1186/1475-2875-11-337

[41] Dorn A, Vippagunta SR, Matile H, Bubendorf A, Vennerstrom JL, Ridley RG. A comparison and analysis of several ways to promote haematin (haem) polymerisation and an assessment of its initiation in vitro. Biochem Pharmacol, 1998;55:737–747. DOI: 10.1016/S0006-2952(97)00509-1

[42] Hoang AN, Ncokazi KK, de Villiers KA, Wright DW, Egan TJ. Crystallization of synthetic haemozoin (beta-haematin) nucleated at the surface of lipid particles. Dalton Trans, 2010;39:1235–1244. DOI: 10.1039/b914359a

[43] Hoang AN, Sandlin RD, Omar A, Egan TJ, Wright DW. The neutral lipid composition present in the digestive vacuole of *Plasmodium falciparum* concentrates heme and mediates beta-hematin formation with an unusually low activation energy. Biochemistry (Mosc), 2010;49:10107–10116. DOI: 10.1021/bi101397u

[44] Choi CYH, Schneider EL, Kim JM, Gluzman IY, Goldberg DE, Ellman JA, et al. Interference with heme binding to histidine-rich protein-2 as an antimalarial strategy. Chem Biol, 2002;9:881–889. DOI: 10.1016/S1074-5521(02)00183-7

[45] Chugh M, Sundararaman V, Kumar S, Reddy VS, Siddiqui WA, Stuart KD, et al. Protein complex directs hemoglobin-to-hemozoin formation in *Plasmodium falciparum*. Proc Natl Acad Sci USA, 2013;110:5392–5397. DOI: 10.1073/pnas.1218412110

[46] Jani D, Nagarkatti R, Beatty W, Angel R, Slebodnick C, Andersen J, et al. HDP—a novel heme detoxification protein from the malaria parasite. PLoS Pathog, 2008;4:e1000053. DOI: 10.1371/journal.ppat.1000053

[47] Nakatani K, Ishikawa H, Aono S, Mizutani Y. Identification of essential histidine residues involved in heme binding and hemozoin formation in heme detoxification protein from *Plasmodium falciparum*. Sci Rep, 2014;4:6137. DOI: 10.1038/srep06137

[48] Sullivan DJ, Gluzman IY, Goldberg DE. Plasmodium hemozoin formation mediated by histidine-rich proteins. Science, 1996;271:219–222. PMID: 8539625

[49] Chou AC, Fitch CD. Heme polymerase—modulation by chloroquine treatment of a rodent malaria. Life Sci, 1992;51:2073–2078. PMID: 1474861

[50] Ridley RG, Dorn A, Matile H, Kansy M. Heme polymerization in malaria—reply. Nature, 1995;378:138–139. DOI: 10.1038/378138b0

[51] Pisciotta JM, Coppens I, Tripathi AK, Scholl PF, Shuman J, Bajad S, et al. The role of neutral lipid nanospheres in *Plasmodium falciparum* haem crystallization. Biochem J, 2007;402:197–204. DOI: 10.1042/BJ20060986

[52] Pathak MA, Fitzpatrick TB. The evolution of photochemotherapy with psoralens and Uva (Puva)—2000 Bc to 1992 Ad. J Photochem Photobiol B: Biol, 1992;14:3–22. DOI: 10.1016/1011-1344(92)85080-E

[53] Parsons BJ. Psoralen photochemistry. Photochem Photobiol, 1980;32:813–821. DOI: 10.1111/j.1751-1097.1980.tb04061.x

[54] Spikes JD. Photodynamic action: From paramecium to photochemotherapy. Photochem Photobiol, 1997;65:142S–147S. DOI: 10.1111/j.1751-1097.1997.tb07977.x

[55] Dougherty TJ, Gomer CJ, Henderson BW, Jori G, Kessel D, Korbelik M, et al. Photodynamic therapy. J Natl Cancer Inst, 1998;90:889–905. DOI: 10.1093/jnci/90.12.889

[56] von Tappeiner H, Jesionek A. Therapeutic trials with fluorescent substances. (in German). Munch Med Wochenschr, 1903;50:2042–2044.

[57] Taub AF. Photodynamic therapy in dermatology: history and horizons. J Drugs Dermatol, 2004;3:S8–S25. DOI: 10.1007/s10103-009-0716-x

[58] Azzouzi AR, Lebdai S, Benzaghou F, Stief C. Vascular-targeted photodynamic therapy with TOOKAD(R) Soluble in localized prostate cancer: standardization of the procedure. World J Urol, 2015;33:937–944. DOI: 10.1007/s00345-015-1535-2

[59] Shishkova N, Kuznetsova O, Berezov T. Photodynamic therapy in gastroenterology. J Gastrointest Cancer, 2013;44:251–259. DOI: 10.1007/s12029-013-9496-4

[60] Hillemanns P, Petry KU, Soergel P, Collinet P, Ardaens K, Gallwas J, et al. Efficacy and safety of hexaminolevulinate photodynamic therapy in patients with low-grade cervical intraepithelial neoplasia. Lasers Surg Med, 2014;46:456–461. DOI: 10.1002/lsm.22255

[61] Azaïs H, Schmitt C, Tardivel M, Kerdraon O, Stallivieri A, Frochot C, et al. Assessment of the specificity of a new folate-targeted photosensitizer for peritoneal metastasis of epithelial ovarian cancer to enable intraperitoneal photodynamic therapy. A preclinical study. Photodiagnosis Photodyn Ther, 2016;13:130–138. DOI: 10.1016/j.pdpdt.2015.07.005

[62] Stallivieri A, Baros F, Jetpisbayeva G, Myrzakhmetov B, Frochot C. The interest of folic acid in targeted photodynamic therapy. Curr Med Chem, 2015;22:3185–3207. DOI: 10.2174/0929867322666150729113912

[63] Friedberg JS, Mick R, Culligan M, Stevenson J, Fernandes A, Smith D, et al. Photodynamic therapy and the evolution of a lung-sparing surgical treatment for mesothelioma. Ann Thorac Surg, 2011;91:1738–1746. DOI: 10.1016/j.athoracsur.2011.02.062

[64] Costa L, Faustino MAF, Neves M, Cunha A, Almeida A. Photodynamic inactivation of mammalian viruses and bacteriophages. Viruses-Basel, 2012;4:1034–1074. DOI: 10.3390/v4071034

[65] Calzavara-Pinton P, Rossi MT, Sala R, Venturini M. Photodynamic antifungal chemotherapy. Photochem Photobiol, 2012;88:512–522. DOI: 10.1111/j.1751-1097.2012.01107.x

[66] Aspiroz C, Cebamanos BF, Rezusta A, Paz-Cristobal P, Dominguez-Luzond F, Diaz JG, et al. Photodynamic therapy for onychomycosis. Case report and review of the literature. Rev Iberoam Micol, 2011;28:191–193. DOI: 10.1016/j.riam.2011.03.004

[67] Jiblaoui A, Leroy-Lhez S, Ouk TS, Grenier K, Sol V. Novel polycarboxylate porphyrins: synthesis, characterization, photophysical properties and preliminary antimicrobial study against Gram-positive bacteria. Bioorg Med Chem Lett, 2015;25:355–362. DOI: 10.1016/j.bmcl.2014.11.033

[68] Lyon JP, Moreira LM, de Moraes PCG, dos Santos FV, de Resende MA. Photodynamic therapy for pathogenic fungi. Mycoses, 2011;54:E265–E227. DOI: 10.1111/j.1439-0507.2010.01966.x

[69] Richter PR, Strauch SM, Azizullah A, Häder DP. Chlorophyllin as a possible measure against vectors of human parasites and fish parasites. Front Environ Sci, 2014;2:18. DOI: 10.3389/fenvs.2014.00018

[70] Alves E, Faustino MAF, Neves M, Cunha A, Nadais H, Almeida A. Potential applications of porphyrins in photodynamic inactivation beyond the medical scope. J Photochem Photobiol, B, 2015;22:34–57. DOI: 10.1016/j.jphotochemrev.2014.09.003

[71] Barbieri A. Fluorescent sensitizers as larvicides. Photodynamic action of light. (in Spanish). Riv Malariol, 1928;7:456–463.

[72] Pimprikar GD, Georghiou GP. Mechanisms of resistance to diflubenzuron in the housefly, *Musca domestica (L)*. Pestic Biochem Physiol, 1979;12:10–22. DOI: 10.1016/0048-3575(79)90089-0

[73] Robinson JR. Photodynamic insecticides—a review of studies on photosensitizing dyes as insect control agents, their practical application, hazards, and residues. Residue Rev, 1983;88:69–100. DOI: 10.1007/978-1-4612-5569-7_2

[74] Abdel-Kader MH, Eltayeb TA, Photodynamic control of malaria vector, noxious insects and parasites, in: H.M. Abdel-Kader (Ed.) Photodynamic Therapy: From Theory to

Application, Springer Berlin Heidelberg, Berlin, Heidelberg, 2014. p. 269–291. DOI: 10.1007/978-3-642-39629-8_13

[75] Rebeiz CA, Juvik JA, Rebeiz CC. Porphyric insecticides. 1. Concept and phenomenology. Pestic Biochem Physiol, 1988;30:11–27. DOI: 10.1016/0048-3575(88)90055-7

[76] Rebeiz CA, Juvik JA, Rebeiz CC, Bouton CE, Gut LJ. Porphyric insecticides. 2. 1,10-Phenanthroline, a potent porphyric insecticide modulator. Pestic Biochem Physiol, 1990;36:201–207. DOI: 10.1016/0048-3575(90)90011-P

[77] Lucantoni L, Magaraggia M, Lupidi G, Ouedraogo RK, Coppellotti O, Esposito F, et al. Novel, meso-substituted cationic porphyrin molecule for photo-mediated larval control of the dengue vector *Aedes aegypti*. PLoS Negl Trop Dis, 2011;5:e1434. DOI: 10.1371/journal.pntd.0001434

[78] Fabris C, Ouedraogo RK, Coppellotti O, Dabire RK, Diabate A, Di Martino P, et al. Efficacy of sunlight-activatable porphyrin formulates on larvae of *Anopheles gambiae* M and S molecular forms and *An. arabiensis*: a potential novel biolarvicide for integrated malaria vector control. Acta Trop, 2012;123:239–243. DOI: 10.1016/j.actatropica.2012.05.011

[79] Stallivieri A, Le Guern F, Vanderesse R, Meledje E, Jori G, Frochot C, et al. Synthesis and photophysical properties of the photoactivatable cationic porphyrin 5-(4-N-dodecylpyridyl)-10,15,20-tri(4-N-methylpyridyl)-21H,23H-porphyrin tetraiodide for anti-malaria PDT. Photochem Photobiol Sci, 2015;14:1290–1295. DOI: 10.1039/C5PP00139K

[80] Peterson LR. Squeezing the antibiotic balloon: the impact of antimicrobial classes on emerging resistance. Clin Microbiol Inf, 2005;11:4–16. DOI: 10.1111/j.1469-0691.2005.01238.x

[81] Pereira Rosa L, da Silva FC. Antimicrobial photodynamic therapy: a new therapeutic option to combat infections. J Med Microb Diagn, 2014;3:Art 158. DOI: 10.4172/2161-0703.1000158

[82] Sperandio FF, Huang Y-Y, Hamblin MR. Antimicrobial photodynamic therapy to kill Gram-negative bacteria. Recent Patents Anti-Infect Drug Disc, 2013;8:108–120. DOI: 10.2174/1574891X113089990012

[83] Maisch T, Szeimies R-M, Jori G, Abels C. Antibacterial photodynamic therapy in dermatology. Photochem Photobiol Sci, 2004;3:907–917. DOI: 10.1039/B407622B

[84] Perni S, Prokopovich P, Pratten J, Parkin IP, Wilson M. Nanoparticles: their potential use in antibacterial photodynamic therapy. Photochem Photobiol Sci, 2011;10:712–720. DOI: 10.1039/C0PP00360C

[85] Adolfo Vera DM, Haynes MH, Ball AR, Dai T, Astrakas C, Kelso MJ, et al. Strategies to potentiate antimicrobial photoinactivation by overcoming resistant

phenotypes. Photochem Photobiol, 2012;88:499–511. DOI: 10.1111/j. 1751-1097.2012.01087.x

[86] Denis TGS, Dai T, Izikson L, Astrakas C, Anderson RR, Hamblin MR, et al. All you need is light antimicrobial photoinactivation as an evolving and emerging discovery strategy against infectious disease. Virulence, 2011;2:509–520. DOI: 10.4161/viru.2.6.17889

[87] Tim M. Strategies to optimize photosensitizers for photodynamic inactivation of bacteria. J Photochem Photobiol B: Biol, 2015;150:2–10. DOI: 10.1016/j.jphotobiol. 2015.05.010

[88] Craig RA, McCoy CP, Gorman SP, Jones DS. Photosensitisers—the progression from photodynamic therapy to anti-infective surfaces. Expert Opin Drug Deliv, 2015;12:85–101. DOI: 10.1517/17425247.2015.962512

[89] Nakonechny F, Nisnevitch M, Nitzan Y, Firer MA, New techniques in antimicrobial photodynamic therapy: scope of application and overcoming drug resistance in nosocomial infections, in: A. Méndez-Vilas (Ed.) Science Against Microbial Pathogens: Communicating Current Research and Technological Advances, Volume 2, Formatex Research Center, 2011. p. 684–691. DOI: 10.1016/j.biomaterials. 2007.06.015

[90] Ryskova L, Buchta V, Slezak R. Photodynamic antimicrobial therapy. Cent Eur J Biol, 2010;5:400–406. DOI: 10.2478/s11535-010-0032-2

[91] Wainwright M. Photodynamic antimicrobial chemotherapy (PACT). J Antimicrob Chemother, 1998;42:13–28. DOI: 10.1093/jac/42.1.13

[92] Souza E, Medeiros AC, Gurgel BC, Sarmento C. Antimicrobial photodynamic therapy in the treatment of aggressive periodontitis: a systematic review and meta-analysis. Lasers Med Sci, 2016;31:187–196. DOI: 10.1007/s10103-015-1836-0

[93] Carpenter BL, Situ XC, Scholle F, Bartelmess J, Weare WW, Ghiladi RA. Antiviral, antifungal and antibacterial activities of a BODIPY-based photosensitizer. Molecules, 2015;20:10604–10621. DOI: 10.3390/molecules200610604

[94] Chang J-E, Oak C-H, Sung N, Jheon S. The potential application of photodynamic therapy in drug-resistant tuberculosis. J Photochem Photobiol B: Biol, 2016;150:60–65. DOI: 10.1016/j.jphotobiol.2015.04.001

[95] Dai T, Huang Y-Y, Hamblin MR. Photodynamic therapy for localized infections—state of the art. Photodiagnosis Photodyn Ther, 2009;6:170–188. DOI: 10.1016/j.pdpdt. 2009.10.008

[96] Baptista MS, Wainwright M. Photodynamic antimicrobial chemotherapy (PACT) for the treatment of malaria, leishmaniasis and trypanosomiasis. Braz J Med Biol Res, 2011;44:1–10. DOI: 10.1590/S0100-879X2010007500141

[97]   Deda DK, Budu A, Cruz LN, Araki K, Garcia CRS. Strategies for development of antimalarials based on encapsulated porphyrin derivatives. Mini-Rev Med Chem, 2015;14:1055–1071. DOI: 10.2174/1389557515666150101094829

[98]   Jori G, Coppellotti O. Inactivation of pathogenic microorganisms by photodynamic techniques: mechanistic aspects and perspective applications. Antiinfect Agents Med Chem, 2007;6:119–131. DOI: 10.2174/187152107780361652

[99]   Wainwright M. The development of phenothiazinium photosensitisers. Photodiagnosis Photodyn Ther, 2005;2:263–272. DOI: 10.1093/jac/42.1.13

[100]   Almeida A, Cunha A, Faustino MAF, Tome AC, Neves MGPMS, Chapter 5 Porphyrins as Antimicrobial Photosensitizing Agents, in: Photodynamic Inactivation of Microbial Pathogens: Medical and Environmental Applications, The Royal Society of Chemistry, 2011. p. 83–160. DOI: 10.1039/9781849733083-00083

[101]   Lindholm PF, Annen K, Ramsey G. Approaches to minimize infection risk in blood banking and transfusion practice. Infect Disord Drug, 2011;11:45–56. DOI: 10.2174/187152611794407746

[102]   Castro E, Chagas and other protozoan diseases, in: Isbt Science Series, Volume 2, No 1: State of the Art Presentations, 2007. p. 1–5. DOI: 10.1111/j. 1751-2824.2007.00062.x

[103]   Reddy HL, Doane SK, Keil SD, Marschner S, Goodrich RP. Development of a riboflavin and ultraviolet light-based device to treat whole blood. Transfusion (Malden, MA, U. S.), 2013;53:131S–136S. DOI: 10.1111/trf.12047

[104]   Goodrich RP, Platz MS. The design and development of selective, photoactivated drugs for sterilization of blood products. Drug Future, 1997;22:159–171. DOI: 10.1358/dof. 1997.022.02.400935

[105]   LeBlanc D, Story R, Gross E. Laser-induced inactivation of *Plasmodium falciparum*. Malar J, 2012;11:Art267. DOI: 10.1186/1475-2875-11-267

[106]   Guttmann P, Ehrlich P. On the effect of methylene blue in malaria. (in German). Berlin Klin Woch, 1891;28:953–956.

[107]   Rounds DE, Opel W, Olson RS, Sherman IW. The potential use of laser energy in the management of malaria. Biochem Biophys Res Commun, 1968;32:616–623. DOI: 10.1016/0006-291X(68)90282-9

[108]   Smith OM, Dolan SA, Dvorak JA, Wellems TE, Sieber F. Merocyanine-540-sensitized photoinactivation of human erythrocytes parasitized by *Plasmodium falciparum*. Blood, 1992;80:21–24. PMID: 1611086

[109]   Das BS, Das DB, Satpathy RN, Patnaik JK, Bose TK. Riboflavin deficiency and severity of malaria. Eur J Clin Nutr, 1988;42:277–283. PMID: 3293996

[110] Traunmuller F, Ramharter M, Lagler H, Thalhammer F, Kremsner PG, Graninger W, et al. Normal riboflavin status in malaria patients in Gabon. Am J Trop Med Hyg, 2003;68:182–185. PMID: 12641409

[111] Akompong T, Ghori N, Haldar K. In vitro activity of riboflavin against the human malaria parasite *Plasmodium falciparum*. Antimicrob Agents Chemother, 2000;44:88–96. DOI: 10.1128/AAC.44.1.88-96.2000

[112] Keil SD, Kiser P, Sullivan JJ, Kong AS, Reddy HL, Avery A, et al. Inactivation of *Plasmodium* spp. in plasma and platelet concentrates using riboflavin and ultraviolet light. Transfusion, 2013;53:2278–2286. DOI: 10.1111/trf.12079

[113] ISLA. Anti-microbial photodynamic therapy as a new treatment option for malaria. 2015. Available from: http://www.isla-laser.org/research-group/en/current/current-projects/

[114] Sigala PA, Crowley JR, Henderson JP, Goldberg DE. Deconvoluting heme biosynthesis to target blood-stage malaria parasites. Elife, 2015;4:e09143. DOI: 10.7554/eLife.09143

[115] Wachowska M, Muchowicz A, Firczuk M, Gabrysiak M, Winiarska M, Wanczyk M, et al. Aminolevulinic acid (ALA) as a prodrug in photodynamic therapy of cancer. Molecules, 2011;16:4140–4164. DOI: 10.3390/molecules16054140

[116] Smith TG, Kain KC. Inactivation of *Plasmodium falciparum* by photodynamic excitation of heme-cycle intermediates derived from d-aminolevulinic acid. J Infect Dis, 2004;190:184–191. DOI: 10.1086/421503

[117] Martiney JA, Cerami A, Slater AF. Inhibition of hemozoin formation in *Plasmodium falciparum* trophozoite extracts by heme analogs: possible implication in the resistance to malaria conferred by the beta-thalassemia trait. Mol Med, 1996;2:236–246. PMID: 8726466

[118] Begum K, Kim HS, Kumar V, Stojiljkovic I, Wataya Y. In vitro antimalarial activity of metalloporphyrins against *Plasmodium falciparum*. Parasitol Res, 2003;90:221–224. DOI: 10.1007/s00436-003-0830-9

[119] Alves E, Iglesias BA, Deda DK, Budu A, Matias TA, Bueno VB, et al. Encapsulation of metalloporphyrins improves their capacity to block the viability of the human malaria parasite *Plasmodium falciparum*. Nanomed Nanotechnol Biol Med, 2015;11:351–358. DOI: 10.1016/j.nano.2014.09.018

[120] Abada Z, Cojean S, Pomel S, Ferrie L, Akagah B, Lormier AT, et al. Synthesis and antiprotozoal activity of original porphyrin precursors and derivatives. Eur J Med Chem, 2013;67:158–165. DOI:10.1016/j.ejmech.2013.06.002

[121] Grellier P, Santus R, Mouray E, Agmon V, Maziere JC, Rigomier D, et al. Photosensitized inactivation of *Plasmodium falciparum* and Babesia divergens-infected erythrocytes in whole blood by lipophilic pheophorbide derivatives. Vox Sang, 1997;72:211–220. DOI: 10.1046/j.1423-0410.1997.7240211.x

[122] Lustigman S, BenHur E. Photosensitized inactivation of *Plasmodium falciparum* in human red cells by phthalocyanines. Transfusion, 1996;36:543–546. DOI: 10.1046/j. 1537-2995.1996.36696269514.x

[123] Zhao XJ, Lustigman S, Kenney ME, BenHur E. Structure-activity and mechanism studies on silicon phthalocyanines with *Plasmodium falciparum* in the dark and under red light. Photochem Photobiol, 1997;66:282–287. DOI: 10.1111/j. 1751-1097.1997.tb08656.x

[124] Loh CCY, Suwanarusk R, Lee YQ, Chan KWK, Choy KY, Renia L, et al. Characterization of the commercially-available fluorescent chloroquine-BODIPY conjugate, LynxTag-CQ(GREEN), as a marker for chloroquine resistance and uptake in a 96-well plate assay. Plos One, 2014;9:Art. e110800. DOI: 10.1371/journal.pone.0110800

[125] Fu Y, Klonis N, Suarna C, Maghzal GJ, Stocker R, Tilley L. A phosphatidylcholine-BODIPY 581/591 conjugate allows mapping of oxidative stress in *P. falciparum*-infected erythrocytes. Cytometry A, 2009;75A:390–404. DOI: 10.1002/cyto.a.20704

[126] Wissing F, Sanchez CP, Rohrbach P, Ricken S, Lanzer M. Illumination of the malaria parasite *Plasmodium falciparum* alters intracellular pH—implications for live cell imaging. J Biol Chem, 2002;277:37747–37755. DOI: 10.1074/jbc.M204845200

[127] Basilico N, Monti D, Olliaro P, Taramelli D. Non-iron porphyrins inhibit beta-haematin (malaria pigment) polymerisation. FEBS Lett, 1997;409:297–299. DOI: 10.1016/S0014-5793(1097)00533-00534.

[128] Slater AF, Swiggard WJ, Orton BR, Flitter WD, Goldberg DE, Cerami A, et al. An iron-carboxylate bond links the heme units of malaria pigment. Proc Natl Acad Sci U S A, 1991;88:325–329. PMID: 1988933

[129] Monti D, Vodopivec B, Basilico N, Olliaro P, Taramelli D. A novel endogenous antima-larial: Fe(II)-protoporphyrin IX alpha (heme) inhibits hematin polymerization to beta-hematin (malaria pigment) and kills malaria parasites. Biochemistry (Mosc), 1999;38:8858–8863. DOI: 10.1021/bi990085k.

[130] Bhat AR, Athar F, Van Zyl RL, Chen C-T, Azam A. Synthesis and biological evaluation of novel 4-substituted 1-{[4-(10,15,20-triphenylporphyrin-5-yl)phenyl]methyli-dene}thiosemicarbazides as new class of potential antiprotozoal agents. Chem Biodiv-ers, 2008;5:764–776. DOI: 10.1002/cbdv.200890073

[131] Cole KA, Ziegler J, Evans CA, Wright DW. Metalloporphyrins inhibit beta-hematin (hemozoin) formation. J Inorg Biochem, 2000;78:109–115. DOI: 10.1016/S0162-0134(1099)00216-00210.

[132] Ziegler J, Pasierb L, Cole KA, Wright DW. Metalloporphyrin probes for antimalarial drug action. J Inorg Biochem, 2003;96:478–486. DOI: 10.1016/S0162-0134(03)00253-8

[133] Chemaly SM, Chen C-T, van Zyl RL. Naturally occurring cobalamins have antimalarial activity. J Inorg Biochem, 2007;101:764–773. DOI: 10.1016/j.jinorgbio.2007.01.006

[134] Rodriguez M, Bonnet-Delpon D, Begue JP, Robert A, Meunier B. Alkylation of manganese(II) tetraphenylporphyrin by antimalarial fluorinated artemisinin derivatives. Bioorg Med Chem Lett, 2003;13:1059–1062. DOI: 10.1016/S0960-894X(03)00076-3

[135] Benoit-Vical F, Robert A, Meunier B. Potentiation of artemisinin activity against chloroquine-resistant *Plasmodium falciparum* strains by using heme models. Antimicrob Agents Chemother, 1999;43:2555–2558. PMID: 10508044

[136] Benoit-Vical F, Robert A, Meunier B. In vitro and in vivo potentiation of artemisinin and synthetic endoperoxide antimalarial drugs by metalloporphyrins. Antimicrob Agents Chemother, 2000;44:2836–2841. DOI: 10.1128/AAC.44.10.2836-2841.2000

[137] El Chaar M, Atwal S, Freimanis GL, Dinko B, Sutherland CJ, Allain JP. Inactivation of *Plasmodium falciparum* in whole blood by riboflavin plus irradiation. Transfusion, 2013;53:3174–3183. DOI: 10.1111/trf.12235

[138] Owusu-Ofori S, Kusi J, Owusu-Ofori A, Freimanis G, Olver C, Martinez CR, et al. Treatment of whole blood with riboflavin and UV light: impact on malaria parasite viability and whole blood storage. Shock, 2014;44:33–38. DOI: 10.1097/SHK. 0000000000000280

8

Identifying Antimalarial Drug Targets by Cellular Network Analysis

Kitiporn Plaimas and Rainer König

Abstract

Malaria is one of the most deadly parasitic infectious diseases and identifying novel drug targets is mandatory for the development of new drugs. To find drug targets, metabolic and signaling networks have been constructed. These networks have been investigated by graph theoretical methods. Furthermore, mechanistic models have been set up based on stoichiometric equations. At equilibrium, production and consumption of internal metabolites need to be balanced leading to a large set of flux equations, and this can be used for metabolic flux simulations to identify drug targets. Analysis of flux variability and knockout simulations were applied to detect potential drug targets whose absence reduces the predicted biomass production and hence viability of the parasite in the host cell. Furthermore, not only the parasite was studied, but also the interaction between the host and the parasite, and, based on experimental expression data, stage-specific metabolic models of the parasite were developed, particularly during the red-blood cell stage. In this chapter, these various network-based approaches for drug target prediction will be explained and summarized.

Keywords: network-based analysis, drug targets, flux balance analysis, malaria

1. Introduction

Network-based analysis has become an important tool in biomedical research. It facilitates the investigation and understanding of a system as a whole, not only its single components. For this, first the networks need to be constructed and then investigated employing different analysis or modeling techniques. According to the applied methodological approaches to analyze these networks, one may distinguish cellular network models for signal transduction, gene regulation and metabolism. The network constructions based on information are compiled from databases and are assembled in an automated way often followed by manual refinement. Network-based models have been applied to study the cellular mechanisms of a large variety of diseases elucidating, for example, tumor growth, malfunctioning of the differentiation of immune cells, or identifying drug targets of invasive pathogens [1, 2]. To find drug targets for the treatment of malaria, metabolic and signaling networks have been constructed and intensively investigated. This chapter will introduce the reader into the basic principles of constructing and applying such cellular networks. It then leads through the application of these systems biology approaches to predict drug targets followed by a small section exemplarily showing an experimental validation for these predictions.

2. Construction of cellular networks

Proteins are involved in all cellular functions. These cellular processes can be put up as cellular networks, which describe associations among these proteins and other cellular compounds such as metabolites and nucleic acids. These cellular networks can conceptually be divided into three distinct parts: the cell signaling, the transcriptional regulatory network, and the metabolic network. The best observed and modeled network is the metabolic network while the complex system of signal transduction is rather captured statistically investigating the experimental information about proteins and their expressed genes of network models basing on protein-protein interactions [3]. The transcriptional regulatory network links transcriptional regulators to their target genes [4]. The simplest form of a network is a network represented by an undirected graph $G = (V, E)$ consisting of nodes V and edges (connections, links) E between these nodes. Each node $i \in V$ represents a unique cellular entity such as enzymes, genes, and proteins, while each edge $(i, j) \in E$ represents an observed interaction between two nodes i and j. A metabolic network model can be constructed as a bipartite graph consisting of two disjoint sets of nodes (reaction and metabolite nodes, see **Figure 1**) [5]. The direction of edges in the metabolic networks is given by the flux from the substrate to the product of a biochemical reaction. An edge indicates that a metabolite is either a substrate or a product of a reaction. The distinction between substrates and products of a reaction is only possible if the graph is directed, that is, if the set of edges E consists of ordered pairs of vertices. This distinction is often useful when modeling metabolic fluxes but may be neglected in simpler models [6]. As a bipartite graph, the metabolic network can be represented as an adjacency matrix of $m \times n$ dimensions, where m is the number of metabolites and n is the number of reactions. More specific models of metabolic networks concerning the stoichiometry can also be represented as an adjacency matrix using stoichiometric coefficients of chemical reactions as weights for the edges between metabolites and reactions. As shown in **Figure 1**, our small example network consists of three reactions (R1, R2, and R3) and six metabolites (A, B, C, D, E, and F):

R1:	A	⇔	B
R2:	2 B + C	→	E + F
R3:	2 E	→	B + D

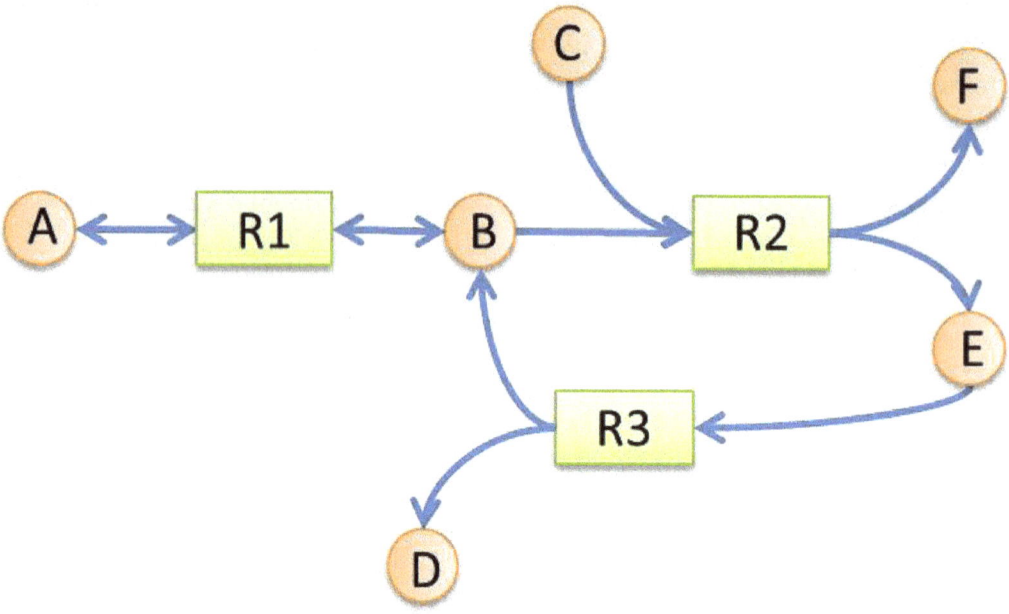

Figure 1. Graphical view of a metabolic network model as a bipartite graph consisting of two disjoint sets of nodes (reactions and metabolites). This network consists of three reactions (R1, R2 and R3) and six metabolites (A, B, C, D, E, F). R1 is a reversible reaction, the other reactions are irreversible.

The stoichiometric matrix or the adjacency matrix containing stoichiometric coefficients of each reaction equation is

$$
s = \begin{bmatrix} -1 & 0 & 0 \\ 1 & -2 & 1 \\ 0 & -1 & 0 \\ 0 & 0 & 1 \\ 0 & 1 & -2 \end{bmatrix}
$$

where the rows correspond to metabolites A, B, C, D, E, and F, and the columns correspond to reactions R1, R2, and R3, respectively. R1 is a reversible reaction. Metabolic networks for *Plasmodium spp* can be constructed using the databases PlasmoCyc [7], Malaria Parasite Metabolic Pathways (MPMP) [8], The Kyoto Encyclopedia of Genes and Genomes (KEGG), http://www.genome.jp/kegg/, and from models in the literature [9]. Unspecific compounds such as water, ATP, ADP, etc., may be discarded for these rather general models but need to be considered for more detailed models when, for example, employing flux balance analysis (see below). Cellular networks can be analyzed mechanistically or statistically by their topological features. In the following, we explain briefly some of these topological features.

3. Topological features for statistical analyses of cellular networks

Several computational techniques have been developed to identify essential genes and drug targets *in silico* for a therapy against malaria. To construct an undirected graph for metabolism, the network representation of a reaction-pair network can be used instead of a bipartite graph. In this representation, enzymes are linked if there is at least one metabolite, which is produced by one of the enzymes and which serves as a substrate for the other. For these simple networks, the network topology can be described by characteristic properties. Similarly, protein interaction networks can be analyzed to get specific characteristics for signal transduction [3, 10, 11]. These characteristics either hint directly to essential genes (serving as drug targets) or can be used when comparing the full network with a network in which one of the nodes (enzymes or signaling proteins) is targeted by a drug.

3.1. Diameter and density of a network

The diameter of a network is the largest distance of all shortest paths between two nodes (reactions, signaling molecules) in the network. The density of a network is the ratio of the edges (links, connections) between two reactions divided by all possible edges of all reactions. These two properties can be used to determine the robustness of a network. In recent studies, a reaction was said to be essential if the mutated or targeted network showed a larger diameter after removing the reaction [12, 13].

3.2. Scale-freeness of networks

Networks can be distinguished by their degree distributions where the degree of a node $v \in V$ is defined as the number of edges between v and its adjacent nodes. Many degree distributions of naturally occurring networks follow power laws [6] $P(k) \sim k^{-\gamma}$ where $\gamma > 0$ is a constant depending on the network and is usually in the range of 2–3. P is the probability to draw a node with degree k. Networks with a power law distribution are also called *scale-free* networks [6, 14]. Basically, these scale-free networks consist of few highly connected vertices, so-called *hubs*, and many less connected vertices [15]. Most real-world networks including metabolic networks are approximately scale-free networks [6]. **Figure 2** shows the degree distribution of the metabolic network of *Plasmodium falciparum*, which is fitted by a power-law distribution. Scale-free networks generally have a small diameter [16], as in particular the highly connected nodes connect nodes within only a few links. Additionally, these networks are highly connected [17]. The benefit of such a highly connected and scale-free architecture is its robustness against single "attacks," that is, a failure of a single node in the system, as it is statistically more probable that vertices with lower degrees are hit from which the general structure of the network is not affected. The scale-free topology provides robustness to the network with increases flexibility to random perturbations where the loss of individual nodes usually has no effect on the overall network topology. Nevertheless, such a network is susceptible to targeted attacks at highly connected critical hubs [18], and mutations affecting hubs are more likely to cause a defect [17].

3.3. Clustering coefficient

The clustering coefficient is used to estimate the local density of links (edges) in the network. It describes the connectedness among neighbors and helps to estimate the probability of local alternative paths of signaling or metabolic fluxes (e.g., after targeting). The clustering coefficient of a node v is defined as the ratio of the number of connecting edges among all neighbors

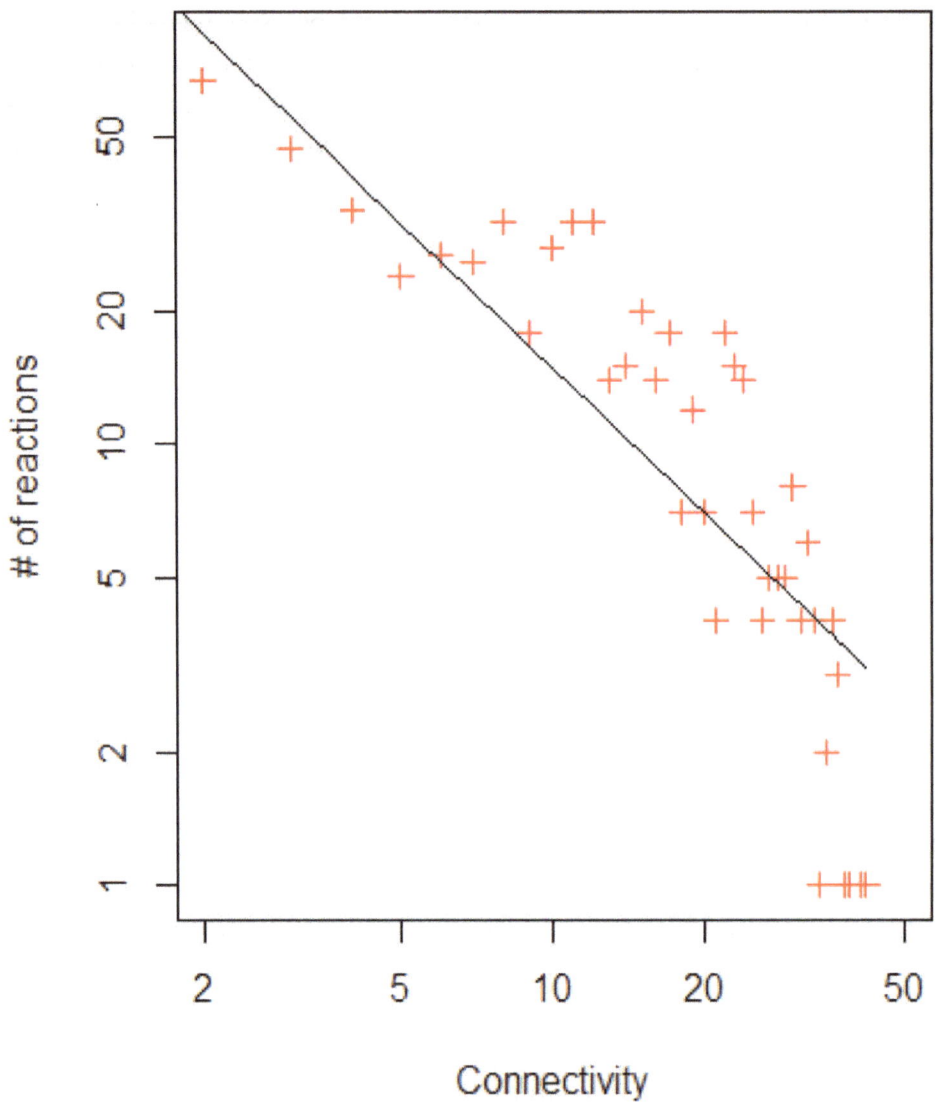

Figure 2. Degree distribution of the metabolic network of *P. falciparum* using the (most suitable) network of [13].

of v and the total number of edges among them that could be possible. This means, if all neighbors are connected among themselves, the clustering coefficient becomes one, if none of the neighbors is connected with any other neighbor, it is zero [6, 19, 20]. In **Figure 3**, the observed reaction in dark has three neighbors and two edges among its neighbors. Having three neighbors, there are six possible connections among neighbors. Thus, the clustering coefficient of the observed reaction in this example can be computed as $\frac{2}{6} = \frac{1}{3}$.

3.4. Centrality

Descriptors for *node centrality* are quite powerful for describing the potential of essentiality of a node. They describe not only the impact of the node to its direct vicinity but also the contribution of a node to the global structure of the network. The simplest of all centrality measures is the connectivity, or degree k, which is just the number of links connecting the node with other nodes. In a cellular network, the degree is commonly used to describe an important node as it

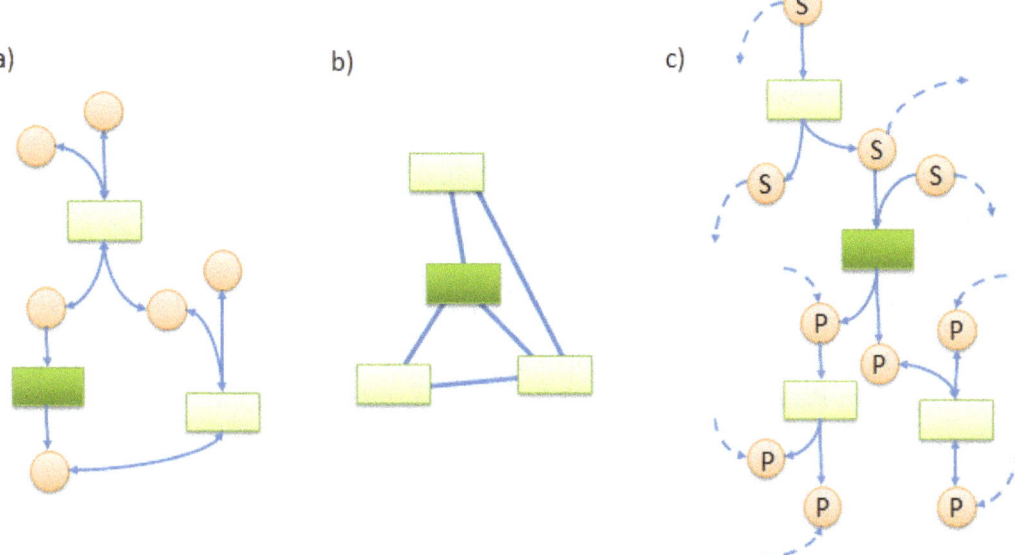

Figure 3. Illustration of the concepts of the topology features. Circles represent metabolites, rectangles reactions, arrows directions of the metabolic flux, lines represent links between two neighboring reactions and dark rectangles represent the investigated reactions. (a) The observed reaction is a chokepoint because it is the only reaction consuming the upstream metabolite. (b) The metabolic network in a reaction-pair representation for computing the clustering coefficient. The observed reaction has three neighbors (degree of 3) and there are two links among these neighbors. Therefore, the clustering coefficient for this observed reaction is 1/3. (c) Graphical illustration of the way to compute producibility of the observed reaction from its substrates (S) to its products (P). Possible alternative pathways to consume substrates S for producing products P are represented by dashed arrows. The percentage of the products that can be produced from the substrates is the producibility of the observed reaction.

is known that often essential genes are nodes in the network with a high degree (so-called hubs). Another commonly used centrality measure is betweenness centrality. Betweenness centrality is the frequency of a node to be part of the shortest paths connecting all pairs of nodes in the network [21].

3.5. Choke points and load points

In metabolic networks, Samal *et al.* found out that most reactions identified as essential are involved in the consumption or production of metabolites with low connectivity [22]. This is because these nodes are more likely to be the limiting factor for consuming or producing these metabolites. In the extreme case, an enzyme is the only enzyme, which consumes or produces a certain compound. Blocking such a reaction may cause severe effects to the cell as, for example, it may cause an assembly of toxic compounds, which cannot be degraded anymore or a lack of substrates for important processes further downstream of the enzyme. Hence, a choke point reaction was defined as a reaction that uniquely consumes or produces a certain metabolite in the metabolic network [23, 24]. This concept has been successfully applied to identify drug targets for *Plasmodium spp.* [24, 25]. Load scores are defined as hot spots in the metabolic network (enzymes or metabolites) based on the ratio of the number of shortest paths (connecting any two enzymes or metabolites in the whole network) passing through a metabolite or enzyme and the number of nearest neighbor links [23].

3.6. Producibility (by deviations)

A reaction is determined to be potentially essential when basically the mutated network cannot yield the products of the reaction from upstream substrates of the reaction using other pathways linking the substrates to the products (see **Figure 3**). The percentage of the products that can be produced from the substrates, the so-called "producibility," can be used to examine the essentiality of the observed reaction [13].

3.7. Applying these topology-based methods to predict drug targets for *Plasmodium* spp.

The concept of choke points and load points was successfully applied to estimate the essentiality of an enzyme in *Plasmodium* [23, 24, 26]. Yeh *et al.* initially applied a chokepoint analysis for *P. falciparum*. Strikingly, they found that 87% of known drug targets with biological evidence are chokepoints according to their analysis [24]. In line, they identified three targets of clinically proven malaria drugs, dihydrofolate reductase, dihydropteroate synthase, and 1-deoxy-D-xylulose 5-phosphate reductoisomerase as chokepoints. Rahman and Schomburg performed a chokepoint and load score analysis for several other organisms [23, 26]. In Fatumo *et al.*, we performed a chokepoint analysis together with our developed producibility concept to obtain a more reliable list of potential drug targets in *P. falciparum*. For example, we identified deoxyhypusine synthase involved in spermidine metabolism, which is a known drug target in *P. falciparum*, *Anopheles stephensi*, and *Trypanosoma evansi* [27]. This enzyme was detected by intersecting the predicted targets from a chokepoint and a producibility analysis [26].

Protein-protein interactions were inferred by a high-throughput method (yeast-2-hybrid) and assembled for a signaling network of *P. falciparum*. This has been performed for the first time by Suthram in 2005 identifying conserved proteins, pathways, and interactions [28]. The network was then analyzed by using a network alignment approach comparing the networks across organisms, by using various graph theoretical measures and an *in silico* knock-out strategy to identify potential drug targets [11, 12, 28, 29]. With this, conserved pathways and proteins between organisms were identified hinting for essentiality. The study showed that a few interactions were conserved among the analyzed organisms, demonstrating that the protein interaction network of *Plasmodium* is distinctively different from the others. Interestingly, a conserved protein complex was found in calmodulin-mediated endocytosis. Indeed, inhibition of calmodulin resulted in attenuated growth [30] and reduced chloroquine extrusion in malarial parasites diminishing drug resistance to chloroquine [31]. Additionally, endocytosis was found to be related to these mechanisms [32]. Thus, the proximity of calmodulin to the formation of endocytic vacuoles in *Plasmodium* provides an interesting link to discover strategies coping drug resistance mechanisms of *Plasmodium* [28].

Recently, Bhattacharyya and Chakrabarti analyzed a large-scale protein-protein interaction network of *Plasmodium* and identified potential drug targets using various graph theoretical measures such as centrality measures. They also used an *in silico* knock-out strategy to study the perturbation due to a loss of a protein in the network [12]. With this, approximately 270 proteins of *P. falciparum* were identified as potential drug targets including proteins, which play crucial roles in intra-pathogen network integrity, stage specificity but also interact with various human proteins involved in multiple metabolic pathways within the host cell. Most of the housekeeping proteins were found to be potential targets [12].

Interactions between the human host and the parasite have been intensively studied [11–13, 33]. The comparison of several reconstructed network models has been performed to find the best suitable reconstruction for detecting drug targets *in silico*. This was performed on a metabolic network reconstruction based on automatically inferred enzymes and compared with a reconstructed model that based only on enzymes whose coding genes were known. These networks were analyzed with criteria for defining essential enzymes including chokepoints, betweenness centrality, connectivity, and the diameter of the networks. Comparing the modeling results with a comprehensive list of known drug targets for *P. falciparum* showed that the most suitable network model was constructed using only enzymes from the parasite alone, which coding genes were known [13].

Chen *et al.* developed a network-based approach to predict malaria-associated genes by a random walk algorithm [33]. They first constructed separate gene networks of the human genome and of the parasite genome and then connected them with known host-pathogen protein interactions. Known malaria target genes were used as the seeds (a set of nodes at which the search started) in a random walk algorithm to prioritize genes. The random walk algorithm then iteratively explored the global structure of the network starting at a set of nodes (seeds) to estimate the probability of a node being reached from the seeds. These probability scores can be viewed as the influential impact over the network imposed by the set of seed nodes. Finally, all the genes were ranked according to their probability scores. Manually examining the top 50 predicted human genes, interesting proteins such as TLR4 and P53 were found to be associated with malaria [33].

4. *In silico* modeling using flux balance analysis to identify drug targets

Flux balance analysis (FBA) is a computational approach to estimate the quantitative flux of metabolites through a mechanistic model of metabolism. Thereby, it is possible to predict the growth rate of an organism or the rate of production of an important metabolite [9, 34–36]. Biochemical stoichiometric equations are used to assemble a set of constraints to limit the feasible search space. The idea is that, at equilibrium, production and consumption of internal metabolites are balanced. This leads to a large set of equations in which the net production flux equals the net consumption flux for each internal metabolite. Additionally, allowable fluxes of any reaction are bounded at plausible maximum and minimum fluxes. Bounds may also be taken from the literature. These balances and bounds define the space of allowable flux distributions of a system, that is, the allowed combinations of fluxes for each reaction. To get a phenotype or modeling prediction from these constraints, an optimization criterion is put up. For example, in the case of predicting growth, the objective is to optimize biomass production which is the rate at which metabolic compounds are converted into the physiological portions of biomass constituents most importantly of nucleic acids, amino acids and lipids. Together with the constraints, this is mathematically formulated as a system of linear equations which is solved using linear programming based programs. Flux variability and knockout simulations are analyzed to detect potential drug targets whose absence reduces the biomass production and hence viability of the parasite in the host cell. By simulating a reconstructed metabolic network of an organism of interest, first a "wildtype" model is investigated and the growth rate of the wildtype under specific bounds (or conditions) obtained. Performing a single gene (or reaction) knockout/deletion under the same condition by limiting its corresponding fluxes to zero (knockout simulation), the fluxes are calculated simulating an organism effected to a drug (targeting the deleted enzyme) and the growth rate is compared to the wildtype. A knocked out gene (or reaction) is predicted to be essential under the given condition if the mutant model yields a much lower growth rate compared to the wildtype. Flux balance analysis is a widely used and well-established technique to assess the essentiality of genes and hence potential drug targets [9, 34–36]. The beauty of this approach is that it does not depend on specific enzymatic parameters for each enzyme like their Michaelis Menten constants, etc., but are rather basing on simple stoichiometric equations. To some extent, the only experimental parameters are the boundary conditions. The drawback is that often several solutions can come out which are mathematically equally good, but physiologically very different leading to follow-up analyses of each of these solutions. Nevertheless, the approach was used for several genome-scale metabolic network constructions, followed by flux simulations of the inner metabolites of *Plasmodium* spp. to identify drug targets. It also enables to embed the metabolism of *Plasmodium* spp. into the metabolism of its environment, for example, human red blood cells [9]. Furthermore, experimental data on a systems view can be embedded using microarray or sequencing based gene expression data and with this, stage-specific metabolic models of the parasite were developed, particularly during the red-blood cell stage [9]. To better understand flux balance analysis and its potential, we will give a brief introduction into the mathematical secrets of it in the next section (which can be skipped without losing the track to understand the subsequent sections).

4.1. Flux balance analysis formulation

Let s_{ij} be the stoichiometric coefficient of metabolite i in reaction j, which specifies the number of metabolites produced or consumed by reaction j. $s_{ij} > 0$ indicates that reaction j produces metabolite i, while $s_{ij} < 0$ indicates that reaction j consumes metabolite i. $s_{ij} = 0$ means that metabolite i does not participate in reaction j. For example, considering a reaction $A + 2B \rightarrow C$, the stoichiometric coefficients of A, B, and C are −1, −2, and 1, respectively. The stoichiometric coefficients s_{ij} can be combined into the so-called *stoichiometric matrix* $S = (s_{ij})$. A rate of concentration change of a metabolite can be formulated by the set of system equations:

$$\frac{dx_i}{dt} = \sum_j s_{ij} v_j \tag{1}$$

where x_i is the concentration of metabolite i, s_{ij} is the stoichiometric coefficient, and v_j is the consumption/production rate of reaction j. Based on the assumption of mass conservation at steady state in the cell, internal metabolite concentrations are constant over time. Therefore, the concentration change of each internal metabolite i is zero, which means $\frac{dx_i}{dt} = 0$. With this assumption, equation (1) can be formulated as

$$\sum_j S_{ij}v_j = Sv = 0 \qquad (2)$$

where S is the $m \times n$ stoichiometric matrix of m metabolites and n reactions in the network. The vector v represents all reaction rates (also called metabolic fluxes) in the metabolic network. The ranges of individual metabolic fluxes are constrained by $\alpha_j \leq v_j \leq \beta_j$ where α_j and β_j are the minimal and maximal fluxes of reaction j, respectively. These inequality constraints allow reversibility. If a reaction is reversible, the flux of the reaction v_j can either be negative or positive. A positive flux indicates the forward direction while a negative flux indicates a backward direction. If we want to block a reaction (knockout simulation), we can constrain the flux of this reaction to be equal to zero ($v_j = 0$). In addition, the benefit of these inequality constraints is to simulate metabolic capabilities under certain conditions such as a glucose minimal medium condition, which we can model by constraining the flux of the glucose uptake rate in a specific range of values and set the uptake rates of all other carbon source to zero. Finally, the set or subspace of vector v that satisfies all constrains and the ranges of individual metabolic fluxes is a set of feasible fluxes covering all feasible capabilities of the metabolic network under the given specific condition. Using an optimization criterion, such as to optimize the biomass of the cell yields then only one or a few out of these solutions. The biomass production rate can be defined by a reaction or several reactions that produce the metabolic building blocks of a cell (e.g., amino acids and nucleotides) or macromolecules that form the biomass in a physiological composition. The physiological biomass composition of a given organism comprises the relative amounts of the important molecules and can be found in the literature [9, 36]. The flux of the biomass production is associated with the specific growth rate of an organism. Finally, the obtained growth rate of the mutant (with a reaction knocked out) is compared to the growth rate of the wildtype to predict a gene or an enzyme to be essential. This section was taken from Ref. [37].

4.1.1. Applying FBA to predict drug targets

FBA has been widely used to predict essential genes of the human malaria parasite *P. falciparum* [9, 36, 38]. A metabolic network reconstruction of *P. falciparum* was developed with 1001 reactions and 616 metabolites [36]. The model allowed predicting the phenotype (growth) of experimental gene knockouts. Validating the predictions with drug inhibition assays yielded approximately 90% accuracy. Several modifications on the linear programming implementation were studied to make the static FBA model more realistic. For example, gene expression profiles of the malaria parasite were integrated into metabolic models [9, 36, 38]. In the study of Plata *et al.* [36], the maximum flux of the associated reactions was constrained by their expression level while Huthmacher *et al.* [9] used a method proposed by Shlomi *et al.* [39]. This method is a modification to flux balance analysis (FBA) by adding binary variables for each reaction. These binary variables act like an on/off switch according to the expression level. The mathematical objective is to maximize the number of non-zero fluxes for the reactions with switched-on-state. Dholakia *et al.* analyzed many available *omics* resources of stage-specific expression and used pathway tools from the BioCyc database to analyze flux distributions with respect to gene expression for identifying drug targets, and in particular in the erythrocytic stage-specific metabolism of the parasite. Based on the FBA approach, Plata *et al.* identified 40 enzymatic drug targets. All of these enzymes had no or very low sequence similarity to human proteins which made them more attractive as this facilitated designing drugs targeting these enzymes and not human host factors. This set of genes consisted of six genes associated with isoprenoid metabolism, three genes involved in nucleotide metabolism, and the rest of genes related to CoA, shikimate, and folate biosynthesis. In addition, one of predicted essential genes, nicotinate nucleotide adenylyltransferase, was selected to be tested further in an experimental assay. This enzyme has been known for anti-microbial development [40] but not in *Plasmodium* spp. yet. Thus, in Plata et al., the experimental validation was done in *P. falciparum* by inhibiting this enzyme by a small-molecule inhibitor from [41] resulting in blocking host cell escape and reinvasion by arresting the parasites in the trophozoite growth stage [36]. Hence, FBA allowed the construction of stage-specific metabolic networks for different stages of the parasites and gave the opportunity to find drug targets for these stages. Additionally, also host-parasite interactions can be studied using FBA [9]. In the study by Huthmacher et al. [9], a host-parasite network was constructed and the metabolic fluxes for each blood life cycle stage were predicted employing gene expression data of the different stages. Knock-out simulations identified 307 indispensable metabolic reactions for the parasite. Of 57, 35 experimentally validated essential enzymes were recovered. Another set of 16 enzymes were predicted, if additionally assuming that nutrient uptake from the host cell is limited and all reactions catalyzed by the inhibited enzyme are blocked. An interesting modification to flux balance analysis was developed by a two-stage flux balance analysis to identify drug targets by comparing the differences of fluxes between a drug treated and untreated condition [42]. This approach was applied to find drug targets in *Plasmodium*, which is described in more detail in the next section.

4.2. Finding multiple drug targets to treat a drug resistant *Plasmodium* strain

Recently, Phaiphinit et al. reconstructed the metabolic network of *P. falciparum* in the human host red blood cell using flux balance analysis [35]. This model was used to analyze two specific metabolic models: a model for the parasite when having invaded the red blood cell without any treatment and, in turn, the treated situation, when a drug like chloroquine acts by inhibiting the hemozoin formation causing a high production rate of harmful heme. The process of identifying target combinations consisted of two main steps (**Figure 4**):

Step 1—Developing two multi-cellular metabolic models: The model was constructed for the situation of the parasite being inside the red blood cell of the human host. All metabolites of the parasite in exchange with the external environment were taken from the red blood cell. To find potential reactions which could harm *P. falciparum* by getting exposed to severe toxicity, the flux distribution of the multi-cellular metabolic model was calculated for two conditions. The first condition was the untreated situation where the parasite was able to get rid of toxins from hemoglobin degradation after consuming hemoglobin from the red blood cell. The second condition mimicked the treated situation in which the toxins could not be degraded. The difference in flux distributions between the two conditions was assumed to be the effect from the drug which disturbed the parasite.

Step 2—Finding the optimal drug target: The reactions in the parasite which were disturbed from the drug in the treated situation may suit as drug targets for a combined treatment, or if

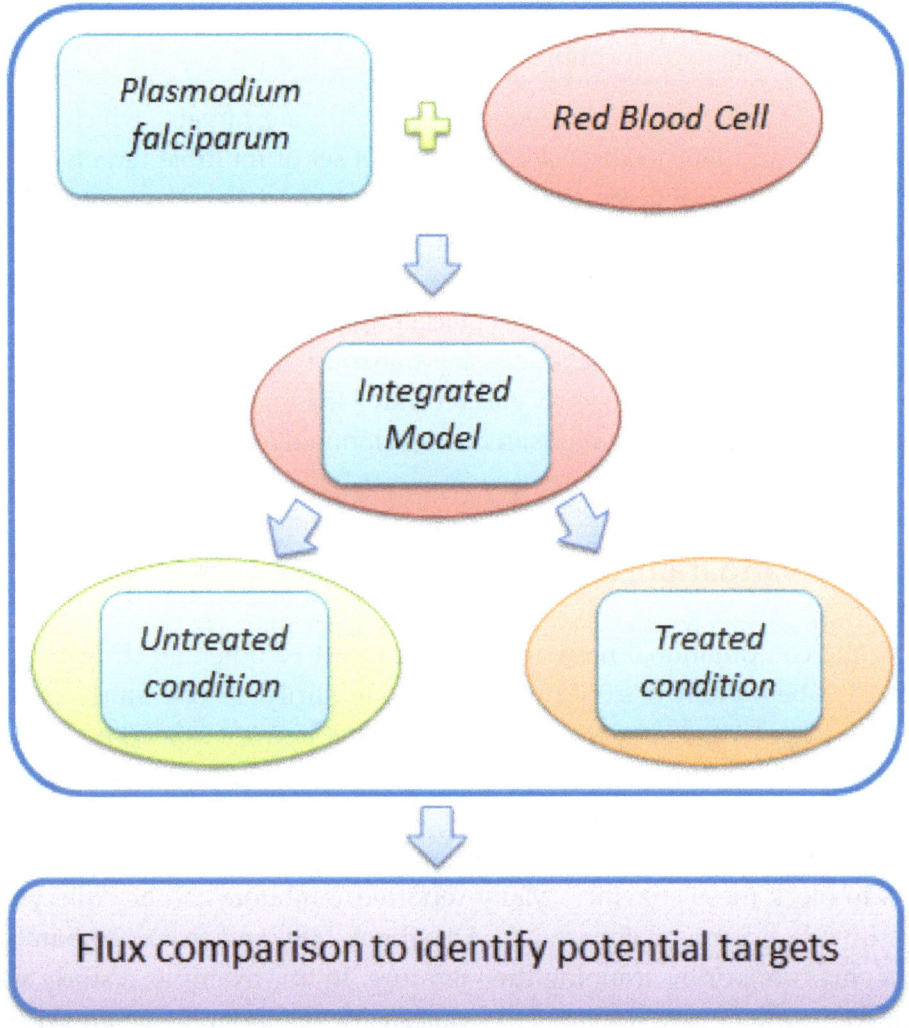

Figure 4. The workflow to identify drug targets by the comparison of treated and untreated conditions. First, *in silico* models of *Plasmodium falciparum* and the human red blood cell are combined as an integrated model. This integrated model is characterized by two specific conditions (treated and untreated). The flux rates of all reactions in both situations are compared to identify a set of potential drug targets.

the parasite gets resistant to the first drug (chloroquine). In particular, reactions for which no flux was predicted in the treated scenario were promising targets because they may have a similar treatment effect when targeted compared to the original drug and may suit as drug targets against strains which are resistant to the first drug.

FBA was used to get the flux distributions for the untreated and the treated conditions. For the untreated condition, the objective was to maximize the production rate of biomass according to Ref. [36], including the Na^+/K^+ ratio based potential at the ATPase, which plays an important role for the homeostasis of red blood cells [43, 44]. In the treated condition, the drug usually inhibits the detoxification process of the parasite harming the parasite due to the toxicity of free heme. Thus, during the treated condition, the (toxic) flux of heme production should be an additional objective to ensure that the toxic flux is not zero when identifying reactions or enzymes to be blocked during the treatment. The flux distributions of both models were then compared to obtain a list of candidate targets by the criteria that the reactions with zero fluxes in the treated condition but non-zero fluxes in the untreated condition could be potential targets for inhibiting heme detoxification.

With this method, 23 enzymes were identified as candidate targets, which mostly were in pyruvate metabolism and the citrate cycle. The optimal set of multiple targets for blocking the detoxification was a set of a heme ligase, adenosine transporter, myo-inositol 1-phosphate synthase, ferrodoxim reductase-like protein, and the guanine transporter. Purine transporters have been known as the major route of purine into the parasitized red blood cell. In the development of anti-malarial drugs, inhibitors targeting purine transport are of pharmaceutical interest and are investigated. Likewise, adenosine transport and its inhibitor have been studied in infected and uninfected human erythrocytes recently [45]. In summary, this shows an efficient way to identify useful target combinations in the development of novel antimalarial drugs [35].

5. Experimental validation, a case study

Typically, after the computational network analysis, a list of potential drug targets is assembled and needs to be validated experimentally. Exemplarily, in one study of a topological network analysis, 22 potential targets were proposed [26]. Using a refined network comprising also the host enzymes led to a refined set of the five potential drug targets (glutamyl–tRNA (gln) amidotransferase, hydroxyethylthiazole kinase, deoxyribose–phosphate aldolase, pseudouridylate synthase, and deoxyhypusine synthase) [46]. The next step was to find effective inhibitors to block these enzymes. Many reported inhibitors can be collected from databases like the Brenda Enzyme database [47], Drugbank [48], and from companies like Sigma (http://www.sigma.com), or by scanning the literature. In this example, a study was found, in which Jahn and coworkers used 6-diazo-5-oxonorleucine (DON) to be an effective inhibitor of glutamyl-tRNA(Gln) amidotransferase in *Chlamydomonas reinhardtii* [49]. Accordingly, an experimental viability assay (IC_{50} analysis) was performed and showed that DON suits as a valid agent against *P. falciparum* (laboratory strain Dd2) in *Plasmodium* infected blood cultures. Strikingly, this was confirmed by an *in vivo* study using *Plasmodium berghei* infected Swiss albino mice. All treated mice survived whereas all untreated died [45].

6. Conclusions

Even though the number of deaths caused by malaria has diminished considerably, it is still a challenge to treat the effected patients and clear off the pathogen after infection. In particular, there are increasingly more strains getting resistant against common treatments, and hence there is a striking demand to find new targets for therapy.

The computational approaches introduced here show some convincing results. However, it needs to be shown that these predictions are experimentally confirmed and finally make their way from the bench to the bedside.

Various techniques of network-based analyses to identify potential drug targets of *Plasmodium* have been described in more detail including the construction of cellular networks, the analysis of topological features, as well as *in silico* models based on flux balance analysis. To construct a network, one needs to consider the network types which are suitable to find the targets of interest. Moreover, the consideration of the interactions between host and pathogen makes the network more realistic, but, however, also more complex to obtain drug targets. Analyzing topological features seems to be a comfortable way to retrieve interesting targets; however, the *in silico* models using flux balance may reflect much more detailed relations of the biochemical reactions in a cell. All of the methods described in this chapter provided promising results, some with experimental evidence. It is to be noted that they have been widely used for a large variety of other organisms as well.

Even though all these presented concepts have the very same aim to find a target, their results are quite heterogeneous lists of different predicted drug targets, some of them validated by experimental assays. As a future aspect, a data and method integration needs to be performed leading to a *consistent* set of targets independent from the data it bases on, and, at its best, being consistent with a larger set of experimental data sets and validations.

Author details

Kitiporn Plaimas[1,2] and Rainer König[3,4*]

*Address all correspondence to: rainer.koenig@uni-jena.de

1 AVIC Research Center, Department of Mathematics and Computer Science, Faculty of Science, Chulalongkorn University, Bangkok, Thailand

2 Omics Sciences and Bioinformatics Center, Faculty of Science, Chulalongkorn University, Bangkok, Thailand

3 Integrated Research and Treatment Center, Center for Sepsis Control and Care (CSCC), Jena University Hospital, Jena, Germany

4 Network Modeling, Leibniz Institute for Natural Product Research and Infection Biology — Hans Knöll Institute, Jena, Germany

References

[1] Ahn YY, et al., Metabolic network analysis-based identification of antimicrobial drug targets in category A bioterrorism agents. PLoS One, 2014. **9**(1): p. e8519.

[2] Peng Q, Schork NJ, Utility of network integrity methods in therapeutic target identification. Front Genet, 2014. **5**: p. 12.

[3] Acencio ML, Lemke N, Towards the prediction of essential genes by integration of network topology, cellular localization and biological process information. BMC Bioinformatics, 2009. **10**: p. 290.

[4] Luscombe NM, et al., Genomic analysis of regulatory network dynamics reveals large topological changes. Nature, 2004. **431**(7006): pp. 308–312.

[5] König R, Eils R, Gene expression analysis on biochemical networks using the Potts spin model. Bioinformatics, 2004. **20**(10): pp. 1500–1505.

[6] Barabasi AL, Oltvai ZN, Network biology: understanding the cell's functional organization. Nat Rev Genet, 2004. **5**(2): pp. 101–113.

[7] Karp PD, et al., Expansion of the BioCyc collection of pathway/genome databases to 160 genomes. Nucleic Acids Res, 2005. **33**(19): pp. 6083–6089.

[8] Ginsburg H, Progress in in silico functional genomics: the malaria metabolic pathways database. Trends Parasitol, 2006. **22**(6): pp. 238–240.

[9] Huthmacher C, et al., Antimalarial drug targets in Plasmodium falciparum predicted by stage-specific metabolic network analysis. BMC Syst Biol, 2010. **4**: p. 120.

[10] Gursoy A, Keskin O, Nussinov R, Topological properties of protein interaction networks from a structural perspective. Biochem Soc Trans, 2008. **36**(Pt 6): pp. 1398–1403.

[11] Swann J, et al., Systems analysis of host-parasite interactions. Wiley Interdiscip Rev Syst Biol Med, 2015. **7**(6): pp. 381–400.

[12] Bhattacharyya M, Chakrabarti S, Identification of important interacting proteins (IIPs) in *Plasmodium falciparum* using large-scale interaction network analysis and in-silico knockout studies. Malar J, 2015. **14**: p. 70.

[13] Fatumo S, et al., Comparing metabolic network models based on genomic and automatically inferred enzyme information from Plasmodium and its human host to define drug targets in silico. Infect Genet Evol, 2011. **11**(4): pp. 708–715.

[14] Barabasi AL, Albert R, Emergence of scaling in random networks. Science, 1999. **286** (5439): pp. 509–512.

[15] Almaas E, Biological impacts and context of network theory. J Exp Biol, 2007. **210**(9): pp. 1548–1558.

[16] Milgram S, Small-world problem. Psychol Today, 1967. **1**(1): pp. 61–67.

[17] Zhu X, Gerstein M, and Snyder M, Getting connected: analysis and principles of biological networks. Genes Dev, 2007. **21**(9): pp. 1010–1024.

[18] Albert R, Jeong H, and Barabasi AL, Error and attack tolerance of complex networks. Nature, 2000. **406**(6794): pp. 378–382.

[19] Wagner A, Fell DA, The small world inside large metabolic networks. Proc Biol Sci, 2001. **268**(1478): pp. 1803–1810.

[20] Zur H, Ruppin E, and Shlomi T, iMAT: an integrative metabolic analysis tool. Bioinformatics, 2010. **26**(24): pp. 3140–3142.

[21] Estrada E, Protein bipartivity and essentiality in the yeast protein-protein interaction network. J Proteome Res, 2006. **5**(9): pp. 2177–2184.

[22] Samal A, et al., Low degree metabolites explain essential reactions and enhance modularity in biological networks. BMC Bioinformatics, 2006. **7**: p. 118.

[23] Rahman SA, Schomburg D, Observing local and global properties of metabolic pathways: 'load points' and 'choke points' in the metabolic networks. Bioinformatics, 2006. **22**(14): pp. 1767–1774.

[24] Yeh I, et al., Computational analysis of *Plasmodium falciparum* metabolism: organizing genomic information to facilitate drug discovery. Genome Res, 2004. **14**(5): pp. 917–924.

[25] Bonday ZQ, et al., Import of host delta-aminolevulinate dehydratase into the malarial parasite: identification of a new drug target. Nat Med, 2000. **6**(8): pp. 898–903.

[26] Fatumo S, et al., Estimating novel potential drug targets of *Plasmodium falciparum* by analysing the metabolic network of knock-out strains in silico. Infect Genet Evol, 2009. **9**(3): pp. 351–358.

[27] Moritz E, et al., The efficacy of inhibitors involved in spermidine metabolism in *Plasmodium falciparum, Anopheles stephensi* and *Trypanosoma evansi*. Parasitol Res, 2004. **94**(1): pp. 37–48.

[28] Suthram S, Sittler T, Ideker T, The Plasmodium protein network diverges from those of other eukaryotes. Nature, 2005. **438**(7064): pp. 108–112.

[29] Kelley BP, et al., PathBLAST: a tool for alignment of protein interaction networks. Nucleic Acids Res, 2004. **32**(Web Server issue): pp. W83–W88.

[30] Scheibel LW, et al., Calcium and calmodulin antagonists inhibit human malaria parasites (*Plasmodium falciparum*): implications for drug design. Proc Natl Acad Sci U S A, 1987. **84**(20): pp. 7310–7314.

[31] Sanchez CP, et al., Evidence for a substrate specific and inhibitable drug efflux system in chloroquine resistant *Plasmodium falciparum* strains. Biochemistry, 2004. **43**(51): pp. 16365–16373.

[32] Hoppe HC, et al., Antimalarial quinolines and artemisinin inhibit endocytosis in Plasmodium falciparum. Antimicrob Agents Chemother, 2004. **48**(7): pp. 2370–2378.

[33] Chen Y, Xu R, Network-based gene prediction for *Plasmodium falciparum* malaria towards genetics-based drug discovery. BMC Genomics, 2015. **16**(Suppl 7): p. S9.

[34] Orth JD, Thiele I, Palsson BO, What is flux balance analysis? Nat Biotechnol, 2010. **28**(3): pp. 245–248.

[35] Phaiphinit S, et al., In silico multiple-targets identification for heme detoxification in the human malaria parasite *Plasmodium falciparum*. Infect Genet Evol, 2016. **37**: pp. 237–244.

[36] Plata G, et al., Reconstruction and flux-balance analysis of the *Plasmodium falciparum* metabolic network. Mol Syst Biol, 2010. **6**: p 408.

[37] Plaimas K, Computational Analysis of the Metabolic Network of Microorganisms to Detect Potential Drug Targets, Doctoral thesis, Heidelberg University, 2011.

[38] Dholakia N, Dhandhukia P, Roy N, Screening of potential targets in *Plasmodium falciparum* using stage-specific metabolic network analysis. Mol Divers, 2015. **19**(4): pp. 991–1002.

[39] Shlomi T, et al., Network-based prediction of human tissue-specific metabolism. Nat Biotechnol, 2008. **26**(9): pp. 1003–1110.

[40] Magni G, et al., NAD(P) biosynthesis enzymes as potential targets for selective drug design. Curr Med Chem, 2009. **16**(11): pp. 1372–1390.

[41] Sorci L, et al., Targeting NAD biosynthesis in bacterial pathogens: structure-based development of inhibitors of nicotinate mononucleotide adenylyltransferase NadD. Chem Biol, 2009. **16**(8): pp. 849–861.

[42] Li Z, Wang RS, Zhang XS, Two-stage flux balance analysis of metabolic networks for drug target identification. BMC Syst Biol, 2011. **5**(Suppl 1): p. S11.

[43] Mauritz JM, et al., The homeostasis of *Plasmodium falciparum*-infected red blood cells. PLoS Comput Biol, 2009. **5**(4): p. e1000339.

[44] Wiback SJ, Palsson BO, Extreme pathway analysis of human red blood cell metabolism. Biophys J, 2002. **83**(2): pp. 808–818.

[45] Quashie NB, Ranford-Cartwright LC, de Koning HP, Uptake of purines in *Plasmodium falciparum*-infected human erythrocytes is mostly mediated by the human equilibrative nucleoside transporter and the human facilitative nucleobase transporter. Malar J, 2010. **9**: p. 36.

[46] Plaimas K, et al., Computational and experimental analysis identified 6-diazo-5-oxonorleucine as a potential agent for treating infection by *Plasmodium falciparum*. Infect Genet Evol, 2013. **20**: pp. 389–395.

[47] Schomburg I, Chang A, Placzek S, Sohngen C, Rother M, Lang M, Munaretto C, Ulas S, Stelzer M, Grote A, et al., BRENDA in 2013: integrated reactions, kinetic data, enzyme function data, improved disease classification: new options and contents in BRENDA. Nucleic Acids Res, 2013. **41**(Database issue): pp. D764–D772.

[48] Wishart DS, Knox C, Guo AC, Cheng D, Shrivastava S, Tzur D, Gautam B, Hassanali M, DrugBank: a knowledgebase for drugs, drug actions and drug targets. Nucleic Acids Res. 2008. **36**(Database issue): pp. D901–D906.

[49] Jahn D, Kim YC, Ishino Y, Chen MW, Soll D. Purification and functional characterization of the Glu–tRNA(Gln) amidotransferase from Chlamydomonas reinhardtii. J Biol Chem, 1990. **265**: pp. 8059–8064.

9

The Next Vaccine Generation Against Malaria: Structurally Modulated *Plasmodium* Antigens

José Manuel Lozano Moreno

Abstract

Challenges for obtaining more effective malaria vaccines depend on precise selection of antigenic motifs and understanding the complexity of *Plasmodium* spp. life cycle. Naturally expressed antigens are characterized for being weak immunogenic when tested as vaccine components, thus these have to be strategically modified to render them immunogenic. A molecular clue in this pursuit is provided by the chemical peptide-bond processing by peptidases, which follows a multistep pathway including ephemeral high energy molecular complexes known as transition states. Thus, we have proposed non-natural peptide-bond isosteres as transition states mimetics, and therefore, stabilizing these high-energy states with site-directed designed immuno-mimetics have demonstrated being a rational approach for stimulating antibody populations harboring multiple functional capacities. Therefore, peptide-bond substitutes constitute a coherent pathway towards obtaining selected immuno-active compounds from specific plasmodial molecular objectives. Chemical strategies for synthesizing peptido-mimetics and antimalarial selected trials lead us to assess a number of peptide-bond substitutes for obtaining immuno-active and structurally defined molecules. *Plasmodium* antigens expressed on merozoite, sporozoite and gametocyte stages have been selected as targets and subsequently modified based on the presence of either a high-binding motif or a potential HLA-reading frame. This new family of immuno-mimetics is and efficient neutralizing antibody inducers when tested in *in vitro* and *in vivo* experiments, thus representing a new generation of malaria vaccine components.

Keywords: malaria, synthetic vaccine, non-natural elements, immuno-mimetic, functional antibody

1. Introduction

Malaria is spreading from old *Plasmodium* colonized territories to other zones of the earth where this lethal disease did not exist before covering about 45% of the planet. Over decades an important number of public health trials for malaria eradication and control have been conducted with a limited success. Malaria is caused by *Plasmodium* spp. to a susceptible human being and is transmitted by the *Anopheles* female mosquito bite and is responsible of 660,000 deaths and around 219 million new cases annually (a range of 154–289 million) especially in children younger than 5 years of age and pregnant women inhabitants of endemic and high transmission areas [1–3].

A number of difficulties inherent to many causes among the pathogen resistance to antimalarials, poor coverage of public health programs and natural human host genetic restrictions make the finding of an effective malaria vaccine be an urgent need.

Malaria vaccine development has constituted a big challenge for researchers, up-to-date about 236 vaccine candidate prototypes are being tested. Approaches based on strategies such as immunization with irradiated sporozoites of *Plasmodium* spp., as well as DNA-based immunogens besides recombinantly expressed antigens such as RTS,S formulated in different vehicles and strong adjuvant systems and prototype delivery systems such as virosomes besides to the most promising strategy constituted by synthetic peptides representing subunit multistage immunogens formulated in human allowed adjuvants represent the main attempts for immuno-prophylaxis [2].

Plasmodium spp. express a number of antigens, more than 100 in its different life cycle stages and most of them have been regarded as vaccine targets such as the so-named merozoite surface antigens 1–10 (MSP1–MSP10), erythrocyte binding antigens EBA-140 and EBA-175, the ring-infected erythrocyte surface antigen (RESA-155), the apical membrane antigen AMA-1 among many others from the merozoite stage including a number of organelle's proteins. Besides the circumsporozoite surface protein (CSP), sporozoite threonine and asparagine-rich protein (STARP), the sporozoite and liver stage antigen (SALSA), the liver stage antigen (LSA) are some representative antigens of the sporozoite stage and the classical Pfs48/45, GSA and Pbs25/28 from gametocytes have been regarded as the targets for transmission blocking vaccines [4].

Natural immunity to malaria is related to hemoglobin structure, some disorders such as thalassemia confer resistance to *Plasmodium falciparum* while Duffy negative RBC constitutes the mechanisms associated to malaria resistance to *Plasmodium vivax*. Immune response against a natural malaria infection is nonspecific and has a weak effect on protection. Innate immunity mediated by NK and non-related auto antibody B-cells as well as the INF-gamma response to infected red blood cells act as a primary line of defense against *Plasmodium* infection. In the adaptative immunity step CD4+, dendritic cells, macrophages, gamma delta T cells and NKT cells are able to detect the parasite and participate in the immune defense. Besides natural immunity to this disease, an effective malaria vaccine can be proposed for a strong stimulation of antibody B-cells. However, at is has been demonstrated that most *Plasmodium* native-derived sequences are proven to be poorly immunogenic and non-protection inducers against malaria. In order to understand this problem, Patarroyo have established a strategy based on selection of non-polymorphic regions of selected antigens and a subsequent rational mutation of those residues belonging to red blood cells and hepatic cells binding motifs allow modified active antigens [4], however, most clinical trials worldwide which have been performed with the above mentioned malaria vaccine candidates have failed to achieve significant protection levels, evidencing intrinsic difficulties for developing a potent fully protective vaccine formulation. Perhaps pathogens including *Plasmodium* spp. have evolved complex mechanisms to recognize, block and destroy natural-presented antigens as vaccines as well as others related to antigen structure modulation.

Our group has introduced in this pursuit some non-natural elements to be incorporated into synthetic antigens with the aim of governing both antigen presentation as well as specific B-cells for functional neutralizing antibody stimulation. Some of these non-natural elements included capture sequences for stimulating antigen degradation and others for the peptide-bond structure modulation. Peptide-bond isosteres included reversal configuration thereof, urea motifs and reduced amide as peptide-bond surrogates all constituting a novel immunogen family herein named as immuno-mimetics.

Once strategically incorporated into selected antigens, produced peptide-bond surrogates overcome non-desirable properties of native non-modified antigens such as cytotoxicity and hemolytic profiles, besides prolonging these new molecules half-life and a remarkably strong immuno-stimulating activity that can be associated to the newly introduced freedom degrees to the 3D structure of immuno-mimetics.

Also, we have consolidated the female BALB/c animal model for malaria vaccine candidate testing based on controlled challenging performed to immunized animals with two rodent malaria strains, being those *Plasmodium berghei ANKA* and *Plasmodium yoelii*-17XL. Additionally, passive transferring antibodies into infected animals have proven to be efficient for malaria disease control and parasite clearance.

2. Global health statistics, economical and environment determinants

In 2015, time for fulfillment of the millennium development goals (MDGs) was getting closer to the end, and a consequent protocol comprising 17 sustainable development goals (SDGs) constitute the next step. In its annual report, World Health Organization (WHO) analyzed 15 years of advances of those proposed MDG and evaluated the next challenges for the coming years.

As reported in world health statistics 2015 issued by the WHO [1], undernutrition was the main cause of mortality in an assessed 45% of all deaths of children under 5 years of age. In the 1990–2013 period, the estimate of underweight children in third-world countries decreased from 28 to 17%, and a sustainable decreasing rate to 16% was expected for the end of 2015. In spite of those proposed efforts for achievement of MDG, these numbers are not still sufficient to the goals. The proportion of underweight children declined globally from 25% in 1990 to 15% in 2013.

Worryingly, poverty is strongly associated with public health especially to problems related to high transmission of infectious diseases. As observed in **Figure 1A**, among the main causes of deaths among children under 5 years (in neonatal and post-neonatal ages), between 2000 and 2013 are responsibility of infectious diseases, pneumonia, malaria, HIV/AIDS, measles, diarrhea and sepsis are the main reasons of mortality accounting 13 and 35%, respectively. Malaria represents 7% of children mortality mainly in the post-neonatal period between 1 and 59 months of age.

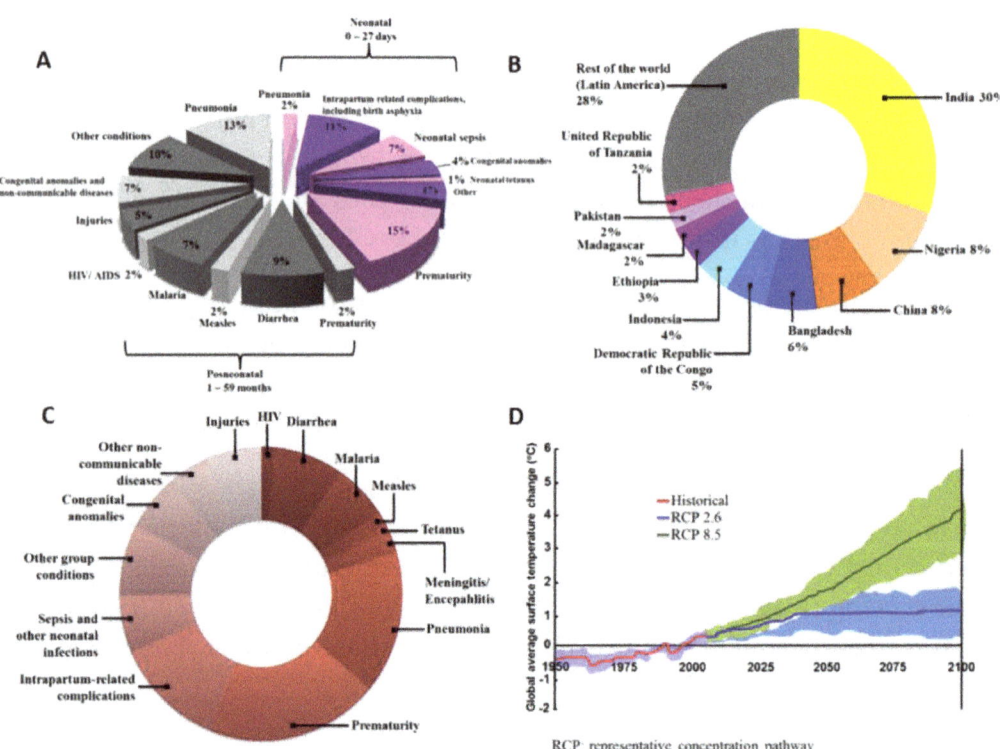

Figure 1. Health statistics and world climate. (A) Causes of deaths among children under 5 years of age. (B) Top 10 countries with largest share of the global extreme poverty. (C) Main causes of child mortality due to transmissible diseases. 5.9 million children under age five died in 2015, nearly 16,000 every day. (D) Climate changes and greenhouse effect. Global average surface temperature changes under two scenarios for considering the global greenhouse gas emissions between years 1950 and 2100. RCP for representative concentration pathway. This figure has been adapted from information provided by WHO [1–3].

In the last year, 836 million of the world population lived on less than US$1.25 daily in comparison with 1.9 billion in 1990. In those the so-named poor countries, 14% of the people lived on less than US$1.25 daily in the same year, regarding the 47% in 1990. Getting closer to an amount of US$2 daily has been difficult at higher poverty levels.

The most inhabited counties of the world such as People's Republic of China and India have been crucial for world reduction in poverty (indeed India remains the earth's country having most extreme poverty; **Figure 1B**) such reduction can be associated to growth of central economic sectors and labors. Other factors such as income transferring, remittances and evolving new demographic profiles have had a lesser impact. However, those efforts have not been enough since one of each seven people in poor countries live on less than US$1.25 daily. In the sub-Saharan countries, more than 40% people are living in extreme poverty in 2015. In the countries having middle-incomes, the 73% of the Earth's poverty is found [3].

Figure 1B displays the top 10 countries with largest share of the global extreme poor, accordingly with WHO classifications, these countries are inhabited by people living on less than US $1.25 per day. Therefore, poverty levels show India 30%, Latin America 28%, China 8% and dramatically 20% represents African countries (Nigeria, Democratic Republic of the Congo, Ethiopia, United Republic of Tanzania, among others). Child mortality was 5.9 million children under age five which died in 2015, nearly 16,000 per day, mainly caused by infectious diseases whose distribution can be observed in **Figure 1C**. Main causes of child death are due to measles, malaria, diarrhea, HIV/AIDS, meningitis/encephalitis, tetanus and sepsis and other neonatal infections besides prematurity among other causes [1–3].

The sustainable development goals (SDGs) also contain ambitious targets for child mortality, with SDG 3.2 seeking to end preventable deaths of newborns and children under five. Those have included local aims for reducing the under-five mortality rates (U5MR) around to 25 deaths per 1000 live births as well as the neonatal mortality rate (NMR) to lower than 12 per 1000 live births, in comparison with a world's U5MR rate of 43 per 1000 live births in the last year, representing 5.9 million deaths of children under 5 years and a NMR rate of 19 per 1000 live births, representing 2.7 million deaths in the first month of life. Main causes of newborn mortality during the last year were prematurity, birth-related complications and neonatal sepsis, while those post-neonatal causes of death were associated to pneumonia, diarrhea, injuries and malaria. Specifically, the so-called Target 4.2 in the document, which encourage for assuring that most children have access to good quality development, heath assistance and care, and basic education join to reducing child mortality while improving a better living quality for childhood in most poor countries [3].

On the other hand, **Figure 1D** displays climate changes and greenhouse effect on earth for a period between 1950 projected to the wear 2100. As described, global average surface temperature change is estimated under two scenarios for turning around global greenhouse gas emissions [1].

The global climate warming is a reality. The average data for the Earth's surface temperature showed a 0.85°C increasing (0.65–1.06) for the 1880–2012 period. Data show that the Earth's north hemisphere had the warmest period from 1983 to 2013, being the highest regarding the last 1400 years. Without any doubt, most causes for this fact can be associated to human activities. Mathematical and predictive algorithms for global warming-cooling allow establishing precise predictions on climate changes over long-time periods, these have included factors such as volcanic activity and gas emissions to the atmosphere. The Intergovernmental Panel on Climate Change's (IPCC) for temperature changing prediction have considered a number of factors and possibilities for future greenhouse gas emissions, which have been termed as representative concentration pathways (RCP). This ranges from RPC 2.6 which considers that global greenhouse gas emissions will reach a highest value between 2010 and

2020, then it significantly decrease after 2020, to RCP 8.5, in which greenhouse gas emissions will continue to increase during the present century. Middle-range positions consider that RCP 4.5 and 6.0 would reach the highest emission values in 2040 and 2080 in consequence [1].

World's predictive temperature changes for 2015–2016 period regarding those recorded between 1986 and 2005 are estimated to vary between 0.3 and 0.7°C. Similarly, increasing temperature ranges for the 2081–2100 period regarding the recorded changes between 1986 and 2005 has been estimated to be 0.3–1.7°C (RCP 2.6) to 2.6–4.8°C (RCP 8.5) (**Figure 1D**). In consequence, the Arctic region's warming rate will increase faster than the world's mean, and that for the land's rate will be higher than the mean for the ocean. Assessed RPCs led to estimate that sea level will growth from 0.26 to 0.82 m by the final of the current age. Earth's surface warming and climate variations will have a deep impact on human living, health and welfare, since obtaining drinking water and the possibility of cultivating the necessary quantities of agricultural products and all resources required for the future world's larger population will be compromised.

3. Malaria: a devastating disease

Malaria is a global disease responsibly of high levels of morbidity and mortality especially in developing countries whose inhabitant populations suffer the consequences of the disease besides the economic impact on these populations. At the beginning of the new millennium, a global strategy for controlling malaria by establishing a global founding for fighting three high impact diseases, i.e., AIDS, tuberculosis and malaria have been proposed by the World Health Organization (WHO) [5]. The 2015 world malaria report from WHO account data from 79 countries affected by this disease reflecting a slight improvement in controlling the disease impact but the problem still remains for a solution. In 2013, diagnosis tests were expanded to most malaria affecting countries and huge steps towards vector control were also conducted. In 2013, the use of insecticides impregnated mosquito nets were promoted and so the amount of populations protected against malaria were increased, thus mortality due to malaria was reduced to 47% between the years 2000 and 2013. However, endemic areas are still far away from reaching a total coverage for malaria control and available founding is each time decreased for managing this important problem. An estimated 278 million people in Africa live in households without a single insecticide mosquito net and 15 million pregnant women have no access to a preventive treatment for malaria. In addition, other diseases affecting these populations alter the development of related campaigns is the case of Ebola whose recent outbreak have conducted to a decreasing in health assistance in those affected zones.

In the last five years, it is estimated that 584,000 deaths due to malaria have occurred (367,000–755,000) of which 78% were children under 5 years of age and 90% came from Africa; today, there are an estimated 3.2 billion people at risk of contracting the disease since are living in areas influenced by the disease, of which 1.2 billion are at high risk (more than 1 into 1000 possibility of acquiring malaria in the year); in the Region of the Americas, it is presumed that the risk is 120 million people in 21 countries in the region [5].

Eradication efforts by public health preventive measures are not sufficiently effective for many reasons, among which are the socioeconomic, demographic and technical policies, emerging resistance to insecticides by the vector and to antimalarial drugs by the parasite [6]. In 2010, vector resistance had been reported in 49 countries around the world of which 39 reported resistance above two or more pyrethroid insecticides. In 2013, this report increased to 82 countries reporting insecticide resistance [3], therefore, to develop an effective vaccine against the disease becomes an urgent need.

By 1967, major efforts were made to find an effective vaccine against human malaria, in one of the most important related studies of the time, 59% protection was achieved after an intravenous challenge of a malaria murine model after being vaccinated with 75,000 live attenuated irradiated sporozoites [7].

Currently among vaccine candidates that are in more advanced clinical trials are the RTS,S and *Pf*SPZ which incorporates the use of non-replicative attenuated sporozoites through controlled radiation [8], which has obtained a dose dependent protection in humans being necessary the application of 1.35×10^5 attenuated sporozoites in five doses [9]. It should be noted that the duration of protective antibodies has not been fully established, thus obtaining a vaccine is not a reality.

As can be observed in **Figure 2**, global malaria spreading accounts for more than 80 countries that are affected by malaria infection (purple background in the map). Besides, insecticide susceptibility status for malaria vectors (*Anopheles* female mosquitoes) demonstrates a resistance increasing to most insecticides concomitant with areas of high transmission of malaria.

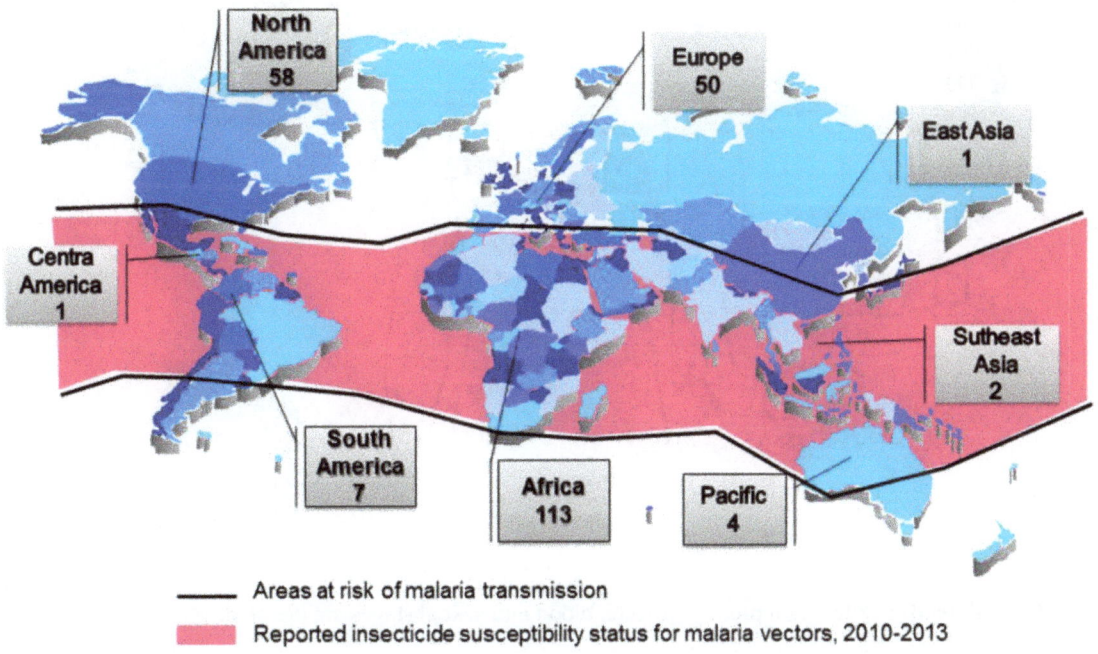

Figure 2. Areas of risk of malaria transmission and ongoing malaria vaccine candidate trials.

4. *Plasmodium* spp. life cycle

A deep knowledge and understanding of the *Plasmodium* parasite life cycle would be a key step towards antigen discovery, and it will establish the molecular basis for a proper immunogen designing to be further tested as a vaccine candidate. The *Plasmodium* spp. belong to the phylum Apicomplexa being the causative agent of malaria, whose clinical and pathological manifestations are associated with asexual erythrocytic stage of the parasite [10].

There are five species of *Plasmodium* causing human malaria, the most lethal disease is caused by *P. falciparum* and followed by *P. vivax*, and less prevalent are *Plasmodium malariae* and *Plasmodium ovale* [11] in 2011 *Plasmodium knowlesi* was included in this list. In Colombia for the year 2014, 356 clinical cases of uncomplicated malaria were reported, 20,074 cases of malaria by *P. vivax*, 19,789 by *P. falciparum*, 17 cases by *P. malariae* and 561 cases of mixed malaria according to data presented by the National Institute of Health (INS) in its weekly report SIVIGILA [12].

Plasmodium parasites have a complex life cycle involving interactions of invertebrates (vector) and vertebrates (mammalian host), besides presenting various stages in intracellular and extracellular environments (**Figure 3**) [13].

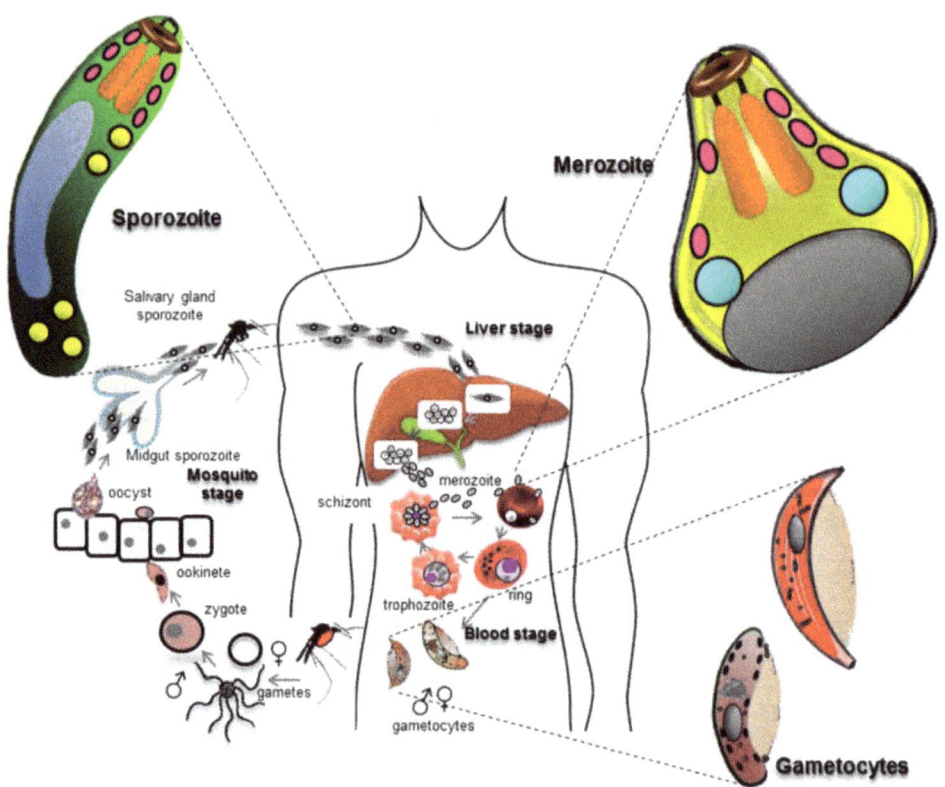

Figure 3. *Plasmodium* **life cycle**. Main pre-erythrocyte, blood and sexual stages are denoted.

In the human host, sporozoites are inoculated by the bite of female *Anopheles* spp. mosquitoes, then invade hepatocytes in a time between 5 and 30 min; within hepatocytes each sporozoite develops a schizont which release between 10,000 ± 30,000 merozoites to blood stream during a period of 2 ± 10 days depending on the parasite specie [14], in the case of *P. vivax* and *P. ovale* also it produces a different stage in the liver called hypnozoite, which is a silent form responsible for the subsequent relapses [11]. During the travel from the skin to the liver, the parasites cross the capillary epithelium in the dermis and enter to blood circulation, cross the hepatic sinusoids epithelium to enter the parenchyma, and this process as the hepatocyte infection are given by activity of the myosin-actin engine located in the plasma membrane of the parasite and its rhoptries, dense granules and micronemes [15].

The invasion of erythrocytes occurs after several steps with multiple interactions between receptor membrane proteins of host cells and parasite protein ligands expressed in its surface as well as in rhoptries and micronemes [16]. The parasite grows and divides in about 72–48 h according to the specie to the schizont stage which contains more than 30 merozoite particles, which are released with the subsequent invasion and replication in healthy erythrocytes [17]. Acquired immune response induced by malaria parasites is complex and varies depending on the level of endemicity, epidemiology, genetic, age of the host, parasitic stage and parasite species. Repeated infections and continued exposure are required to achieve clinical immunity with symptom reduction and reduced number of parasites in an infected individual or inhibition of parasite replication [18].

5. The murine model in the search for vaccine candidates against malaria

The mouse model has been widely used in the study on malaria, and it has been regarded as a practical model for experimental studies since its genetical features regarding human beings such as homology and similarity at the protein structure level, physiology and life cycle besides of owning a malaria transmission vector (*Anopheles stephensi*) that can be maintained under defined laboratory [19].

Due to this, there are several *Plasmodium* strains that infect rodent models by malaria (*P. berghei, P. yoelii, P. chabaudi, P. vincker*), and their experimental behavior can be extrapolated due to the fulfillment of a standard life cycle under controlled conditions. The two most commonly employed strains in malaria vaccine discovery are the *P. yoelii* and *P. berghei*, which have high similarity with the clinical symptoms and pathology developed by *P. falciparum* in relation to those stages of cerebral malaria, placental malaria, severe malaria and organ damage as liver, kidney and lung [20]. The *P. berghei* infection model has allowed demonstrating the role of interferon in response to parasite replication in the liver, and this participation was then demonstrated in *P. falciparum* [20].

The rodent malaria infection by *P. yoelii* has allowed to demonstrate that humans immunized with the *Pf*CS protein from the parasite sporozoite stage, induced antibodies that cross-react with *P. yoelii*, as well as mice immunized with *Py*CSP stimulated antibodies that cross-react with *P. falciparum*; therefore, this model evidenced its usefulness as a predictive tool for immune response against certain malarial antigens since there are a 70% of genome similarity between *P. yoelii and P. falciparum* [14]. This similarity associate at least 3300 orthologous genes of *P. yoelii* with 5268 genes of *P. falciparum* [21]. Although the erythrocytic cycle of *P. berghei* and *P. yoelii* takes place more rapidly (24 and 18 h, respectively) compared to those developed in *P. falciparum* (36–48 h) and *P. vivax* (48 h), differences in tropism for invasion of reticulocytes in the case of *P. yoelii* and *P. berghei* are not presented in *P. falciparum* and the genetic similarity between these *Plasmodium* is quite important, and so the rate of increase in parasitemia levels is similar during the first 3–4 days after inoculation *in vitro* as well as the parasite growth [22]. Also, *in vivo* conditions and clinical symptoms associated to the disease are presented in terms of fever, malaise, splenomegaly and breathlessness related with red blood cells rupture which differ of symptoms present in infections with other strains such as *P. chabaudi* where in contrast the infection is associated with hypothermia [23]. The production and regulation in the cytokines expression are no exception to the similarity between the mouse model and a malaria human infection since *P. yoelii* and *P. berghei* replicate many events that can be correlated between both of the infection types [24, 25].

In studies at the level of liver infection cycle were found that about 654 (92%) of proteins in *P. yoelii* correlated with orthologous sequences present in *P. falciparum* and 66% of the genes in the *P. yoelii* transcriptome have orthologues in *P. falciparum* [26]. Also in this stage of infection, it has been possible to obtain *in vivo* images in models of infection with *P. berghei* in mice, these have shown details of hepatocyte invasion by *Plasmodium* which were not yet known in humans, as well as the fact that sporozoites can recognize heparan-sulfate proteoglycans besides that *P. yoelii* infection models have been conducted to tests the oxidative stress in the liver induced by infected erythrocytic forms [27].

Bearing in mind, the possibilities offered by murine infection models, we have conducted an important amount of experiments in order to test a variety of chemically modified antigens as potential vaccine components.

In spite of impressive economic and political efforts conducted by WHO and other non-government organizations for malaria eradication and control, based on insecticide treatment of bed-nets (mainly DTT), use of new formulations of artemisinin and other antimalarials for treatment of infected patients and teaching about an appropriate water and environment care to inhabitants of malaria high-transmission areas, among other strategies, malaria still remains as one of the most important health problems for developing countries. Contrary to those expectations, most of these strategies have failed for malaria control, mainly due to novel and powerful biological evolution of antimalarials-resistance mechanisms developed by *Plasmodium* parasites, joint to the continuous mosquito adaptation and colonization of new environments and territories, climate changing and global warming due to non-controlled gas emissions to the atmosphere. Therefore, hopes for controlling this lethal disease are based on developing more efficient preventive strategies and highly potent malaria vaccines.

Up-to-date, about 236 including chemoprophylaxis and malaria vaccines clinical trials are being conducted worldwide, most of them have been completed showing a limited success (as shown in **Figure 2**). Most conducted studies have been focused on vaccine candidates aimed to block three different potential targets, being the transmission-blocking approach the first (gametocyte-derived proteins such as Pf25 and Pf125); secondly, those candidates directed against *Plasmodium* liver-malaria stages (considering proteins such as Circumsporozoite surface protein (CSP), liver stage antigen (LSA), sporozoite and liver stage antigen (SALSA), Thrombospondin-related anonymous protein (TRAP) and others) and vaccine candidates directed against malaria blood stages (classical merozoite protein targets are Merozoite surface proteins 1-10 (MSP-1-10), apical membrane antigen-1 (AMA-1), ring-infected erythrocyte surface antigen (RESA-155), serine repeat antigen (SERA), Erythrocyte binding antigen 175 (EBA-175) among others).

As recently mentioned by Birkett in 2015, the European Medicines Agency announced a positive opinion for the malaria vaccine candidate most advanced in development, RTS,S/AS01, which provides modest protection against clinical malaria in all conducted trials, but in spite of its poor efficacy later in 2016, this product was recommended by WHO for large-scale trials in moderate to high malaria transmission areas [28]. As observed in **Figure 2**, 113 trials of pharmaceutical products among antimalarials and vaccine formulations are being conducted in Africa in high-transmission malaria regions by immunizing mainly with modified or attenuated sporozoite NF54 strain malarial parasites or other products such as the so-named biological *Pf*SPZ vaccine all of them formulated on strong adjuvant systems such as AS01 as can be observed in the web site ClinicalTrials.gov, a service of the U.S. National Institutes of Health [29].

Due to the moderate success conducted in the last three decades of researching for finding highly potent vaccines for preventing malaria, the field is open for new ideas regarding the discovery of strategies for developing structurally modulated molecular probes which address the *Plasmodium* complex molecular mechanisms involved in parasite detection, facing the challenge of demonstrating protective efficacy profiles and parasite clearance capacity, so those would enter the pathway of being regarded as components of novel vaccine formulations.

6. Current status of *P. vivax* vaccine progress

Morbidity to malaria outside of the sub-Saharan Africa still remains meaningful causing more than 50% of malaria cases, especially in the Americas and Pacific-Asia where poverty and public health systems are associate to multiple problems. The complex *P. vivax* biology and its ability to differentiate into latent forms called hypnozoites which appear longtime later to produce erythrocyte infective forms, prompt occurrence of macro and micro gametes previous to clinical manifestations are seeming, and thus a short evolution cycle into the mosquito makes useless using standard tools to control *P. vivax*. Simultaneously to decreasing in global incidence, some dramatic changes in pathogen infective species have been reported by *P. vivax* being currently the prevalent *Plasmodium* spp. in those mentioned world regions.

For multiple reasons, the epidemiologic spreading of malaria due to *P. vivax* is being regarded as careless. However, turning on attention to malaria caused by *P. vivax* has to be a priority when thinking in a vaccine against malaria. Most approaches for a *P. vivax* malaria vaccine candidate have considered orthologous sequences among the most predominant *Plasmodium* species as being *P. falciparum* and *P. vivax* especially antigens of both pre-erythrocyte and erythrocyte stages. Among a number of vaccine candidates, the VMP001/AS01 targets the CSP antigen of *P. vivax*. This has been assessed in controlled human malaria infection (CHMI) studies but proven to be unsuccessful with poor protection capacity. Another candidate, which is a recombinantly expressed on appropriate virus, targets the TRAP antigen and currently is currently in study and another prototype vaccine candidate is based on using the strategy of attenuated sporozoites.

On the other hand, the most focused *P. vivax* erythrocyte-stage antigen is the Duffy binding protein (DBP), which is considered crucial for red blood cell (RBC) invasion; however, the DBP non-conserved character establishes an important hindrance. Importantly, time of protection against malaria would be more relevant for a *P. vivax* vaccine regarding a *P. falciparum* vaccine due to *P. vivax* disease incidence is not focused in given populations as it is for *P. falciparum*. Hepatic *P. vivax*-stages also contribute to reinforce this problem complexity [30, 31].

Therefore, developing potent *P. vivax* vaccines would depend on several key aspects among establishing a continuous *P. vivax*—culture in enriched reticulocyte media or specific growth factors aimed to reproducing parasite infections, also appropriate animal models for vaccine candidate testing and most importantly the right selection of multi antigen formulations in human adjuvants and delivery systems, thus peptido-mimetics would play a role in this pursuit.

7. The meaning of being non-visible to α/β-TCR of T lymphocytes

It is well known the fact that the T-cell receptor sees antigen on the surface of cells associated with an MHC class I or II molecule. Therefore, activating humoral and cell-mediated immune responses requires factors such as cytokines and costimulatory molecules expressed by Th cells. A fine and specific regulation of Th has to be highly regulated in order to avoid any self-reactivity would conduct to auto-immune disorders. In order to ensure the Th-cells activation and regulation, these have to recognize a given antigen that is being presented in the MHC class-II context which is located on an antigen presenting cell (APC) surface. As it is known, these professional presenting cells among macrophages, dendritic cells and B lymphocytes harbor two relevant features: (1) surface expression of class-II (MHC-II) molecules, and (2) recruitment of costimulatory molecules as signals for activation of Th-cells.

Antigen-presenting cells first internalize antigen, and then display a part of that antigen on their membrane bound to a MHC-II molecule. The TH cell recognizes and interacts with the antigen–MHC-II molecule complex on the membrane of the antigen-presenting cell. Immune system is prepared for antigen presentation by stabilizing MHC-II molecules in the endoplasmic reticulum bound to an endogen invariant Ii chain which is later cleaved to a small peptide called class II-associated invariant chain peptide (CLIP) which remains bound to the MHC-II molecule to be then replaced by a given antigen-peptide assisted by a chaperone molecule named HLA-DM in endosomal compartments. Therefore, the antigen-MHC-II bimolecular complex will travel to the APC membrane surface to be presented to T-cell receptors (TCR) of

T-lymphocytes to establish and stabilize in consequence specific ternary complexes able to trigger CD4+TH cell proliferation and so an immune response.

As mentioned one of the main functions of CLIP is to prevent the binding of self-peptide fragments prior to the MHC II localization within the endosome-lysosome, a consensus primary structure of CLIP is [87]PVSKMRMATPLLMQA[101], which is able to a proper interaction with a HLA-II molecule by anchoring-specific residues to the so-named pockets 1, 3, 4 and 9 of the MHC-II molecule in such a way that its entire structure will remain buried into the HLA-II molecule. The CLIP-HLA-II (CLIP: HLA-DR3) molecular complex is shown in **Figure 4**. As observed, the endogenous peptide is hidden into the presenting HLA-II molecule, and the possibility of being recognized by any TCR is completely abolished, and so an auto-reactive immune response will not take place, thus if a given pathogen can develop immune response evasion mechanisms based on its ligands structure features, it would be desirable to its convenience to resemble the most relevant structure characteristics of CLIP to avoid be recognized by TCRs [32].

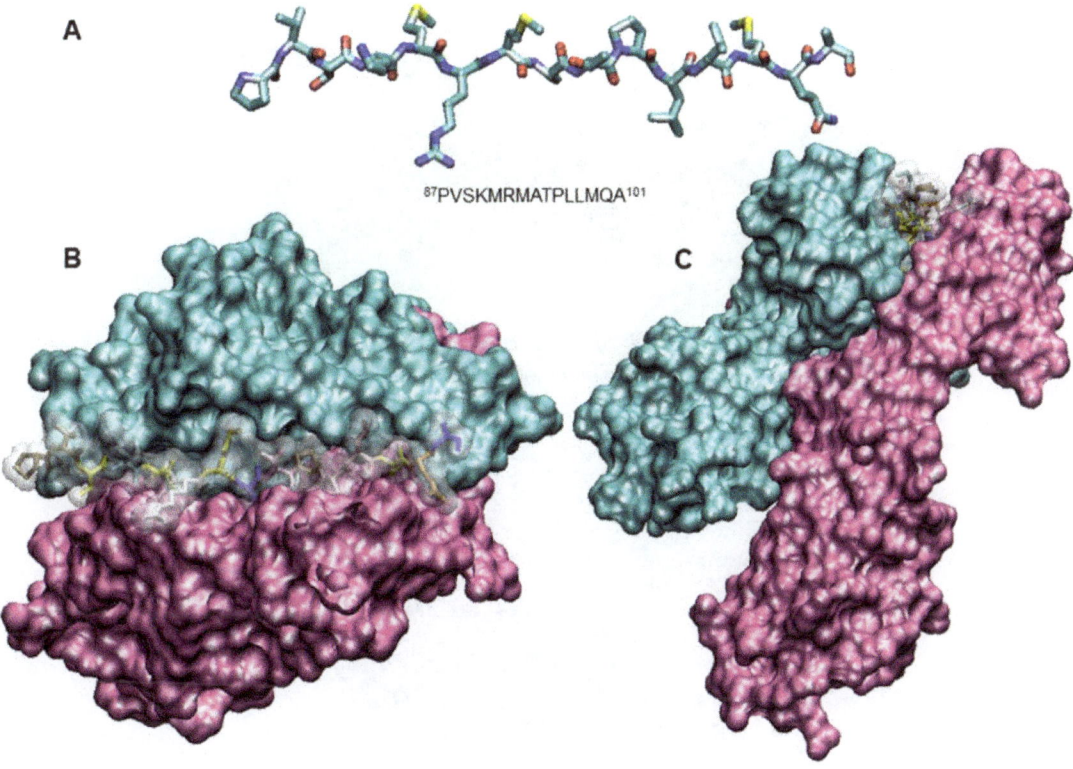

Figure 4. An endogen peptide-MHC-II bimolecular complex. The endogenous invariable Ii-chain cleaved CLIP product ([87]PVSKMRMATPLLMQA[101]) complexed to a HLA-DR3 allele. Coordinates of the CLIP-HLA-DR3 complex from the protein data bank (PDB) coded 1A6A corresponded to the structure determined by X-ray diffraction at a 2.75 Å resolution, was downloaded and molecular modeled with the visual molecular dynamics (VMD1.7ŋ) software of the University of Illinois at Urbana-Champaign. Color code representation for HLAII α-chain in purple, β-chain in cyan, HA peptide is represented in amino acid id code [32].

8. How to become recognized by a TCR-T lymphocyte

Influenza hemagglutinin (HA) or hemagglutinin is a glycoprotein found on the surface of influenza viruses. Its role is to bind the influenza viruses to their target cells through sialic acid, specifically to red blood cells and upper respiratory tract cells [33, 34]. Once the pH has been decreased, a second role of HA is to join the viral cover to formed endosomes. HA is an integral membrane glycoprotein expressed as homo-trimers which seem a barrel-like structure having around 13.5 nm in length. HA is confirmed by three monomers built into a alpha-helical core displaying spherical tips containing those sialic acid-binding motifs. HA is synthesized as monomeric units as precursor forms which are glycosylated and processed on protein maturation, to produce two shorter proteins called HA1 and HA2. The HA monomers are long helical chains attached to the cell membrane by HA2 and capped by HA1. Thus, HA has been responsible for stimulation of neutralizing antibodies which are proven to avoid influenza virus infection to its target cells, thus constituting an important molecular tool for infection control using mechanisms associated to ternary complex stabilization of HA-HLA-II α/β-TCR (CD4$^+$) with specific HLA-DR4 alleles such as DRA*0101 and DRB1*0401 [34].

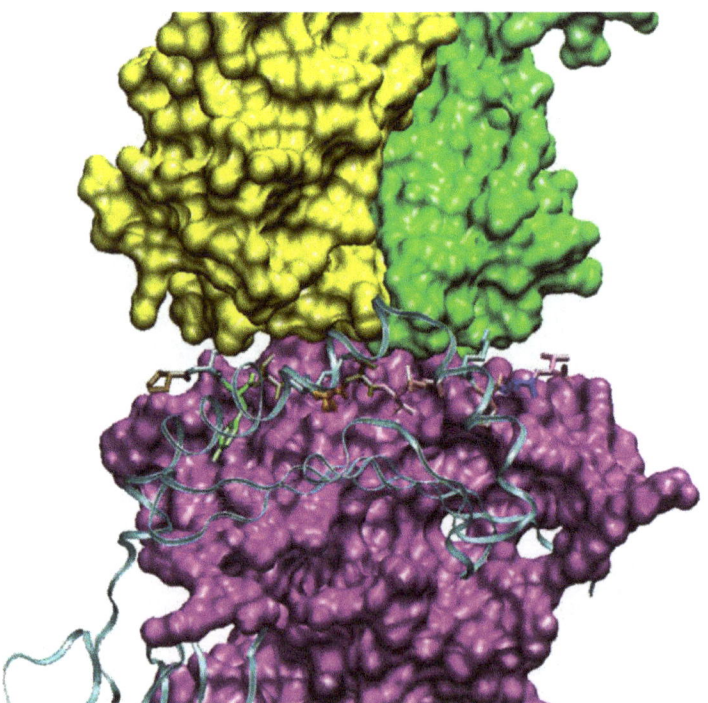

Figure 5. Reactive and T-lymphocyte proliferation upon a stabilized ternary HA-hemagglutinin-HLAII-TCR complex. Coordinates of the human T-cell receptor (TCR) HA1.7, influenza hemagglutinin peptide, and major histocompatibility complex class II molecule, HLA-DR4 (DRA*0101 and DRB1*0401) were downloaded from the protein data bank (PDB) whose code 1J8H corresponded to structure obtained by X-ray diffraction at a 2.40 Å resolution, and then was molecular modeled with the visual molecular dynamics (VMD1.7ή) software of the University of Illinois at Urbana-Champaign. Color code representation for HLAII α-chain in purple, β-chain in cyan, HA peptide is represented in amino acid id code, TCR α-chain in yellow and β-chain in green [34].

Figure 5 recreates the 3D structure of the HA-hemagglutinin-HLAII-TCR ternary complex. As observed, the HA306–318 peptide backbone whose amino acid sequence is PKYVKQNTL-KLAT anchor-specific residues into the HLA-II 1, 3, 4 and 9 pockets and clearly expose some residues in positions 5, 8 and 7 to be recognized by α/β-TCR chains and so stabilizing the molecular complex. However, the HA peptide binds promiscuously and can be presented by most of the frequently occurring DR alleles. Therefore, CD4+ T-lymphocyte proliferation would lead a subsequent neutralizing antibody production able to block the influenza virus infection, being this molecular interaction an effective mechanism effectively used for the immune response. As this a number of similar immuno-reactive complexes have been described [35–40].

9. New modified vaccine components containing non-natural elements considering chiral and topochemical constraints

Current prototype vaccines against malaria are failed to the goal of protecting any individual living in high risk malaria transmission areas even the most promising such as RTS,S which have less than 30% effectivity. As discussed above, the complex life cycle of *Plasmodium* parasites besides human genetic restrictions and immune mechanisms associated with protection makes obtaining an effective malaria vaccine a challenge. Therefore, obtaining new immunogens as vaccines and other molecular systems having potential application in malaria therapy would have to be with precisely selecting relevant antigens which would be submitted for steps of redesigning, production, formulation and *in vitro* tested before assayed in animal models; thus, after proven to be effective have to cross the border line for human clinical trials.

The aim of our research is to produce back-bone modified immunogenic antigens which included non-natural elements such as chiral and peptide-bond substitutions directed to modulate the antigen 3D structure and stimulation of neutralizing antibodies. Our approach is based on low-polymorphic sequences of *Plasmodium* which are then modified into immu-nological relevant motifs as well as strategically including lysosomal substrates to stimulate processing and presentation steps on vaccinated individuals. Therefore, we have analyzed and produced representative modified immunogens based on a number of native sequences belonging to different stages of *Plasmodium* which upon vaccination of animal models have proven to be effective against malaria infection and parasite clearance [41–43].

One of our first approaches for antigen peptide backbone modification consisted in introducing topochemical elements into the selected antigen primary structure, which consisted in two key features, first the amino acids chirality and second the peptide backbone space orientation. As represented in **Figure 6A**, the N-terminus low polymorphic region of the *Pf*MSP1[42-61] native sequence (GYSLFQKEKMVLNEGTSGTA) was the base for evaluating the above described considerations. Thus, chirality impact on immunogenic properties was tested by introducing local and global L- and D-amino acid substitutions, and the peptide backbone orientation influence was assessed by reversing the primary structure but upholding its native composi-tion. Therefore, a set of peptido-mimetic analogues were designed and synthesized and subsequently tested. As observed, the experimental group consisted in the *Pf*MSP1[42-61] native sequence, entirely made of ʟ-amino acids; its chiral D-analogue which preserved the sequence and was built with ᴅ-amino acids (represented in lowercase letters); another so-named *Retro* analogue sequence, which was constructed with ᴅ-amino acids and reversing the sequence orientation and an analogue called *Retro-inverso*, which was synthesized with ʟ-amino acids and reversing the peptide sequence orientation. Also punctual or partially D-substitutions were include in the experimental group. CD profiles for the four molecules reflected interesting spectrophotometric properties, thus when comparing the native L-sequence (black line) with its D-enantiomer (red line), their CD profiles behave as specular images of one another as displayed in **Figure 6B**. Similarly, CD profile for the L-native sequence compared with that of the **Retro-inverso** analogue (green line), behave as mirror images of each other bearing in mind that both were made with only ʟ-amino acids, but having opposite peptide backbone orientation.

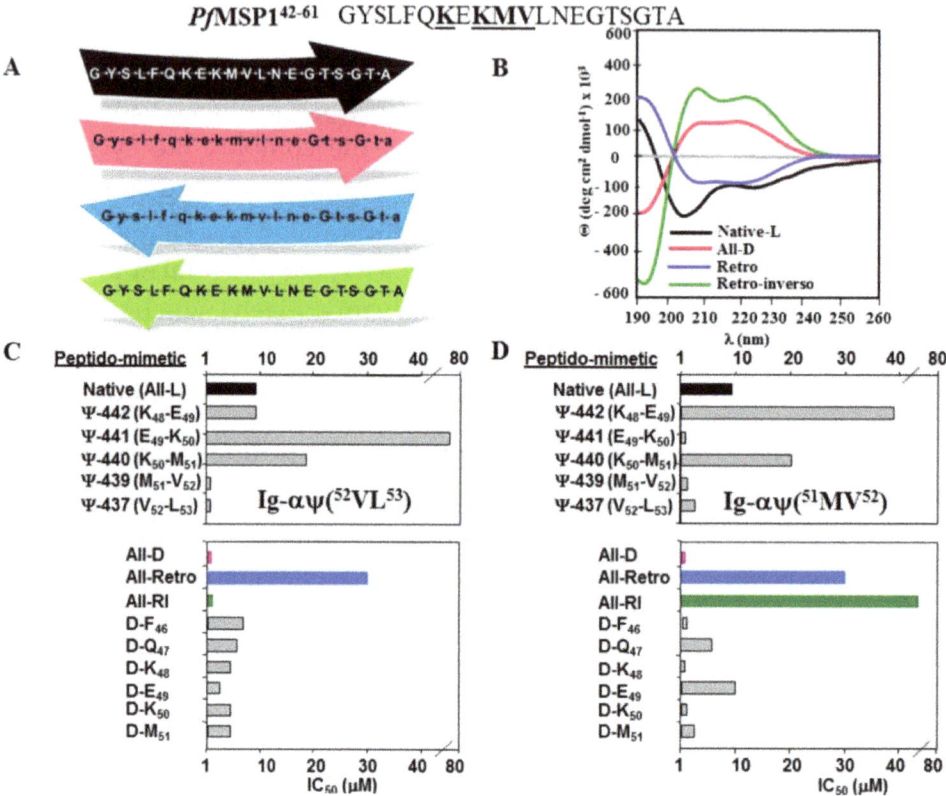

Figure 6. Chiral and topochemical peptido-mimetic designing. (A) Molecular peptido-mimetic design based on the N-terminus *Pf*MSP1⁴²⁻⁶¹ peptide. The native sequence is represented in capital letters for ʟ-amino acids, D-enantiomer represented by lowercase letters purple highlighted, Retro-sequence is constituted by ᴅ-amino acids in lowercase letters blue highlighted and the so-named Retro-inverso peptidomimetic is confirmed by ʟ-amino acids green highlighted. **(B)** Circular dichroism secondary structure patterns for *Pf*MSP1⁴²⁻⁶¹ peptido-mimetics. Used color code was black line for the native sequence, purple for its D-enantiomer, blue line for the Retro-analogue and green line for the Retro-inverso peptido-mimetic. Competition ELISA was used for the *Pf*MSP1⁴²⁻⁶¹ peptide mapping with monoclonal antibodies coded Ig-αψ-437(⁵²V-L⁵³) and Ig-αψ-439(⁵¹M-V⁵²) as shown in **(C)** and **(D)**, respectively. IC50 μM values represent the average of data obtained in triplicate.

CD patterns for the D-enantiomer and the *Retro-inverso* analogue had a close relationship regarding the all-*L* native sequence. On the other hand, CD profiles for the all-D-enantiomer (red line) and the *Retro*-analogue (blue line) behaved as specular images of each other, keeping in mind that these molecules are made of only D-amino acids, having the second a reversed backbone regarding the first. Interestingly, CD patterns of both, the L-*native* sequence and *Retro*-analogue resemble each other but are opposite to the CD profile of the D-enantiomer. Therefore, a partial conclusion emerged from these findings, independently of the amino acid composition; backbone orientation seemed to play a key role for the 3D structure properties of the antigen molecule.

In order to test the unique recognition of an antibody stimulated by a reduced amide peptido-mimetic in which the oxygen atom of the carbonyl group (–R–CO–NH–R'–) of a relevant peptide-bond was replaced with two hydrogen atoms to lead an analogue being the reduced form of it and herein named reduced amide peptido-mimetic ψ(–R–CH$_2$–NH–R'–). Thus, two monoclonal immunoglobulins (mAb) were produced, one directed to *Pf*MSP1[42-61] modified between the -[52]V-L[53]- and another directed to the -[51]M-V[52]- amino acid pairs, respectively, which herein are named as **Igα-ψ-VL[52-53]** and **Igα-ψ-MV[51-52]**. Both mAbs possess inhibitory capacities in both *in vitro* and *in vivo* malaria infections by *P. falciparum* as well as *P. yoelii* and *P. berghei* as elsewhere published [42]. Also our experiments allowed to a fine mapping of the MSP-1 N-terminus portion using monoclonal and polyclonal antibodies induced by reduced amide peptido-mimetics of the *Pf*MSP1[42-61] peptide and so we identified the antigen epitope whose amino acid sequence is [51]MVLNEGTSGTA[61] as elsewhere reported [44].

Therefore, a whole set of *Pf*MSP1[42-61] modified analogues were used in competition assays for their ability to bind these mAbs. As observed in **Figure 6C** and **D**, the non-modified native sequence (all-L) bound at a 10 µg/mL while their inducer modified peptido-mimetics did it at a 1 µg/mL concentration. The reduced amide modification between 49E-K50 residues was an excellent competitor for binding to the **Igα-ψ-MV[51-52]**. Interestingly, the *All*-D-enantiomer and *Retro-inverso* form of the sequence behaved as strong competitors for the **Igα-ψ-VL[52-53]** binding, both of them are built with D-amino acids. In a similar way, most partially made D-substitutions were strong binders to both tested antibodies. Thus, both chirality and back-bone orientation become critical properties for antigen-antibody recognition, considering that natural features have to be resembled in artificially-modified immunogens, as well as preserving the molecule structure topology but most relevant it is an appropriate side-chain space orientation, which will be crucial for binding and functional effects.

In another set of experiments conducted based on the C-terminus low polymorphic portion the MSP1 antigen, the *Pf*MSP1[1282-1301] peptide whose primary structure EVLYLKPLAG-VYRSLKKQLE was the basis for protection capacity assays against malaria in Aotus monkeys immunized with reduced amide peptido-mimetics and partially made D-mutations. Animals were treated in agreement with Colombian and environmental regulations, and those individuals that developed malaria infection after being experimentally challenged with controlled doses of *P. falciparum* were subjected to medication to ensure their health conditions.

As observed in **Figure 7**, a few number of animals vaccinated have controlled the *Plasmodium* parasitemia levels, especially two out of ten vaccinated with the reduced amide ψ-[7]P-L[8] peptido-mimetic and four out of eight with a partial D-substitution in K[6] of the *Pf*MSP-1[1282-1301] sequence.

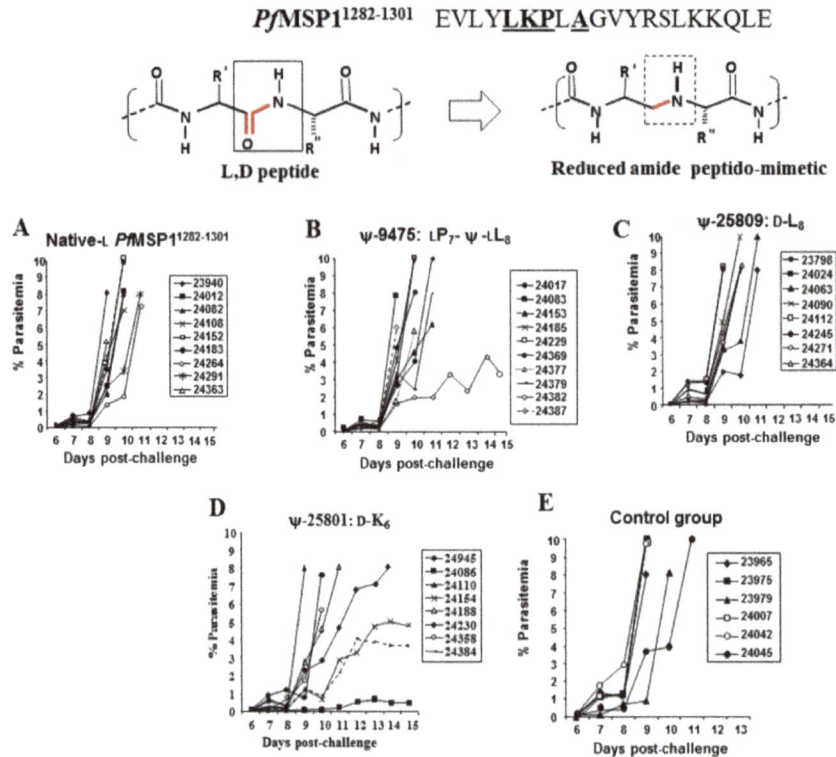

Figure 7. Protection capacity of *Pf*MSP-1/[1282-1301] peptido-mimetics. (A) Aotus monkeys immunized with the *Pf*MSP-1[1282-1301] native sequence. (B) Animal group immunized with the ψ-9475 ([7]P-L[8]) reduced amide peptido-mimetic analogue. (C) Animals immunized with the partially substituted *D*-L[8] analogue. (D) Group of animals immunized with the partially substituted *D*-K[6] analogue. (E) Aotus monkeys immunized with saline solution as the placebo control group.

On the contrary, animals of the placebo-control and those vaccinated with the native sequence became faster infected and did not control the *Plasmodium* parasitemia. Therefore, the evidence supported the relevance of chiral-space occupancy as well as topochemical modifications as being important elements to be considered for malaria vaccine designing.

In order to be consisting with our proposed molecular models, we decided to focus our attention in another relevant *Plasmodium* antigen, the so-named *Pf*MSP-2 surface antigen. Specifically, we have designed and synthesized some reduced amide peptido-mimetics based on the N-terminus *Pf*MSP2[21-40] peptide whose amino acid sequence is KNESKYSNTFIN-NAYNMSIR. Thus, two peptido-mimetic analogues coded ψ-128 and ψ-130 which were modified between the [30]F-I[31] and [31]I-N[32] amino acid pairs, respectively, were obtained and characterized. Our experiments for a fine *Pf*MSP2[21-40] sequence mapping with monoclonal antibodies directed to both modified motifs have revealed a functional epitope whose exact location was [25]KYSNTFIN[32] as previously published [45].

As observed in **Figure 8**, the reactivity patterns of both antibodies by western blot analyses lead to identified native *Pf*MSP2 protein fragments stained at 30.54, 34.21 and 37.90 kDa on a *P. falciparum* FCB-2 membrane protein lysate. Faster polypeptide fragments of *Pf*MSP2 on the SDS-PAGE, could be associated to this antigen cleavage during blood-stage parasite maturation to mature schizonts, previously to merozoite releasing (**Figure 8A**).

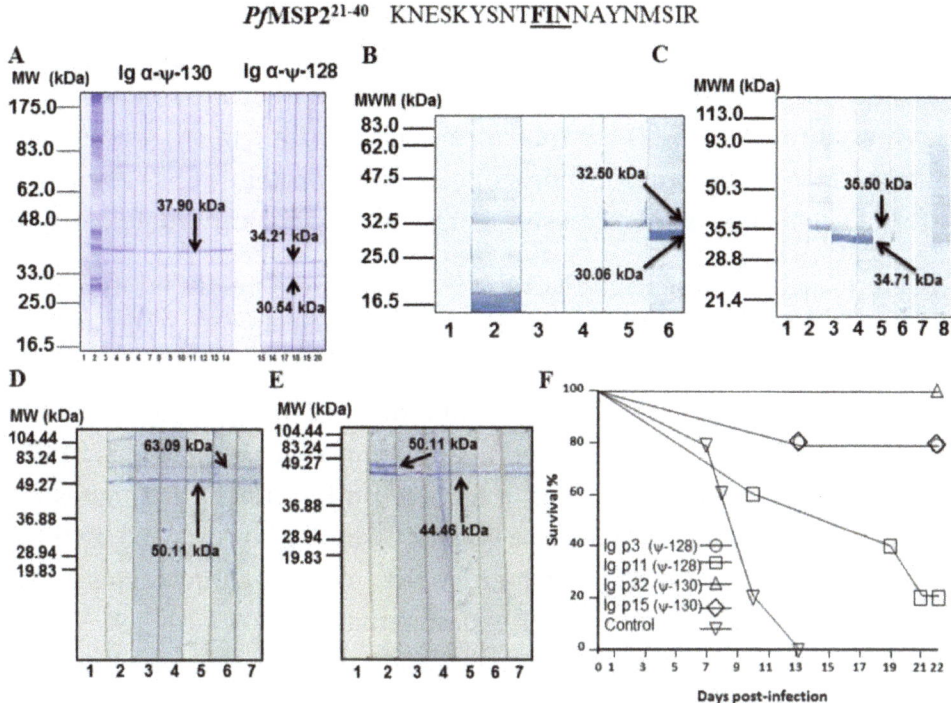

Figure 8. Reactivity and functional properties of *Pf*MSP2²¹⁻⁴⁰ peptido-mimetics. **(A)** *Plasmodium falciparum* FCB-2 membrane protein lysed resolved on a 7.5–15% SDS-PAGE gradient system. **(B)** Recombinant MSP2-(His)₆ protein treated with the Ig-αψ-128 (³⁰F-I³¹) monoclonal antibody. **(C)** Recombinant MSP2-(His)₆ protein treated with the Ig-αψ-130 (³¹I-N³²) monoclonal antibody. **(D)** Surface membrane proteins from blood stages of *P. berghei* treated with the Ig-αψ-128 and Ig-αψ-130 monoclonal antibodies. **(E)** Surface membrane proteins from blood stages of *P. yoelii* treated with the Ig-αψ-128 and Ig-αψ-130 monoclonal antibodies. **(F)** BALB/c mice infected with lethal doses of rodent malaria treated by passive transference of Ig-αψ-128 and Ig-αψ-130 monoclonal antibodies.

In order to verify the antibody reactivity, an *Escherichia coli* recombinantly MSP2 expressed fragment which contained part of the *Pf*MSP2 N-terminus sequence was employed. Hence, the Ig-αψ-128 antibody detected lysate produced bands at 30.06 and 36.50 kDa and the Ig-αψ-130 antibody recognize bands at 34.71 and 35.50 kDa, all polypeptide bands contained the MSP2 recombinantly expressed fragment as compared with the control raw, as shown in **Figure 8B, C** respectively.

Similarly, a lysate composed by membrane proteins from blood stages of *P. berghei* and *P. yoelii* were analyzed for these mAbs recognition. Therefore both Ig-αψ-128 and Ig-αψ-130 antibodies detected bands at 50.11 and 63.09 kDa mobilities for *P. berghei* ANKA and 44.46 and 50.11 kDa for the *P. yoelii* 17XL strain, respectively, as observed in **Figure 8D** and **E**. Besides, functional *in vivo* activity of these antibodies was tested by passive transferring experiments of both into *P. berghei* and *P. yoelii* infected BALB/c mice groups. Most animals survived to the lethal challenging with *Plasmodium* strains and efficiently have controlled parasitemia levels due to the antibody therapeutic activity as it was published and observed in **Figure 8F** [45]. This set of experiments revealed the importance of performing peptide-backbone strategic modifications by introducing non-natural elements into the immunogen primary structure, but its amino acid sequence identity has to be preserved to avoid any non-specific or non-desirable cross-reactive effects.

To obtain a complete landscape of this novel scenario, further scopes of the strategy of obtaining next generations of malaria vaccine candidates based on introducing non-natural elements into immunogens, trials performed in selected antigens of other *Plasmodium* stages, such as those called pre-erythrocytic as well as sexual forms on macro and micro-gamete particles have to be conducted. Hence, the circumsporozoite surface protein (CSP) expressed on pre-erythrocyte forms offers a classical interesting target for vaccine candidate development.

As reported before, a class-I restricted *Pb*CSP[252-260] epitope was identified in the CSP primary structure of *Plasmodium berghei*, a rodent malaria specie [46–49]. Thus, in order to test our hypothesis, we conducted experiments by introducing reduced amide peptide-bond isosteres in a systematic fashion and their subsequent evaluation regarding antibody stimulation and their reactivity was performed. This epitope whose amino acid sequence is SYIPSAEKI was the basis for the molecular designing. Thus, a set of peptido-mimetic analogues were synthesized and characterized. As shown in **Figure 9B** and **C**, antibodies induced by the *Pb*CSP[252-260] native sequence have some reactivity for both sporozoite and gametocytes as analyzed by indirect immunofluorescence assays (IFA) experiments while a stronger reactivity of the modified [257]A-E[258] amino acid pair of *Pb*CSP[257-258] peptido-mimetic-induced antibodies, become evident regarding both sporozoites and gametocytes as observed in **Figure 9E** and **F**. Antibodies of pre-immune sera did not show any reactivity as seen in **Figure 9A** and **D**.

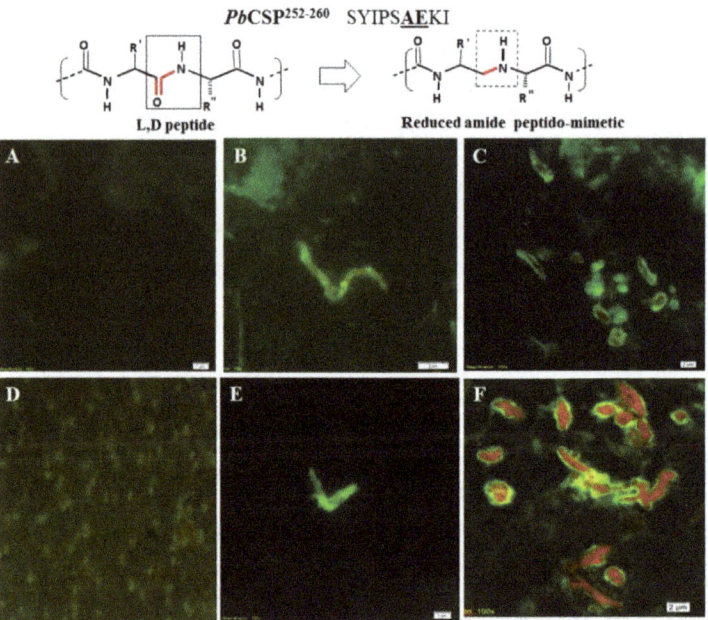

Figure 9. Exploring immunological properties of the restricted class-I *Pb*CSP[252-260] epitope by indirect immunofluorescence assays (IFA). (A) Pre-immune serum of mouse 2. **(B)** *Plasmodium falciparum* sporozoites detected by antibodies induced by the *Pb*CSP[252-260] native peptide post-third boost (mouse 2), image captured at 2 μm. **(C)** Detection of *Plasmodium falciparum* (NF54 strain) gametocytes by antibodies induced by the *Pf*CSP[252-260] native sequence post-third boost (mouse 2), and image recorded at 2 μm. **(D)** Reactivity of pre-immune serum of mouse 23. **(E)** Detection of *Plasmodium falciparum* sporozoites by antibodies to the *Pb*CSP (A–E) peptido-mimetic obtained post-third boost (mouse 23), image recorded at 1 μm. **(F)** Detection of *Plasmodium falciparum* (NF54 strain) gametocytes by antibodies directed to the *Pb*CSP (A–E) peptido-mimetic (mouse 23), and image captured at 2 μm.

The proposed hypothesis has been confirmed by challenging it in different molecular scenarios, all based on analysis of different antigens derived from different *Plasmodium* species and stages and proved in *in vivo* and *in vitro* assays. Thus, an emerging conclusion states the importance of a careful and strategic molecular designing of potential malaria vaccine candidates which consider the antigen global structure modulation but preserving their specific fingerprint represented by their amino acid sequence.

Aimed to understand a possible structure-immunological activity relationship, a subsequent set of nuclear magnetic resonance NMR and molecular dynamic *in silico* experiments lead us to compare in all cases, both the native antigen, as well as their modified derivatives regarding their 3D structure properties. Thus, generated data are presented in **Figure 10**, in which either native antigen backbone conformation is overlapped with that of its functional representative peptido-mimetics or polypeptide conformations of homologue proteins in two *Plasmodium* species are compared.

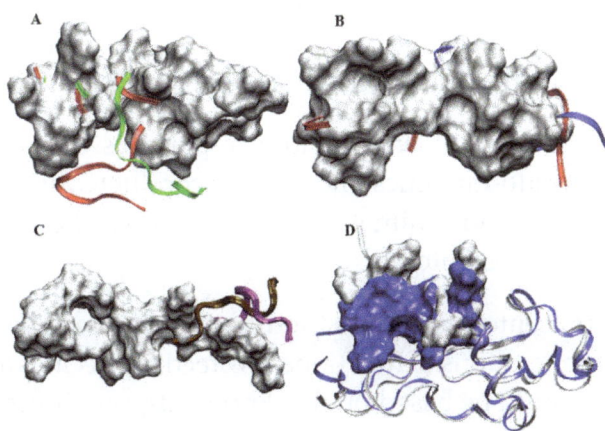

Figure 10. Structure-immunological activity relationship. Overlapped backbone of native and modified peptido-mimetic analogues were organized as follow. **(A)** Accessible solvent surface of the *Pf*MSP1[42-61] native sequence in white and ψ-437 in red ribbons and ψ-439 in blue ribbons. **(B)** Accessible solvent surface of the *Pf*MSP1[1282-1301] native sequence, ψ-9473 in blue ribbons and ψ-9475 in red ribbons. **(C)** Accessible solvent surface of the *Pf*MSP2[21-40] native sequence, ψ-128 in purple ribbons and ψ-130 in ochre ribbons. **(D)** Accessible solvent surfaces in white for *Pf*CSP and blue for *Pb*CSP. The [308]SYIPSAEKI[316] class-I restricted epitope is highlighted.

As observed in **Figure 10A**, overlapped 3D conformations of the *N*-terminus *Pf*MSP1[42-61] peptide whose solvent accessible surface depicted in white, and two of its peptido-mimetics those coded as ψ-437 ([52]V-L[53]) and ψ-439 ([51]M-V[52]) represented by red and green ribbons, revealed deep structure differences between them. A highly compact α-helix structure present in the native sequence became flexible in its two peptido-mimetic analogues due to a single peptide bond modification, in which the oxygen atom of the –CO–NH– amide function of a specific peptide-bond, was replaced with two hydrogen atoms so leading –CH_2–NH– surrogates.

Similarly, backbone of the low polymorphic C-terminus of the same *Pf*MSP1 antigen specifically the *Pf*MSP-1[1282-1301] peptide fragment (solvent accessible surface in white) was overlapped with its two derive ψ-9473 ([6]K-P[7]) and ψ-9475 ([7]P-L[8]) peptido-mimetics (red and blue ribbons)

[50]. As in the first analyzed case, a highly compact α-helix structure present in the native sequence became flexible in its two peptido-mimetic analogues due to single peptide bond modifications which surely have introduced new freedom degrees to the molecule, as seen in **Figure 10B**.

On the other hand, backbone structural analyses for the PfMSP2$^{21\text{-}40}$ regarding its two ψ-128 (^{30}F-I^{31}) and ψ-130 (^{31}I-N^{32}) reduced amide peptido-mimetics, revealed a close-related behavior regarding the couple of the above discussed examples for a different *Plasmodium* protein, the PfMSP1. **Figure 10C**, displays the β-stranded conformation of the native sequence (solvent accessible surface depicted in white) regarding the more flexible conformations of both of its peptido-mimetics (represented by purple and ochre ribbons).

An interesting observation become evident when backbone of two homologue proteins are overlapped regarding a class-I epitope region, as it was the case of the PfCSP and PbCSP, as shown in **Figure 10D**; consisted in that those overlapped polypeptide conformations, suggest an intermediate molecular state among them, which could be represented by a peptido-mimetic structure probe. Thus, the peptido-mimetic coded PbCSP$^{252\text{-}260}$ which represents a peptide-bond surrogate located between the ^{257}A-E^{258} amino acid pair, thus this strategic peptide-bond replacement could be responsibly of the stimulated cross-reactive antibodies.

Further experiments in this pursuit will explore hypothesis on *in vivo* protection against malaria regarding CSP peptido-mimetics and will be conducted in order to assess the functional inhibitory activity of peptido-mimetics and their antibodies on malaria-infected mice through *Anopheles albimanus* mosquito bites.

The family of the herein presented structural modified compounds constitute molecular tools to be considered for new generations of functional protective vaccines against malaria, as such, future vaccine candidates could be based on this knowledge and outstanding findings.

Acknowledgements

As the author of this work, I am indebted to Prof. Manuel Elkin Patarroyo for his invaluable contribution to my personal view on the malaria vaccine field. Special thanks to the Colombian Science Technology and Innovation Department (Colciencias) (Grant No. 212456934488).

Author details

José Manuel Lozano Moreno

Address all correspondence to: jmlozanom@unal.edu.co

Molecular Mimetism of Infectious Agents, Department of Pharmacy, Universidad Nacional de Colombia, Bogotá, Colombia

References

[1] World health statistics 2015. World health Organization, WHO Press, World Health Organization, 20 Avenue Appia, CH-1211 Geneva 27, Switzerland, pp. 1–161. ISBN 978-92-4-156488-5.

[2] World Malaria Report 2015. WHO global malaria programme, World Health Organization, WHO Press, World Health Organization, 20, Avenue Appia, CH-1211 Geneva 27, Switzerland, pp. 1–244. ISBN 978-92-4-156515-8.

[3] Health in 2015, from Millennium development goals (MDG) to Sustainable Development Goals (SDG), World Health Organization, WHO Press, World Health Organization, 20 Avenue Appia, CH-1211 Geneva 27, Switzerland, pp. 1–206. ISBN 978-92-4-156511-0.

[4] Patarroyo ME, Bermudez A, Patarroyo MA. Structural and immunological principles leading to chemically synthesized, multiantigenic, multistage, minimal subunit-based vaccine development. *Chemical Reviews*. 2011. 111:3459–3507.

[5] World Malaria Report 2014.WHO global malaria programme, World Health Organization, WHO Press. World Health Organization, 20, Avenue Appia, CH-1211 Geneva 27, Switzerland, pp. 1–242. ISBN: 978-92-4-156483-0.

[6] Ridley RG. Malaria: to kill a parasite. *Nature*. 2003. 424:887–889.

[7] Nussenzweg R, Vanderberg J, Most H, Orton C. Protective immunity produced by the injection of X-irradiated sporozoites of *Plasmodium berghei. Nature*. 1967. 216(5111): 160–162.

[8] Hoffman S, Billingsley P, James E, Richman A, Lyevsky M, Li T, Chakravarty S, Gunasekera A, Chattopadhyay R, Li M, Stafford R, Ahumada A, Epstein J, Sedegah M, Reyes S, Richie T, Lyke K, Edelman R, Laurens M, Plowe C, Sim L. Development of a metabolically active, non-replicating sporozoite vaccine to prevent *Plasmodium falciparum* malaria. *Human Vaccines*. 2010. 6(1):97–106.

[9] Seder R, Chang L, Enama M, Zephir K, Sarwa V, Gordon I, Holman L, James G, Billingstey P, Gunasekera A, Richman A, Chakravarty S, Manoj A, velmurugam S, Li NM, Ruben A, Li T, Eappen A, Stafford R, Plummer S, Hendel C, Novik L, Costner M, Mendoza F, Sanders J, Nason M, Richardson J, Murphy J, Davidson S, Lyke K, Laurens M, Roeder M, Tewari K, Epstein J, Sim K, Lenderwood J, Graham B, Hoffman S. Protection against malaria by intravenous immunization with a nonreplicating sporozoite vaccine. *Science*. 2013. 341(6152):1359–1365. doi: 10.1126/science.1241800

[10] Tolia NH, Enemark EJ, Sim BK, Joshua-Tor L. Structural basis for the EBA-175 erythrocyte invasion pathway of the malaria parasite *Plasmodium falciparum. Cell*. 2005. 122(2):183–193.

[11] Carvalho L, Ribeiro D, Goto H. Malaria vaccine: candidate antigens, mechanisms, constraints and prospects. *Scandinavian Journal of Immunology.* 2002. 56:327–343.

[12] INS Colombian National Institute of Health, Routinary Surveillance for Epidemiology Events, Departaments 2014, Sistema Nacional de Vigilancia en Salud Pública SIVIGILA (National system of surveillance in public health), events numbers 460, 470, 480, 490, 495, 2015, URL website: www.ins.gov.co. Accessed February 15th, 2016.

[13] Doolan D. *Plasmodium* immunomics. *International Journal for Parasitology.* 2011. 41(1):3–20. doi:10.1016/j.ijpara.2010.08.002

[14] Doolan DL, Hoffman SL. DNA-based vaccines against malaria: status and promise of the multi-stage malaria DNA Vaccine Operation. *International Journal of Parasitology.* 2001. 31(8):753–162.

[15] Mishra S, Nussenzweig R, Nussenzweig V. Antibodies to *Plasmodium* circumsporozoite protein (CSP) inhibit sporozoite's cell traversal activity. *Journal of Immunological Methods.* 2012. 377:47–52.

[16] Richards J, Arumugam T, Reiling L, Heales J, Hooder A, Fawkes F, Cross N, Langer C, Takeo S, Uboldi A, Thompson J, Gilson P, Coopel P, Siba P, King C, Torii M, Chitnis C, Narum D, Mueller I, Crabb B, Cowman A, Tsuboi T, Beeson J. Identification and prioritization of merozoíte antigens as targets of protective human immunity to *Plasmodium falciparum* malaria for vaccine and biomarker development. *The Journal of Immunology.* 2013. 191:795–809.

[17] Booyle M, Wilson D, Beeson J. New approaches to studying *Plasmodium falciparum* merozoíte invasion and insights into invasion biology. *International Journal for Parasitology.* 2013. 43:1–10.

[18] Meraldi V, Romero J, Kensil C, Corradin G. A strong CD8+ T cell response is elicited using the syntethic polypeptide from the C-terminus of the circumsporozoite protein of *Plasmodium berghei* together with the adjuvant QS-21; quantitative and phenotypic comparison with the vaccine model of irradiated sporozoites. *Vaccine.* 2005. 23:2801–2812.

[19] Yandar N, Bianco A, Pastorin G, Pratto M, Patarroyo ME and Lozano JM. Immunological profile of a *Plasmodium vivax* AMA-1 N-terminus peptide-carbon nanotube conjugate in an infected *Plasmodium berghei* mouse model. *Vaccine.* 2008. 26(46):5864–5873.

[20] Zuzarte V, Mote M, Vigario A. Malaria infections, what and how can mice tech us. *Journal of Immunological Methods.* 2014. 410:113–122.

[21] Kooij T, Janse C, Waters A. *Plasmodium* post-genomics better the bug you now? *Nature Reviews Microbiology.* 2006. 4:344–357.

[22] Gibbons P, Batty K, Barnett P, Davis T, Itett K. Development of a pharmacodynamics mooter of murine malaria and antimalarial treatment with dihydroartemisinin. *International Journal for Parasitology*. 2007. 37:1569–1576.

[23] Stephens R, Culleton RL, Lamb TJ. The contribution of *Plasmodium chabaudi* to our understanding of malaria. *Trends in Parasitology*. 2012. 28(2):73–82. doi:10.1016/j.pt. 2011.10.006.

[24] Noulin F. Malaria modeling: *in vitro* stem cells vs *in vivo* models. *World J Stem Cells*. 2016. 8(3):88–100. doi:10.4252/wjsc.v8.i3.88.

[25] Li C, Seixas E, Langhorne J. Rodent malarias: the mouse as a model for understanding, immune responses and pathology induced by the erythrocytic stage of the parasite. *Medical Microbiology Immunology*. 2001. 189:115–126.

[26] Doolan D. *Plasmodium* immunomics. *International Journal for Parasitology*. 2011. 41:3–20.

[27] Shaw TN, Stewart-Hutchinson PJ, Strangward P, Dandamudi DB, Coles JA, Villegas-Mendez A, Gallego-Delgado J, van Rooijen N, Zindy E, Rodriguez A, Brewer JM, Couper KN, Dustin ML. Perivascular arrest of CD8+ T cells is a signature of experimental cerebral malaria. *PLoS Pathogens*. 2015. 11(11):e1005210. doi:10.1371/journal.ppat.1005210.eCollection 2015.

[28] Birkett AJ. Status of vaccine research and development of vaccines for malaria. Vaccine. 2016. 34:2915–2920. http://dx.doi.org/10.1016/j.vaccine.2015.12.074.

[29] US National Institutes of Health; Malaria vaccines. In: ClinicalTrials.gov [Internet]. Bethesda (MD): National Library of Medicine (US). 2000- [cited 2016 September 5]. Available from: http:// clinicaltrials.gov/ct2/results?term=malaria+vaccine.

[30] Vekemans J. Major global vaccine challenges: recent progress on malaria vaccine development, Chapter 19. In: Bloom BR, Lambert PH (eds.) The Vaccine Book, 2nd edn. Academic Press is an imprint of Elsevier Inc., London, 2016, pp. 385–396, 597, ISBN 978-0-12-802174-3.

[31] Mueller I, Shakri AR, Chitnis CE. Development of vaccines for *Plasmodium vivax* malaria. *Vaccine*. 2015. 33:7489–7495.

[32] Ghosh P, Amaya M, Mellins E, Wiley DC. The structure of an intermediate in class II MHC maturation: CLIP bound to HLA-DR3. *Nature*. 1995. 378(6556):457–462.

[33] Russell RJ, Kerry PS, Stevens DJ, Steinhauer DA, Martin SR, Gamblin SJ, Skehel JJ. Structure of influenza hemagglutinin in complex with an inhibitor of membrane fusion. *Proceedings of the National Academy of Sciences of the United States of America*. 2008. 105(46): 17736–17741.

[34] Hennecke J1, Wiley DC. Structure of a complex of the human alpha/beta T cell receptor (TCR) HA1.7, influenza hemagglutinin peptide, and major histocompatibility complex class II molecule, HLA-DR4 (DRA*0101 and DRB1*0401):

insight into TCR cross-restriction and alloreactivity. *Journal of Experimental Medicine*. 2002. 195(5):571–581.

[35] García-Guerrero E, Pérez-Simón JA, Sánchez-Abarca LI, Díaz-Moreno I, De la Rosa MA, Díaz-Quintana A. The dynamics of the human leukocyte antigen head domain modulates its recognition by the T-cell receptor. *PLoS One*. 2016. 11(4):e0154219.

[36] Xia Z, Chen H, Kang SG, Huynh T, Fang JW, Lamothe PA, Walker BD, Zhou R. The complex and specific pMHC interactions with diverse HIV-1 TCR clonotypes reveal a structural basis for alterations in CTL function. *Science Report*. 2014. 4:4087.

[37] De Oliveira DB, Harfouch-Hammoud E, Otto H, Papandreou NA, Stern LJ, Cohen H, Boehm BO, Bach J, Caillat-Zucman S, Walk T, Jung G, Eliopoulos E, Papadopoulos GK, van Endert PM. Structural analysis of two HLA-DR-presented autoantigenic epitopes: crucial role of peripheral but not central peptide residues for T-cell receptor recognition. *Molecular Immunology*. 2000. (14):813–825.

[38] Wiertz E, van Gaans-van den Brink J, Hoogerhout P, Poolman J. Microheterogeneity in the recognition of a HLA-DR2-restricted T cell epitope from a meningococcal outer membrane protein. *European Journal of Immunology*. 1993.23(1):232–239.

[39] Wucherpfennig KW. The structural interactions between T cell receptors and MHC-peptide complexes place physical limits on self-nonself discrimination. *Current Topics in Microbiology and Immunology*. 2005. 296:19–37.

[40] Murray JS, Fois SD, Schountz T, Ford SR, Tawde MD, Brown JC, Siahaan TJ. Modeling alternative binding registers of a minimal immunogenic peptide on two class II major histocompatibility complex (MHC II) molecules predicts polarized T-cell receptor (TCR) contact positions. *Journal of Peptide Research*. 2002. 59(3):115–122.

[41] Lozano JM, Espejo F, Ocampo M, Salazar L, Tovar D, Barrera N, Guzmán F, Patarroyo ME. Mapping the anatomy of a *Plasmodium falciparum* MSP-1 epitope using pseudo-peptide-induced mono- and polyclonal antibodies and CD an NMR formation analysis. *Journal of Structural Biology*. 2004. 148:110–122.

[42] Lozano JM, Espejo F, Vera R, Vargas L, Rojas J, Lesmes L, Torres E, Cortes J, Silva Y, Patarroyo ME. Protection against malaria induced by chirally modified *Plasmodium falciparum*'s MSP-1$_{42}$ pseudopeptides. *Biochemical and Biophysical Research Communications*. 2005. 329:1053–1066.

[43] Lozano JM, Salazar L, Rivera Z, Patarroyo ME. What is Hidden Behind peptide bond restriction and α-carbon asymmetry of conserved antigens? Peptide bond isosters and chirally transformed pseudopeptides as novel elements for synthetic vaccines and therapeutic agents against malaria. *Current Organic Chemistry*. 2006. 10(4):433–456.

[44] Lozano JM, Lesmes LP, Gallego GM, Patarroyo ME. Protection against malaria is conferred by passive transferring rabbit F(ab)2' antibody fragments, induced by

Plasmodium falciparum MSP-1 site-directed designed pseudopeptide-BSA conjugates assessed in a rodent model. *Molecular Immunology*. 2011. 48(4):657-69.

[45] Lozano JM, Guerrero YA, Alba MP, Lesmes LP, Escobar JO, Patarroyo ME. Redefining an epitope of a malaria vaccine candidate, with antibodies against the N-terminal MSA-2 antigen of *Plasmodium* harboring non-natural peptide-bonds. *Amino Acids*. 2013. 45, 4913–4935.

[46] Romero P, Corradin G, Luescher IF, Maryanski JL. H-2Kd-restricted antigenic peptides share a simple binding motif. *Journal of Experimental Medicine*. 1991. 174:603–612.

[47] Maryanski JL, Lüthy R, Romero P, Healy F, Drouet C, Casanova JL, Jaulin C, Kourilsky P, Corradin G. The interaction of antigenic peptides with the H-2Kd MHC class I molecule. *Seminars in Immunology*. 1993. 5(2):95–104.

[48] Guichard G, Calbo S, Muller S, Kourilsky P, Briand JP, Abastado JP. Efficient binding of reduced peptide bond pseudopeptides to major histocompatibility complex class I molecule. *Journal of Biological Chemistry*. 1995. 270(44):26057–26059.

[49] Bongfen SE, Ntsama PM, Offner S, Smith T, Felger I, Tanner M, Alonso P, Nebie I, Romero JF, Silvie O, Torgler R, Corradin G. The N-terminal domain of *Plasmodium falciparum* circumsporozoite protein represents a target of protective immunity. *Vaccine*. 2009. 27(2):328–335.

[50] Lozano JM, Alba MP, Vanegas M, Silva Y, Torres-Castellanos J, Patarroyo ME. MSP-1 malaria pseudopeptide analogues: biological, immunological and three-dimensional structure significance. *Biological Chemistry*. 2003. 384:72–81.

10

Approaches, Challenges and Prospects of Antimalarial Drug Discovery from Plant Sources

Ifeoma C. Ezenyi and Oluwakanyinsola A. Salawu

Abstract

Nearly 3.3 billion people globally are at risk of malaria, with 1.2 billion being at high risk. Children under 5 years of age and pregnant women in sub-Saharan Africa still account for a higher percentage of malaria-related mortalities, despite recent reports of decline in malaria mortalities in Africa. Majority of these deaths are caused by *Plasmodium falciparum*, a lethal malaria parasite which has developed resistance to different classes of antimalarial drugs and is responsible for complicated, severe disease. To forestall the debilitating impact of the disease and provide safe and effective alternative therapies, medicinal plants have been explored as a source of new antimalarials. The isolation of quinine and artemisinin from plants present medicinal plants as a robust source of effective antimalarials. In this chapter, we review the different approaches employed in antimalarial discovery from plants, different classes of plant antimalarial compounds and their proposed mechanisms of action. Compounds that show potential for further development based on their high efficacy and selectivity are also highlighted. Common obstacles encountered in the process of antimalarial drug discovery from plant sources are identified and prospects for the identification of new, effective antimalarial components from plant sources are also discussed.

Keywords: Antiplasmodial screening, Antimalarial, Medicinal plants, *Plasmodium falciparum*, Selectivity

1. Introduction

Malaria has remained a leading cause of mortality in close to 100 countries where nearly 2.4 billion people reside, almost half of whom are located in sub-Saharan Africa. With continuous malaria transmission all year round and increasing rates of human movement in disease-endemic areas, a high burden of antimalarial use in these areas has contributed to global malaria burden [1]. Exposure of parasites to suboptimal antimalarial drug concentrations favors the selection of parasites with traits that enable them to survive in the presence of the drug [2]. Over time, the most lethal strain of the malaria parasite, *Plasmodium falciparum*, has developed resistance to many classes of antimalarial drugs and this contributes to the development of severe malaria complications which can be fatal without prompt treatment. Other less lethal strains, *P. ovale* and *P. vivax*, can exist as latent hypnozoites in the liver which can initiate a relapse months to years after the initial infection [3]. With increased global warming, it has been predicted that the geographic area covered by the malaria vector, *Anopheles* will increase species and this will cause wider transmission of malaria parasites that are resistant to most of the antimalarials presently available [4]. Thus, it has become necessary to develop versatile, robust alternatives to current antimalarial regimens that would be effective against all malaria parasite strains. Within the last decade, efforts have been made to identify new strategies to prevent and treat malaria [5]. Plants have been identified as a robust source for antimalarial drug discovery and interestingly, cinchona alkaloids (such as quinine and quinidine) and artemisinin obtained from plants are still clinically relevant today for the treatment of severe malaria [6].

In order to fast-track the development of effective, alternative medicines from medicinal plants, appropriate pre-clinical studies that confirm their safety and efficacy are required to provide sound experimental data that establish an evidence base. The development of effective medicines from plants is not without its challenges and efforts should be made to address these especially with novel approaches to preclinical screening and clinical testing. Conventional drug development is very time dependent and cost dependent but is rarely rewarding eventually; as the number of approvals for new drugs has declined in recent years [7]. Hence, we also explore the revisited "reverse pharmacology" paradigm to address this problem and secure the future of antimalarial drug discovery.

1.1. Current status of drug discovery from plant sources

Many medicines used against different diseases including cancer, diabetes, hypertension, neurodegenerative disorders and infectious diseases have been sourced from a plant or designed based on scaffolds of compounds isolated from plants. The latest of these include artemether (antimalarial), galantamine (for Alzheimer's disease), nitisinone (for tyrosine-associated metabolic disorder) and tiotropium (anticholinergic), which have all recently been introduced in the United States or are currently involved in late-phase clinical trials [8]. Drug discovery from medicinal plants involves a multi-thronged approach that includes, but is not limited to traditional medicine practitioners, botanists, medicinal chemists, pharmacologists and molecular biologists. Conventionally, plants are selected either randomly or based on their claimed historical medicinal relevance and subjected to sequential extraction and purification steps. This can be very tedious and time-consuming and more effective methods for identifying new lead molecules from plants have been explored. These include chemoinformatics and bioinformatics as tools for in silico drug discovery [9], systems/polypharmacology approach which integrates oral bioavailability tests, druggability, blood-brain barrier permeation, target identification and network analysis owing to the complex composition of medicinal plant extracts and their diverse physiological effects [10]. High throughput pharmacological screens and genetic manipulation have also been applied to discover new drug leads from plants, in which plants extracts are screened against an array of receptors with or without gene manipulation and compared to existing drugs [11].

2. Approaches in antimalarial drug discovery

Six major approaches to antimalarial drug discovery have been identified and reviewed, including the investigation of natural products [12]. A plant-based approach is particularly useful in resource-poor, malaria-endemic areas where nearly one-fifth of patients rely on herbal remedies to treat malaria and febrile illnesses [13]. The choice of plants for antimalarial drug discovery may be based on both random and empirical methods to explore biodiversity or through studies guided by traditional use of the plant in the treatment of fever. The latter ethnopharmacological approach has been recognized to give higher success rates for finding active compounds, as over 50% of extracts from ethnomedicinal plants were active in vivo and/ or in vitro [14].

2.1. Ethnopharmacology-based plant selection and extraction

Herbal medicines have played a pivotal role in health and disease management for many centuries. Different ancient civilizations, including Mesopotamian, Indian ayurveda, ancient traditional Chinese medicine and Greek unani medicine, show documented evidence for the use of herbs in the treatment of different ailments. In Africa, knowledge of traditional medicine constitutes part of a wholistic system, passed through generations by oral communication and indigenous practices [15]. The scientific exploitation of herbs used ethnomedicinally for pain relief, wound healing and abolishing fevers has resulted in the identification of a wide range of compounds that have been developed as new therapeutics [16].

The major role of ethnopharmacology is to discover new plant-derived compounds based on the traditional use of medicinal plants. The knowledge on the use of plants for fevers and other symptoms of malaria is used to guide the selection of plants to be subjected to antimalarial screening and isolation of active constituents. This is a favored and conservative approach in drug discovery as historical use of a plant as medicine increases the possibility that safe and pharmacologically active compounds would be isolated from it.

2.2. Preclinical efficacy studies

2.2.1. In vitro assays

In vitro cultures of asexual forms of *P. falciparum* are generally maintained in leukocyte-free erythrocytes at 2–5% hematocrit, in Roswell Park Memorial Institute (RPMI) culture medium supplemented with 5–10% human serum at 37°C under reduced oxygen conditions [17]. Advantages associated with this assay are the small amount of test sample required and its flexibility, as it has been adapted for high — throughput screening of large compound libraries. With latest developments in image processing and automation technology, screening against live parasites in host cells can also be run in 1536-well formats. Also, concentrations producing 50% inhibition (IC_{50}) and 90% inhibition (IC_{90}) can easily be obtained from drug-response curves by nonlinear regression. Drawbacks to these assays include the need for continuous parasite culture and more importantly, the exclusion of host in vivo factors which affect drug disposition and action.

Detection of parasite growth in in vitro assays generally involves the examination of Giemsa-stained smears for viable parasites. This method is very time-consuming, lacks precision and limits rapid, large-scale screening of compounds. Colorimetric determination of parasite lactate dehydrogenase in the presence of nitro blue tetrazolium which is reduced to a formazan derivative has been developed and used successfully [18]. Other methods have been developed which rely on incorporation of radiolabeled metabolic precursors, measurement of dye-stained parasite DNA by fluorimetry or flow cytometry and use of luminometry for genetically modified parasites that express luciferase [19–21]. Fluorescence-based assays that employ DNA-binding fluorophores have also been described, for example, the fluorimetric method described by Benoît et al. [20] in which parasite growth is quantified by stained DNA of viable parasites. Enzyme-linked immunosorbent assays (ELISAs) with monoclonal antibodies which measure P. falciparum–specific antigen histidine-rich protein 2 (HRP2) or Plasmodium lactate dehydrogenase (pLDH) protein as index of parasite growth have also been reported [22].

Culture conditions for other human and nonhuman Plasmodium species are reviewed in detail elsewhere [23]. The culturing of exoerythrocytic sporozoites was elucidated by infecting a primary culture of human hepatocytes with P. falciparum and P. vivax sporozoites [24]. Though promising, this assay is rarely used as production of large number of sporozoites in insects is a rate-limiting step. Only few in vitro assays have been developed for hypnozoites of P. vivax and P. ovale and the monkey malaria parasite P. cynomolgi [25].

2.2.2. In vivo assays

Mouse models of malaria infection using rodent parasites are especially useful for studying the pathological effects of interactions between the host and the parasite. These models predict clinical outcomes of infections such as parasitemia, sequestration of parasitized red blood cells, splenomegaly, pulmonary edema and hematological and biochemical phenomena. Laboratory rodent parasites such as P. berghei and P. yoelii are used for evaluation of plant extracts and compounds [26]. With advances in genetic manipulation, humanized mouse models to study blood- and liver-stage P. falciparum infections in genetically modified mice have been recently reported [27]. These models have also been used in studying cell-mediated immune responses to liver-stage malaria vaccines [28]. Preliminary tests against P. vivax in non-human primate models like Aotus and Saimiri monkeys have also been carried out [29].

2.2.3. Bioactivity-guided studies, compound isolation and identification

In common practice, traditional herbal remedies are prepared in water, either at room temperature or by boiling to obtain a decoction. Alcoholic solvents are also used as they produce higher extract yield and extract a wider variety of chemical components compared to aqueous extraction [30]. Separation and purification processes for antimalarial plant extracts and fractions involve different chromatographic methods. Frequently, as the extract is separated sequentially, antiplasmodial activity is monitored with a high-throughput in vitro bioassay until the compounds responsible for activity are isolated. This method is based on the assumption that antiplasmodial activity is limited to one or few compounds, whereas when such activity is due to different compounds acting synergistically, it may be lost with further separation [31]. Chromatographic procedures commonly employed include flash column, medium- and high-pressure liquid chromatography and centrifugal countercurrent chromatography. The structure of isolated compounds is determined on the basis of their spectroscopic properties using mass spectrometry, ultraviolet and infrared spectroscopy and complete proton and carbon mapping using one- and two-dimensional nuclear magnetic resonance techniques. It has also been possible to use tandem or hyphenated techniques of these spectroscopies for full stereochemical elucidation of constituents without isolation from extracts [32]. The compound obtained is thereafter subjected to further testing, extending to transmission and radical cure assays. Following the selection of a lead compound, it may be optimized by synthesizing chemical derivatives with the desired bioavailability, potency and selectivity before pre-clinical testing for efficacy and safety, preparatory for phase I clinical testing [33].

3. Isolated compounds and antiplasmodial activity

Some examples of identified compounds that exhibit good antimalarial activity *in vitro* are shown in **Table 1**. Criteria adopted for selection of the compounds shown were inhibition of *P. falciparum* growth by 50% at a concentration of either < 5 µg/mL or < 5 µM in vitro, with high selectivity (>100) for the parasite, where selectivity is expressed as

$$Selectivity\left(S\right) = \frac{EC_{50}}{IC_{50}} \tag{1}$$

where EC_{50} = effective concentration required to inhibit cellular growth by 50% and IC_{50} = concentration required to inhibit parasite growth by 50%.

From the compounds shown in **Table 1**, it is evident that a remarkable diversity of plant-derived compounds exists and they can form good templates for the design of novel antimalarials. One example of such is gedunin, a limonoid extracted from the leaves of *Azadirachta indica* with high antiplasmodial activity in vitro. Its antiplasmodial potency was attributed to the α,β-unsaturated ketone group in Ring A of its limonoid backbone, a 7α-acetate group as well as its furan ring [34]. *Dichroa febrifuga* is a popular fever remedy in traditional Chinese medicine and guided studies led to the isolation and identification of febrifugine over 50 years ago [35]. Studies on febrifugine were hindered for a long time because of its toxicity. Some of its derivatives with good antiplasmodial activity have however been shown to exhibit lower toxicity compared with the parent compound [35]. The monoterpene indole alkaloid ellipticine and its isomer olivacine isolated from the bark of *Aspidosperma olivaceum* were shown to possess antiplasmodial effects in addition to its previously reported antitumor properties [36]. The selectivity of the ellipticine and olivacine for the parasitic targets was evident from the high S values (500–1200, ellipticine and 330–390, olivacine) against *P. falciparum* K1 and 3D7 [36]. Ellipticine was shown to be antiplasmodial, by inhibiting heme crystal growth and interacting with parasite DNA. It was speculated that this effect was similar to that of other analogous cryptolepine- and harmane-type indole alkaloids, depending on structural similarity [36]. *Uvaria leptocladon* is a shrub growing in the West Usambara Mountains of Tanzania, where it is used against cerebral malaria [37]. Investigation of the Tanzanian *U. leptocladon* root bark afforded the isolation of the chalcones, uvaretin and diuvaretin, which were shown to possess antiplasmodial activity with $IC_{50} < 5$ µg/mL [38]. Antiplasmodial screening of *Dorstenia barteri* twigs yielded the isolation of the prenylated chalcones, bartericin A ($IC_{50} = 2.15$ µM) and 4-hydroxylonchocarpin ($IC_{50} = 3.36$ µM) which were devoid of toxicity to erythrocytes at concentrations below 20 mM [39]. The authors deduced that the presence of a hydroxylated prenyl group on carbon 5' on Ring B of bartericin A enhanced its antiplasmodial activity compared to a prenyl group at the same position in 4-hydroxylonchocarpin [39]. Lanaroflavone is a biflavonoid isolated from the methanol extract of the aerial part of *Campnosperma panamense* Standl. In vitro screening revealed its highly selective ($S = 159$) antiplasmodial activity ($IC_{50} = 0.48$ µM) [40]. For this compound, it was observed that its C-4‴—O—C-8 interflavonoid linkage was relevant for antiplasmodial activity [40].

A study of species of *Carpesium* genus used as traditional remedies for the treatment of parasite infections led to the identification and isolation of ineupatorolide A, a sesquiterpene from *Carpesium rosulatum*. Of particular interest were its high antiplasmodial activity ($IC_{50} = 0.019$ µM) and selectivity ($S > 1000$) [41]. *Bowdichia nitida* Spruce ex Benth., commonly referred to as "sucupira," is distributed in the Brazilian Amazon and the seeds of this plant are traditionally used for rheumatic arthritis, fever and gouty arthritis [42]. 6α,7β-Diacetoxyvouacapane isolated from a methanol extract of *B. nitida* seeds displayed high activity against *P. falciparum* 3D7 (IC_{50} 0.39 µg/mL) and high selectivity for the parasite, as cytotoxic IC_{50} on COLO 201 cells was higher than 100 µg/mL [42]. Another antiplasmodial compound identified as neosergeolide, a quassinoid obtained from the root and stem of *Picralemma sprucei*, had high antiplasmodial activity (0.002 µM) and was cytotoxic toward selected tumor cell lines at concentrations ranging from 5 to 27 mg/mL [43]. Antiplasmodial activity-aided fractionation of *Piptadenia pervillei* leaves afforded the identification of (+)-catechin-3-gallate and (+)-catechin-5-gallate, which displayed high antiplasmodial effects against *P. falciparum* FcB1 and had no significant cytotoxic effects against the human embryonic lung cells MRC-5 [44].

Other compounds have also been investigated and found highly active against hepatic stage *Plasmodium* species. N-Cyclopentyl-tazopsine, a semisynthetic derivative of a plant-derived morphinan compound, tazopsine, was shown to have specific activity against liver-stage parasites of *P. falciparum* (IC_{50} = 42.4 μM, S = 60) and *P. yoelii* (IC_{50} = 3.3 μM, S = 46) [45]. Its efficacy against hepatic-stage parasites indicates its potential for development as a prophylactic agent.

Compounds	Plant source	Family	Antiplasmodial activity	Source
Gedunin	*Azadirachta indica*	Meliaceae	(Pf D6) 0.039 μg/mL	[34]
			(Pf W2) 0.02 μg/mL	
Febrifugine	*Dichroa febrifuga*	Hydrangeaceae	(Pf W2) 0.53 ng/mL	[35]
			(Pf D6) 0.34 ng/mL	
Ellipticine	*Aspidosperma vargasii*	Apocynaceae	(Pf K1) 0.81 μM	[36]
			(Pf 3D7) 0.35 μM	
Olivacine	*Aspidosperma olivaceum*	Apocynaceae	(Pf K1) 1.4 μM	[36]
			(Pf 3D7) 1.2 μM	
Uvaretin	*Uvaria* spp.	Annonaceae	(Pf K1) 3.49 μg/mL	[37, 38]
Diuvaretin			4.20 μg/mL	
Bartericin A	*Dorstenia barteri*	Moraceae	(Pf W2) 2.15 μM	[39]
4-Hydroxylonchocarpin			3.36 μM	
Lanaroflavone	*Campnosperma panamense*	Anacardiaceae	(Pf K1) 0.48 μM	[40]
Ineupatorolide A	*Carpesium rosulatum*	Asteraceae	(Pf D10) 0.019 μM	[41]
6α,7β-Diacetoxyvouacapane	*Bowdichia nitida*	Leguminosae	(Pf 3D7) 0.97 μM	[42]
Neosergeolide	*Picralima sprucei*	Simaroubaceae	(Pf K1) 0.002 μM	[43]
(+)-Catechin-3-gallate	*Piptadenia pervillei*	Fabaceae	(Pf FcB1) 1 μM	[44]
(+)-Catechin-5-gallate			1.2 μM	

Table 1. Antiplasmodial compounds with high selectivity isolated from plants.

4. Isolated compound classes and intra-parasitic targets

4.1. Alkaloids

This group of plant secondary metabolites represents the largest group of plant secondary metabolites with the highest number of compounds displaying potent antiplasmodial activity. They also serve as good templates for synthesis of many quinolone-based antimalarial drugs. Alkaloids displaying potent antiplasmodial activity occur as steroidal alkaloids, bisbenzylisoquinolines, naphthylisoquinolines, indoloquinolines and indolomonoterpenoid alkaloids, among others. Quinoline alkaloids isolated from the bark of *Cinchona officinalis* including quinine, quinidine, cinchonine and cinchonidine (**Figure 1**) are all highly effective against malaria, with cure rates exceeding 98% in humans [33]. Although quinine is associated with serious side effects, it has remained an important drug to treat severe malaria due to chloroquine resistance. Quinine is schizonticidal against all intraerythrocytic malaria parasites and gametocytocidal for *P. vivax* and *P. malariae*, but not against *P. falciparum* gametocytes [46].

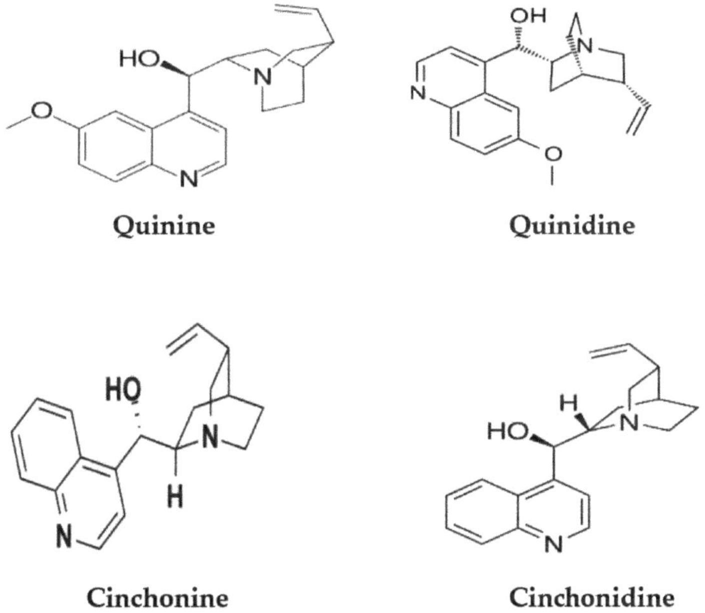

Figure 1. Chemical structures of cinchona alkaloids: quinine, quinidine, cinchonine and cinchonidine.

Although the mechanism of action of quinine has not been fully resolved, it has been reported to exhibit inhibitory effects on heme polymerization and heme catalase activity [47]. Following the success of quinine identification and use, natural antiplasmodial alkaloids have been isolated and reviewed by Kaur et al. [48]. Some alkaloids have been reported to inhibit fatty acid biosynthesis in the parasite [22], while some act as resistance reversers. The monoindole alkaloids strychnobrasiline and malagashanine isolated from Strychnos myrtoides potentiated the effects of chloroquine, quinolones, aminoacridines and halofantrine [49]. Malagashanine has no intrinsic antiplasmodial or cytotoxic action, but aids chloroquine accumulation in drug-resistant parasites by improving chloroquine influx and preventing its efflux from the parasites [50].

4.2. Flavonoids and chalcones

Flavonoids occur ubiquitously in many higher plants where they act as growth regulators and offer protection against plant pathogens [51]. They have been proposed to act by inhibiting the fatty acid biosynthesis (FAS II) pathway, which is present in the parasite's apicoplast but absent in human hosts [52]. The flavonoid, luteolin-7-O-β-D-glucopyranoside, was reported as the first natural product that targets plasmodial FAB I enzyme which regulates the FAS II pathway [53]. Some flavonoids have also been shown to inhibit L-glutamine and myoinositol influx into infected erythrocytes or act by interfering with hemin degradation [54, 55]. In addition, chalcones have been proposed to act by inhibiting cyclin-dependent protein kinases and plasmepsin II [56].

4.3. Terpenes and terpenoids

In recent times, attention has been devoted to this class of compounds especially sesquiterpenoids, following the discovery of the endoperoxide sesquiterpene lactone; artemisinin. These compounds are attractive because some possess intrinsic antiplasmodial activity and offer good starting points for chemical modification into derivatives with desired physicochemical properties and enhanced efficacy. Artemisinin and its derivatives owe their antiplasmodial effects to the presence of an endoperoxide bridge that generates toxic-free radicals when it is broken down (**Figure 2**). Another example of a highly potent antiplasmodial sesquiterpene is ineupatorolide A (**Table 1**).

Apart from the major classes of isolated compounds discussed above, other examples such as xanthones, stilbenes, coumarins, lignans, tannins and steroids have also been reported to exhibit potent antiplasmodial effects [57].

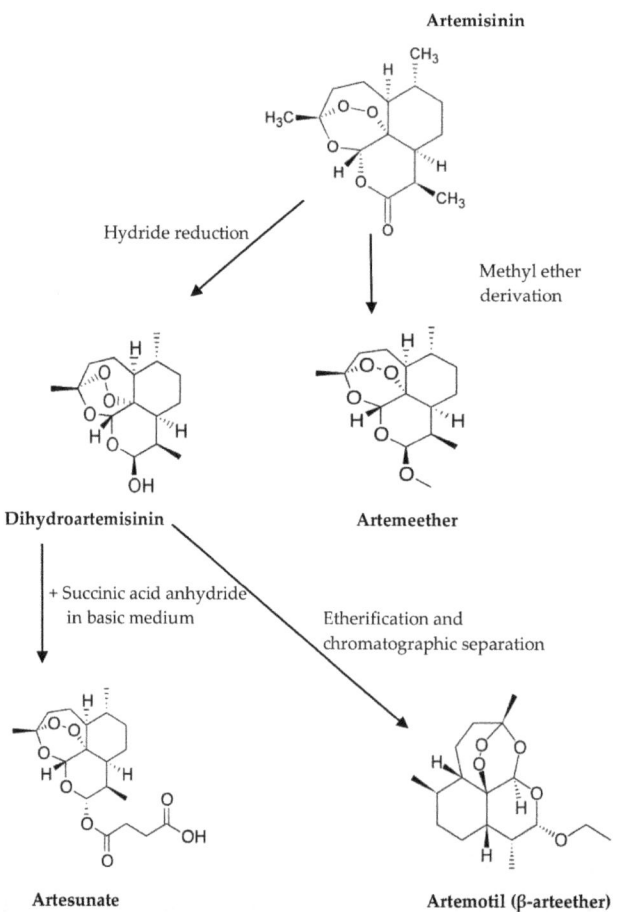

Figure 2. Artemisinin and its chemical derivatives in clinical use.

5. Clinical studies

Literature search revealed only few plant-derived extracts or compounds undergoing clinical studies and these are shown in **Table 2**. Spirotetrahydro β-carbolines (spiroindolones) present a unique group of compounds that share structural similarities with strictosamide, an iridoid indole alkaloid identified in an extract of *Nauclea pobeguinii* stem bark, but also present in *Nauclea latifolia* and *Nauclea officinalis* extracts [58, 59]. A spiroindolone (NITD609, **Figure 3**) displayed low IC_{50} within the range of 0.5–1.4 nM, showed no evidence of diminished potency against drug-resistant strains and was not significantly cytotoxic to mammalian cells [60, 61]. It was also effective against clinical isolates of *P. falciparum* and *P. vivax* (IC_{50} < 10nM) and comparable to artesunate. Additionally, it inhibited gametocyte development in vitro and oocyst development in mosquitoes [60]. *Argemone mexicana* decoction administered orally also produced antimalarial effects that were comparable to artesunate-amodiaquine combination in patients [62].

Plant extract/compound	Stage of clinical development	Mechanism of action
Nauclea pobeguinii [58]	Phase IIb/III	Not known
Argemone mexicana [62]	Phase IIb/III	Not known
NITD609 [60, 61]	Phase IIa	Chemotherapeutic, transmission blocking

Table 2. Plant extracts and natural product–derived compound in clinical development.

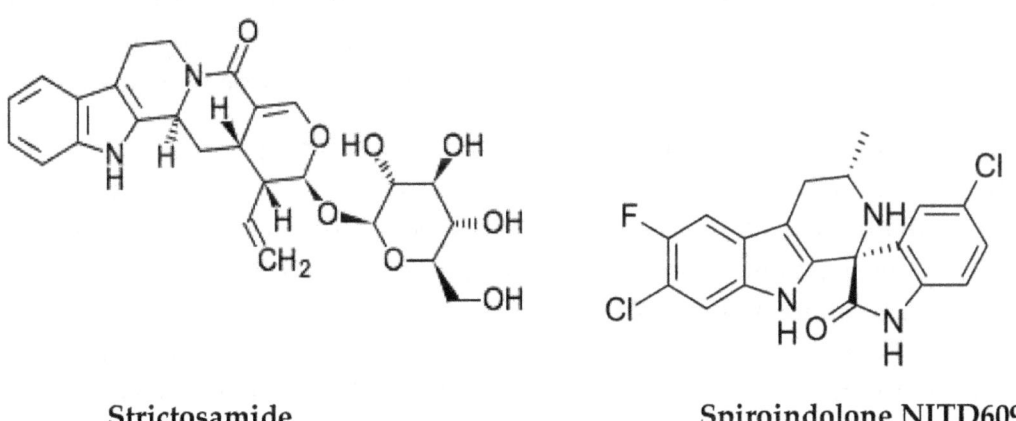

Strictosamide   **Spiroindolone NITD609**

Figure 3. Chemical structures of strictosamine, an iridoid indole alkaloid and structurally similar spiroindolone in clinical development, NITD609.

6. Reverse pharmacology: from bedside to bench

Conventional drug discovery and development is an energy-, time- and resource-demanding venture; hence, the entire process results in minimal success rates. Millions of compounds are involved during initial screening and identified hits are ranked based on potency, ease of synthesis, known limitations to therapeutic use and novelty to determine a possible lead compound [33]. The lead compound is thereafter subjected to preclinical tests and various optimization processes to confer desired chemical and pharmacokinetic properties on it before final clinical testing. After passing through rigorous Phases I-III trials, it may be accorded statutory approval for clinical use. This is very expensive and time-consuming and many pharmaceutical companies are looking for new approaches in drug discovery that will lead to expedited launch of new, effective and safe drugs.

Reverse pharmacology is a science that integrates well-documented clinical experiences and observations toward lead development, through interdisciplinary studies (preclinical, clinical) for drug development [63]. Here, "safety" is the starting point as well-documented evidence of traditional use as medicine. This provides an important basis for further scientific testing. Hence, reverse pharmacology adopts a "bedside to bench" approach, compared to conventional "bench to bedside" drug discovery and development.

The use of *Artemisia annua* as treatment for fever and malaria in traditional Chinese medicine afforded the discovery of artemisinin through a reverse pharmacology approach. Today, artemisinin derivatives like artemether, artesunate, artemether and dihydroartemisinin remain useful antimalarial agents against drug-sensitive and drug-resistant malaria. However, the case of artemisinin is a unique one where artemisinin was identified as an active molecule, as not all traditional medicinal herbal extracts owe their therapeutic effects to a single chemical entity. The effects of some extracts may be due to different phytochemicals acting on different targets or a synergistic effect between different constituents and further separation and purification may lead to a loss of activity [30]. In this case, bioactivity markers should be identified and a standardized formulation of the extract should be prepared and screened using a systems biology approach before consideration for further development.

An example of antimalarial drug development using the reverse pharmacology approach in recent times is seen in the study of a standardized extract of *A. mexicana* for the treatment of malaria [64]. Initially, the authors conducted a retrospective treatment-outcome study to select a candidate for development before a dose-escalating clinical study to identify and choose a dose with desirable safety and efficacy. Next, they carried out a randomized controlled trial for comparison of the selected phytomedicine with conventional first line antimalarial therapy followed by identification of active compounds which could be employed as chemical markers to standardize the phytomedicine. This scheme was used successfully and can be adopted for antimalarial drug development (**Figure 4**). The process of identifying chemical and/or biological markers of efficacy which are used to ensure herbal medicine quality is known as standardization. This is an important step in drug development from herbal medicines, as quantity and quality of secondary metabolites depend on intrinsic factors, environmental factors and biotic factors [65].

It is interesting to note that subsequent to the report on the clinical efficacy of *A. mexicana* [62], three antiplasmodial protoberine-type alkaloids were isolated by conventional methods from an extract of *A. mexicana*, namely, berberine, allocryptopine and protopine, but berberine was found to be cytotoxic relative to the parent extract, while allocryptopine and protopine were more selective for parasites compared to berberine [66] (see **Figure 4**).

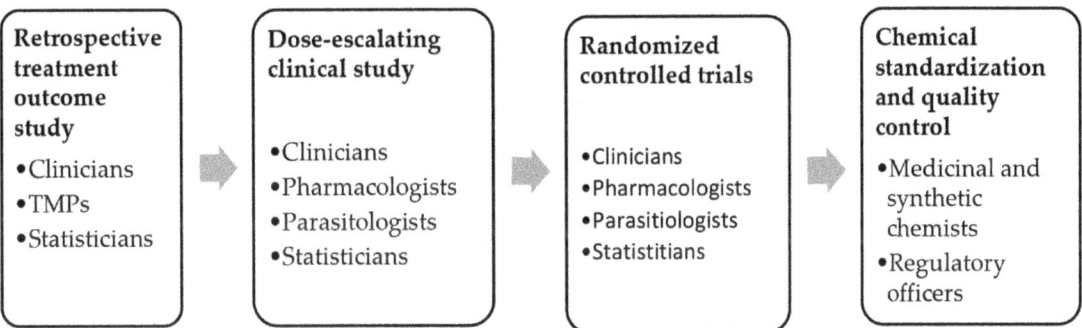

Figure 4. Antimalarial drug development by reverse pharmacology flow chart as described by Willcox et al. [64], showing key personnel involved during each stage of the process.

7. Conclusions

Naturally occurring antiplasmodial compounds in plants show vast chemical diversity but also exist within a complex mixture of other plant secondary metabolites which in itself constitutes a major challenge to efforts in identifying compounds responsible for biological effects. Other problems with plant-based drug discovery process range from the basic ones like sustainable access to plant material, seasonal and environmental variations and legislative issues concerning plant use, to challenges concerning complex fractionation procedures, small quantity of pure compounds and poor pharmacokinetic/physicochemical properties that negatively affect druggability [67]. With an increasing understanding and use of genomics, it is possible that bioactive molecules can be produced more efficiently using plant-cell cultures and genetically modified microbes [68]. This has already been exploited in the production of artemisinin precursors from genetically modified *Saccharomyces cerevisiae* and *Escherichia coli* [69].

Innovative drug discovery through reverse pharmacology or conventional methods especially in resource-constrained remote areas where medicines are urgently needed should be given more attention. There is the need to explore other aspects of the use of plant extracts and compounds as efficacy boosters or drug resistance reversers in combination with conventional therapy [50]. Efficacy screening against the parasite at all stages of development including gametocytes and hypnozoites should be incorporated in preclinical drug testing as they are often overlooked yet useful tools to identify agents that block transmission of resistance and prevent relapse [70]. In the course of literature review, a number of antimalarial compounds reported also displayed significant cytotoxic effects on human cells. Thus, screening for inhibitors against parasite-specific targets in organelles like the apicoplast and pathways such as heme degradation and type II fatty acid biosynthesis would likely identify active leads with highly selective antiplasmodial action.

Author details

Ifeoma C. Ezenyi* and Oluwakanyinsola A. Salawu

*Address all correspondence to: iphie_odike@yahoo.com

Department of Pharmacology and Toxicology, National Institute for Pharmaceutical Research and Development, Idu, Abuja, Nigeria

References

[1] Agusto F. Malaria drug resistance: the impact of human movement and spatial heterogeneity. Bulletin of Mathematical Biology. 2014;76(7):1607–41.

[2] Schneider, P, Chan BHK, Reece SE, Read AF. Does the drug sensitivity of malaria parasites depend on their virulence? Malaria Journal. 2008;7:257.

[3] Collins WE, Jeffery GM. Plasmodium ovale: parasite and disease. Clinical Microbiology Reviews. 2005;18(3):570.

[4] Laporta GZ, Linton Y-M, Wilkerson RC, Bergo ES, Nagaki SS, Sant'Ana DC, et al. Malaria vectors in South America: current and future scenarios (research). Parasites & Vectors. 2015;8:426.

[5] Hemingway J, Shretta R, Wells TNC, Bell D, Djimdé AA, Achee N, et al. Tools and strategies for malaria control and elimination: what do we need to achieve a grand convergence in malaria? PLoS Biology. 2016;14(3):e1002380.

[6] Pasvol G. The treatment of complicated and severe malaria. British Medical Bulletin. 2005;75–76(1):29–47.

[7] Mullard A. 2014 FDA drug approvals: the FDA approved 41 new therapeutics in 2014, but the bumper year fell short of the commercial power of the drugs approved in 2013 (news & analysis). Nature Reviews Drug Discovery. 2015;14(2):77.

[8] Balunas MJ, Kinghorn AD. Drug discovery from medicinal plants. Life Sciences. 2005;78(5):431–41.

[9] Lagunin AA, Goel RK, Gawande DY, Pahwa P, Gloriozova TA, Dmitriev AV, et al. Chemo- and bioinformatics resources for in silico drug discovery from medicinal plants beyond their traditional use: a critical review. Natural Product Reports. 2014;31(11):1585–611.

[10] Liu H, Wang J, Zhou W, Wang Y, Yang L. Systems approaches and polypharmacology for drug discovery from herbal medicines: an example using licorice (report). Journal of Ethnopharmacology. 2013;146(3):773.

[11] Littleton J, Rogers T, Falcone D. Novel approaches to plant drug discovery based on high throughput pharmacological screening and genetic manipulation. Life Sciences. 2005;78(5):467–75.

[12] Rosenthal PJ. Antimalarial drug discovery: old and new approaches. The Journal of Experimental Biology. 2003;206(Pt 21):3735.

[13] Willcox ML, Bodeker G. Traditional herbal medicines for malaria. British Medical Journal. 2004;329(7475):1156.

[14] Carvalho LH, Krettli AU. Antimalarial chemotherapy with natural products and chemically defined molecules. Memórias do Instituto Oswaldo Cruz. 1991;86 (Suppl) 2:181.

[15] Romero-Daza N. Traditional medicine in Africa. Annals of the American Academy of Political and Social Science. 2002;583:173–6.

[16] Harvey AL. Natural products in drug discovery. Drug Discovery Today. 2008;13(19): 894–901.

[17] Trager W. Cultivation of malaria parasites. British Medical Bulletin. 1982;38(2):129–31.

[18] Orjuela-Sánchez P, Duggan E, Nolan J, Frangos John A, Carvalho Leonardo J. A lactate dehydrogenase ELISA-based assay for the in vitro determination of *Plasmodium berghei* sensitivity to anti- malarial drugs. Malaria Journal. 2012;11(1):366.

[19] Jun G, Lee J-S, Jung Y-J, Park J-W. Quantitative determination of *Plasmodium parasitemia* by flow cytometry and microscopy. Journal of Korean Medical Science. 2012;27(10): 1137.

[20] Benoît M, Carla C, Alice Soh Meoy O, Rossarin S, Kanlaya S, Shanshan Wu H, et al. A rapid and robust tri-color flow cytometry assay for monitoring malaria parasite development. Scientific Reports. 2011;1: 118

[21] Hasenkamp S, Wong EH, Horrocks P. An improved single-step lysis protocol to measure luciferase bioluminescence in *Plasmodium falciparum*. Malaria Journal. 2012;11:42.

[22] Cláudio RN, Lucia MXL. Antiplasmodial natural products. Molecules. 2011;16(3):2146–90.

[23] Frederick L. Schuster, Cultivation of Plasmodium spp. Clinical Microbiology Reviews. 2002;15(3):355.

[24] Sattabongkot J, Yimamnuaychoke N, Leelaudomlipi S, Rasameesoraj M, Jenwithisuk R, Coleman RE, et al. Establishment of a human hepatocyte line that supports in vitro development of the exo-erythrocytic stages of the malaria parasites *Plasmodium falciparum* and *P. vivax*. The American Journal of Tropical Medicine and Hygiene. 2006;74(5):708.

[25] Pohlit AM, Lima RB, Frausin G, Silva LF, Lopes SC, Moraes CB, Cravo P, Lacerda MV, Siqueira AM, Freitas-Junior LH, Costa FT. Amazonian plant natural products: perspectives for discovery of new antimalarial drug leads. Molecules. 2013;18(8):9219–40.

[26] Wykes MN, Good MF. What have we learnt from mouse models for the study of malaria? European Journal of Immunology. 2009;39(8):2004–7.

[27] Legrand N, Ploss A, Balling R, Becker PD, Borsotti C, Brezillon N, Debarry J, de Jong Y, Deng H, Di Santo JP, Eisenbarth S, Eynon E, Flavell RA, Guzman CA, Huntington ND, Kremsdorf D, Manns MP, Manz MG, Mention JJ, Ott M, Rathinam C, Rice CM, Rongvaux A, Stevens S, Spits H, Strick-Marchand H, Takizawa H, van Lent AU, Wang C, Weijer K, Willinger T, Ziegler P. Humanized mice for modeling human infectious disease: challenges, progress and outlook (report). Cell Host & Microbe. 2009;6(1):5.

[28] Good MF, Hawkes MT, Yanow SK. Humanized mouse models to study cell-mediated immune responses to liver-stage malaria vaccines. Trends in Parasitology. 2015;31(11):583.

[29] Collins WE, Sullivan JS, Strobert E, Galland GG, Williams A, Nace D, et al. Studies on the Salvador I strain of *Plasmodium vivax* in non- human primates and anopheline mosquitoes. The American Journal of Tropical Medicine and Hygiene. 2009;80(2):228.

[30] Willcox M, Bodeker G, Rasoanaivo P. Traditional Medicinal Plants and Malaria: Volume 4 of the Traditional Herbal Medicine for Modern Times Series Boca Raton, London, New York, Washington, DC: CRC Press, 2004. pp. 381–2.

[31] Phillipson JD. Phytochemistry and medicinal plants. Phytochemistry. 2001;56(3):237–43.

[32] Bringmann G, Messer K, Wolf K, Mühlbacher J, Grüne M, Brun R, et al. Dioncophylline E from Dioncophyllum thollonii, the first 7,3'- coupled dioncophyllaceous naphthylisoquinoline alkaloid. Phytochemistry. 2002;60(4):389–97.

[33] Erika LF, Arnab KC, Elizabeth AW. Antimalarial drug discovery—approaches and progress towards new medicines. Nature Reviews Microbiology. 2013;11(12):849.

[34] Adebayo JO, Krettli AU. Potential antimalarials from Nigerian plants: a review. Journal of Ethnopharmacology. 2011;133(2):289–302.

[35] Jiang S, Zeng Q, Gettayacamin M, Tungtaeng A, Wannaying S, Lim A, et al. Antimalarial activities and therapeutic properties of febrifugine analogs. Antimicrobial Agents and Chemotherapy. 2005;49(3):1169.

[36] Silva LFRe, Montoiaa A, Amorim RCN, Melo MR, Henrique MC, Nunomura SM, et al. Comparative in vitro and in vivo antimalarial activity of the indole alkaloids ellipticine, olivacine, cryptolepine and a synthetic cryptolepine analog. Phytomedicine: International Journal of Phytotherapy & Phytopharmacology. 2012;20(1):71.

[37] Nkunya MHH, Weenen H, Renner C, Waibel R, Achenbach H. Benzylated dihydro-chalcones from Uvaria leptocladon. Phytochemistry. 1993;32(5):1297–300.

[38] Gessler MC, Nkunya MHH, Mwasumbi LB, Heinrich M, Tanner M. Screening Tanzanian medicinal plants for antimalarial activity. Acta Tropica. 1994;56(1), 65–77.

[39] Ngameni B, Watchueng J, Boyom FF, Keumedjio F, Ngadjui BT, Gut J, Abegaz BM, Rosenthal PJ. Antimalarial prenylated chalcones from the twigs of Dorstenia barteri var. subtriangularis. Arkivoc. 2007;13: 116–123.

[40] Weniger B, Vonthron-Sénécheau C, Kaiser M, Brun R, Anton R. Comparative antiplasmodial, leishmanicidal and antitrypanosomal activities of several biflavonoids. Phytomedicine : International Journal of Phytotherapy and Phytopharmacology. 2006;13(3): 176–180.

[41] Moon H-I. Antiplasmodial activity of ineupatorolides A from Carpesium rosulatum. Parasitology Research. 2007;100(5):1147–9.

[42] Matsuno Y, Deguchi J, Hirasawa Y, Ohyama K, Toyoda H, Hirobe C, et al. Sucutiniranes A and B, new cassane-type diterpenes from Bowdichia nitida. Bioorganic & Medicinal Chemistry Letters. 2008;18(13):3774–7.

[43] Silva ECC, Cavalcanti BC, Amorim RCN, Lucena JF, Quadros DS, Tadei WP, et al. Biological activity of neosergeolide and isobrucein B (and two semi- synthetic derivatives) isolated from the Amazonian medicinal plant Picrolemma sprucei (Simaroubaceae). Memórias do Instituto Oswaldo Cruz. 2009;104(1):48.

[44] Ramanandraibe V, Grellier P, Martin MT, Deville A, Joyeau R, Ramanitrahasimbola D, Mouray E, Rasoanaivo P, Mambu L. Antiplasmodial phenolic compounds from Piptadenia pervillei. Planta Medica. 2008;74(4):417–21.

[45] Carraz M, Jossang A, Franetich J-F, Siau A, Ciceron L, Hannoun L, et al. A plant-derived morphinan as a novel lead compound active against malaria liver stages. PLoS Medicine. 2006;3(12):e513.

[46] Achan J, Talisuna AO, Erhart A, Yeka A, Tibenderana JK, Baliraine FN, et al. Quinine, an old anti-malarial drug in a modern world: role in the treatment of malaria (review) (report). Malaria Journal. 2011;10:144.

[47] Bohorquez EB, Chua M, Meshnick SR. Quinine localizes to a non-acidic compartment within the food vacuole of the malaria parasite Plasmodium falciparum (research) (report). Malaria Journal. 2012;11:350.

[48] Kaur K, Jain M, Kaur T, Jain R. Antimalarials from nature. Bioorganic & Medicinal Chemistry. 2009;17(9):3229–56.

[49] Rafatro H, Ramanitrahasimbola D, Rasoanaivo P, Ratsimamanga-Urverg S, Rakoto-Ratsimamanga A, Frappier F. Reversal activity of the naturally occurring chemosensi-

tizer malagashanine in Plasmodium malaria. Biochemical Pharmacology. 2000;59(9): 1053–61.

[50] Ramanitrahasimbola D, Rasoanaivo P, Ratsimamanga S, Vial H. Malagashanine potentiates chloroquine antimalarial activity in drug resistant Plasmodium malaria by modifying both its efflux and influx. Molecular & Biochemical Parasitology. 2006;146(1): 58–67.

[51] Saliba Kevin J, Lehane Adele M. Common dietary flavonoids inhibit the growth of the intraerythrocytic malaria parasite. BMC Research Notes. 2008;1(1):26.

[52] Waller RF, Ralph SA, Reed MB, Su V, Douglas JD, Minnikin DE, et al. A Type II pathway for fatty acid biosynthesis presents drug targets in *Plasmodium falciparum*. Antimicrobial Agents and Chemotherapy. 2003;47(1):297.

[53] Ezenyi I, Salawu O, Kulkarni R, Emeje M. Antiplasmodial activity-aided isolation and identification of quercetin-4'-methyl ether in Chromolaena odorata leaf fraction with high activity against chloroquine-resistant *Plasmodium falciparum*. Parasitology Research. 2014;113(12):4415–22.

[54] Elford BC. l-Glutamine influx in malaria-infected erythrocytes: a target for antimalarials? Parasitology Today. 1986;2(11):309–12.

[55] Frölich S, Schubert C, Bienzle U, Jenett-Siems K. In vitro antiplasmodial activity of prenylated chalcone derivatives of hops (*Humulus lupulus*) and their interaction with haemin. The Journal of Antimicrobial Chemotherapy. 2005;55(6):883.

[56] Rozmer Z, Perjési P. Naturally occurring chalcones and their biological activities. Phytochemistry Reviews. 2016;15(1):87–120.

[57] Bero J, Frédérich M, Quetin-leclercq J. Antimalarial Compounds Isolated from Plants used in Traditional Medicine. Oxford, UK, 2009. pp. 1401–33.

[58] Mesia K, Cimanga RK, Dhooghe L, Cos P, Apers S, Totté J, et al. Antimalarial activity and toxicity evaluation of a quantified *Nauclea pobeguinii* extract. Journal of Ethnopharmacology. 2010;131(1):10–6.

[59] Li N, Cao L, Cheng Y, Meng Z-Q, Tang Z-H, Liu W-J, et al. In vivo anti- inflammatory and analgesic activities of strictosamide from *Nauclea officinalis*. Pharmaceutical Biology. 2014;52(11):1445.

[60] Pelt-Koops JCv, Pett HE, Graumans W, Vegte-Bolmer Mvd, Gemert GJAv, Rottmann M, et al. The spiroindolone drug candidate NITD609 potently inhibits gametocytogenesis and blocks Plasmodium falciparum transmission to anopheles mosquito vector. Antimicrobial Agents and Chemotherapy. 2012;56:3544–4804.

[61] Rottmann M, McNamara C, Yeung BKS, Lee MCS, Zou B, Russell B, et al. Spiroindolones, a potent compound class for the treatment of malaria. Science. 2010;329(5996): 1175.

[62] Graz B, Willcox ML, Diakite C, Falquet J, Dackuo F, Sidibe O, et al. Argemone mexicana decoction versus artesunate-amodiaquine for the management of malaria in Mali: policy and public-health implications. Transactions of the Royal Society of Tropical Medicine and Hygiene. 2010;104(1):33.

[63] Patwardhan B, Vaidya A. Natural products drug discovery: accelerating the clinical candidate development using reverse pharmacology approaches. Indian Journal of Experimental Biology 2010;48: 220–7.

[64] Willcox ML, Graz B, Falquet J, Diakite C, Giani S, Diallo D. A "reverse pharmacology" approach for developing an anti- malarial phytomedicine. Malaria Journal. 2011;10(Suppl 1):S8–S.

[65] Phillipson JD. Phytochemistry and pharmacognosy. Phytochemistry. 2007;68(22):2960–72.

[66] Simoes-Pires C, Hostettmann K, Haouala A, Cuendet M, Falquet J, Graz B, et al. Reverse pharmacology for developing an anti- malarial phytomedicine. The example of Argemone mexicana. International Journal for Parasitology: Drugs and Drug Resistance. 2014;4(3):338–46.

[67] Vederas J. Drug Discovery and Natural Products: End of an Era or an Endless Frontier? Washington: The American Association for the Advancement of Science; 2009. pp. 161–5.

[68] Bologa CG, Ursu O, Oprea TI, Melançon CE, Tegos GP. Emerging trends in the discovery of natural product antibacterials. Current Opinion in Pharmacology. 2013;13(5):678–87.

[69] Zeng Q, Qiu F, Yuan L. Production of artemisinin by genetically-modified microbes. Biotechnology Letters. 2008;30(4):581–92.

[70] Baird JK. Eliminating malaria—all of them. The Lancet. 2010;376(9756):1883–5.

Permissions

The contributors of this book come from diverse backgrounds, making this book a truly international effort. This book will bring forth new frontiers with its revolutionizing research information and detailed analysis of the nascent developments around the world.

We would like to thank all the contributing authors for lending their expertise to make the book truly unique. They have played a crucial role in the development of this book. Without their invaluable contributions this book wouldn't have been possible. They have made vital efforts to compile up to date information on the varied aspects of this subject to make this book a valuable addition to the collection of many professionals and students.

This book was conceptualized with the vision of imparting up-to-date information and advanced data in this field. To ensure the same, a matchless editorial board was set up. Every individual on the board went through rigorous rounds of assessment to prove their worth. After which they invested a large part of their time researching and compiling the most relevant data for our readers.

The editorial board has been involved in producing this book since its inception. They have spent rigorous hours researching and exploring the diverse topics which have resulted in the successful publishing of this book. They have passed on their knowledge of decades through this book. To expedite this challenging task, the publisher supported the team at every step. A small team of assistant editors was also appointed to further simplify the editing procedure and attain best results for the readers.

Apart from the editorial board, the designing team has also invested a significant amount of their time in understanding the subject and creating the most relevant covers. They scrutinized every image to scout for the most suitable representation of the subject and create an appropriate cover for the book.

The publishing team has been an ardent support to the editorial, designing and production team. Their endless efforts to recruit the best for this project, has resulted in the accomplishment of this book. They are a veteran in the field of academics and their pool of knowledge is as vast as their experience in printing. Their expertise and guidance has proved useful at every step. Their uncompromising quality standards have made this book an exceptional effort. Their encouragement from time to time has been an inspiration for everyone.

The publisher and the editorial board hope that this book will prove to be a valuable piece of knowledge for researchers, students, practitioners and scholars across the globe.

List of Contributors

Ken Tucker, Amy R. Noe, Vinayaka Kotraiah, Timothy W. Phares and Gabriel M. Gutierrez
Leidos Life Sciences, Leidos Inc., Frederick, MD, USA

Moriya Tsuji
HIV and Malaria Vaccine Program, Aaron Diamond AIDS Research Center, Affiliate of the Rockefeller University, New York, NY, USA

Elizabeth H. Nardin
Division of Parasitology, Department of Microbiology, New York University School of Medicine, New York, NY, USA

Mariana Conceição de Souza, Tatiana Almeida Pádua and Maria das Graças Henriques
Laboratory of Applied Pharmacology, Farmanguinhos, Oswaldo Cruz Foundation, Rio de Janeiro, RJ, Brazil
National Institute of Science and Technology of Innovation on Diseases of Neglected Populations (INCT-IDPN), Rio de Janeiro, RJ, Brazil

Pratap Parida, Kishore Sarma, Biswajyoti Borkakoty and Pradyumna Kishore Mohapatra
Regional Medical Research Centre, NE Region, Indian Council of Medical Research, Dibrugarh, Assam, India

Sergey Lunev, Fernando A. Batista and Matthew R. Groves
Department of Drug Design, Groningen Research Institute of Pharmacy, University of Groningen, Groningen, The Netherlands

Soraya S. Bosch and Carsten Wrenger
Unit for Drug Discovery, Department of Parasitology, Institute of Biomedical Sciences, University of São Paulo, São Paulo, SP, Brazil

Kamal Hamed
Novartis Pharmaceuticals Corporation, East Hanover, NJ, USA

Kirstin Stricker
Novartis Pharma AG, Basel, Switzerland

Lyazzat Gumarova
Halberg Chronobiology Center, University of Minnesota, Minneapolis, MN, USA

Al-Farabi Kazakh National University, Almaty, Kazakhstan

Germaine Cornelissen
Halberg Chronobiology Center, University of Minnesota, Minneapolis, MN, USA

Borislav D Dimitrov
Primary Care and Population Sciences, University of Southampton, Southampton, UK

Franz Halberg
Halberg Chronobiology Center, University of Minnesota, Minneapolis, MN, USA

Régis Vanderesse and Samir Acherar
Macromolecular Physical Chemistry Laboratory, University of Lorraine, Nancy Cedex, France

Ludovic Colombeau and Céline Frochot
Reactions and Process Engineering Laboratory, University of Lorraine, Nancy Cedex, France

Kitiporn Plaimas
AVIC Research Center, Department of Mathematics and Computer Science, Faculty of Science, Chulalongkorn University, Bangkok, Thailand
Omics Sciences and Bioinformatics Center, Faculty of Science, Chulalongkorn University, Bangkok, Thailand

Rainer König
Integrated Research and Treatment Center, Center for Sepsis Control and Care (CSCC), Jena University Hospital, Jena, Germany
Network Modeling, Leibniz Institute for Natural Product Research and Infection Biology — Hans Knöll Institute, Jena, Germany

José Manuel Lozano Moreno
Molecular Mimetism of Infectious Agents, Department of Pharmacy, Universidad Nacional de Colombia, Bogotá, Colombia

Ifeoma C. Ezenyi and Oluwakanyinsola A. Salawu
Department of Pharmacology and Toxicology, National Institute for Pharmaceutical Research and Development, Idu, Abuja, Nigeria

Index

Lightning Source UK Ltd.
Milton Keynes UK
UKHW051609210922
409191UK00002B/59